Recent Results in Cancer Research 148

Springer

Berlin
Heidelberg
New York
Barcelona
Budapest
Hong Kong
London
Milan
Paris
Santa Clara
Singapore
Tokyo

N. Neymark

Assessing the Economic Value of Anticancer Therapies

With 21 Tables

Springer

Niels Neymark
EORTC Health Economics Unit
Ave. E. Mounier 83, bte 11
B-1200 Brussels
Belgium

ISBN-13: 978-3-642-72125-0 e-ISBN-13: 978-3-642-72123-6
DOI: 10.1007/978-3-642-72123-6

ISSN 0080-0015

Library of Congress Cataloging-in-Publication Data
Neymark, Niels: Assessing the economic value of anti-cancer therapies / N. Neymark. (Recent results in cancer research, ISSN 0080-0015; 148) Includes bibliographical references and index. ISBN 3-540-64030-4 (hardcover: alk. paper) 1. Cancer - Treatment - Economic aspects. 2. Cancer - Treatment - Cost effectiveness. 3. Medical care, Cost of. I. Title. II. Series. [DNLM: 1. Neoplasms - therapy. 2. Cost-Benefit Analysis - methods. 3. Neoplasms - economics. 4. Health Care Costs. W1 RE106P v. 148 1998 / QZ 266 N572a 1998] RC261.R35 vol. 148 [RC270.8] 616.99'4 s-dc21 [338.4'361699406] DNLM/DLC

Softcover reprint of the hardcover 1st edition 1998

Production: PRO EDIT GmbH, Heidelberg
Data conversion: K+V Fotosatz GmbH, Beerfelden

SPIN 10630530 19/3133-5 4 3 2 1 0 – Printed on acid-free paper

Preface

With ever increasing demands on the constrained resources available for health care services, no one involved in decision making in health care can continue to ignore the economic costs of the services provided or the relative value for money offered by the available treatments. Economic evaluation has therefore become an important and indispensable tool for medical decision making, alongside the well-known methods for clinical evaluation.

This is also true for cancer, despite the aura of sanctity often surrounding this dreaded disease and the apparent willingness of the general population to spend large sums in this area and do "everything possible" for the patients. In recent years, articles dealing with assessing the costs and benefits of various cancer treatments have begun to appear in scientific medical and economic journals.

This book provides a comprehensive survey and assessment of the current state of the art of economic evaluations and cost analyses in cancer. It gives an introduction to the methods available for economic evaluations, before surveying and assessing the available publications. Separate chapters are devoted to the most prevalent cancers, and in each chapter the current clinical practice and research problems are summarized in order to provide a background for the economic analyses. At the end, a summary assessment of the literature is provided along with some suggestions for a future research agenda.

Acknowledgements

Several clinical experts from a number of the EORTC cooperative groups have provided me with numerous and invaluable helpful comments during the process of writing this manuscript. I would like to express my gratitude to Dr. Sam Ahmedzai, University of Sheffield, Dr. Michel Bolla, University of Grenoble, Dr. Ben de Pauw, University of Nijmegen, Dr. Giuseppe Giaccone, The Free University Amsterdam, Dr. Martine Piccart, Institut Jules Bordet, Brussels, Dr. Hein van Poppel, University of Leuven and Dr. Jaques Wils, hospital of Roermond for their assistance in improving my understanding of the clinical issues. In addition, Dr. Françoise Meunier, Director General of the EORTC, Brussels, has provided me with very useful comments and suggestions. Needless to say, all remaining misinterpretations or errors remain my sole responsibility.

The EORTC Health Economics Unit was created in the fall of 1993 and has received substantial financial support from the Biomed 1 and 2 programs of the DG XII of the European Commission. The present study originated as a report for the European Commission, related to the first Biomed program and built upon the ongoing Biomed project. The EORTC Health Economics Unit is dedicated to carrying out economic evaluations of treatment alternatives in cancer with the ultimate aim of contributing information relevant for the efficient management of cancer patients, taking outcomes as well as costs into account.

Contents

Introduction

In most of the richer countries of the world, cancer is one of the major killers, along with cardiovascular diseases. Together, these two major groups of diseases are responsible for about two thirds of the annual deaths. Some figures[1] may illuminate the order of magnitude of the problem. For all the types of cancers considered together, the prevalence rate is about 1% of the population and the yearly incidence rate is about 0.5%. It is primarily a disease of the elderly, with an incidence rate for people aged 65 or older more than ten times larger than the incidence for younger people. Almost one tenth of the patients discharged from hospitals have cancer as their primary diagnosis, while the direct medical costs of cancer treatment and care are comparatively low. Most studies show that the share of cancer-related health care services in the yearly direct medical costs borne by the countries concerned is in the order of 5%–7%.

Cancer is a much dreaded disease, partly because of its often hidden, insidious nature and the general impression that in most cases there are no really effective treatments available. Partly, the fear is caused by the common and often serious and very unpleasant adverse effects caused by many of the usual treatment regimens, for instance nausea and vomiting after many forms of chemotherapy. It is not uncommon that patients decline to receive the treatment offered because they consider the expected gain in survival time too modest to justify the anticipated suffering due to adverse effects. There may be an increasing tendency that the conventional treatments offered are refused for this reason. On the other hand, quite the opposite opinion is also frequently heard, i.e., that patients are not willing to accept much of a reduction in expected survival in exchange for an increase in health-related quality of life.

Probably because of the dreadfulness of the disease, there is a widespread willingness on the part of the population to make sacrifices. Thus a large part of the research and treatment activities in cancer are carried out on the basis of private donations and run by private non-profit-making societies, even in countries with an otherwise almost completely publicly funded health care system (e.g., Denmark). These factors combine to establish a cer-

[1] The figures are actually for Sweden, but they are probably representative for many countries.

tain aura of sanctity around treatment and research activities in the cancer field. Any attempt at critically assessing the relative value of cancer treatments and research programs in economic terms will first have to overcome considerable resistance and the feeling that a kind of sacrilege is being committed (see, e.g., Culyer and Jönsson 1993). The powerful positions of many of the charitable cancer research, treatment, and patient support organizations have led some researchers (e.g., Maynard 1993) to refer to a "cancer industry," which is accused of being resistant to change and of pursuing cost-*in*effective treatment strategies, despite a lack of signs of any real breakthrough.

However that may be, recent years have witnessed an increasing cost-consciousness in health care systems all over the world. This is usually interpreted as a consequence of increasing budgetary constraints. Whatever the exact structure of the health care system and its financing mechanisms, the tightening of constraints is believed to be the result of popular resistance to increases in taxes or premiums, the appearance of new and promising, but typically more expensive treatment possibilities and the general aging of the populations, leading to great increases in demand for these new and costlier treatment possibilities. An alternative, and perhaps more relevant, interpretation of the increasing cost-consciousness and interest in ensuring "value for money" is the following: The existence or not of an economic problem is not primarily determined by the fact that very substantial resources are being spent, but rather by the appearance of previously unknown alternatives (see Jönsson and Karlsson 1992 for a similar formulation of the essentials of the economic problem). The cost of treating any given disease is in itself not a very interesting piece of information if only one treatment possibility exists. It is due to the appearance of treatment *alternatives* and the consequent problem of having to choose between several different treatment regimens that an economic problem arises. It then becomes relevant to determine, in a systematic way, the relative value in economic terms of the various treatment alternatives by calculating and comparing their costs and benefits.

The considerable research resources poured into the cancer field during the last decades are now coming to fruition, both in the form of an improved understanding of the basic biological mechanisms and in the development and eventual marketing of innovative products. Many of these are supportive therapies, which aim at allowing an intensification of the delivery of conventional treatment modalities and thereby presumably an improvement of the outcomes. Others, such as gene therapy, are more innovative in their approach. At the same time, the general perception of the aims and outcomes of treatment is (perhaps) changing, as issues other than the mere length of survival have only recently become pertinent in the clinical evaluation of the outcome of cancer treatments. Traditionally, clinicians have considered the length of survival (or sometimes disease-free survival) as the only relevant outcome measure for assessing cancer treatments, despite being well aware of the often severe toxic effects of many anticancer therapies and their probable impact on the patients' quality of life. However, there is increasing consciousness about the negative impact of many anticancer therapies on the patients' well-being or quality of life, and many are questioning the desirability of increasing the length of survival at any price. As for other diseases, there is an increasing interest in assessing the impact of cancer and of the treatment alternatives on patients' quality of life.

The factors mentioned above are among the causes of an increasing academic interest in the "economics of cancer" (see also Goddard and Drummond 1991; Levine et al. 1985; Markman 1988; Rees 1985; Yarbro 1991). Presumably, there is frequently a trade-off between length of survival and quality of life (because of the toxicity of most treatments), and increasingly there is also a choice between old and new treatment regimens with varying resource requirements and outcomes. These choices are examples of *decision problems* in medicine. Economics may be characterized as the *science of choice*[2], and economics may as an academic discipline contribute important information in order to enable rational decision making, inter alia in medical decision problems. This contribution may be achieved by carrying out economic evaluations based on formalized and explicit procedures. Defined very briefly, economic evaluation is a widely applicable economic method concerned with the comparison of two or more alternatives with respect to both their positive and negative impacts or benefits and costs, respectively, as these impacts are generally termed. The following are the essential two characteristics of economic evaluation. It is a comparison according to explicit, systematic, and consistent criteria of (1) two or more alternative ways of achieving a given aim, (2) taking into account both their costs and benefits.

By the simultaneous fulfillment of these two criteria, economic evaluations of medical treatments are distinguishable from two other types of studies common in the medical literature. Randomized, controlled clinical trials are only concerned with assessing the efficacy of the treatments compared, while their costs are generally ignored. On the other hand, studies in which the costs of specific treatments are calculated without any attempt at formally assessing the outcomes of the treatment are increasingly often published in clinical journals. Usually such detailed costing studies comprise only one specific treatment regimen without any explicit comparison with an alternative treatment. Both types of studies may of course provide indispensable information for medical decision making. From an economic point of view, however, rational decision making about the allocation of scarce resources requires information derived from real economic evaluations, in which both

---

[2] In the 1930s, the well-known and acknowledged British economist Lionel Robbins stated this point very concisely: "Economics is the science concerned with the allocation of scarce means among competing ends." An immediate implication of this definition is the central *opportunity cost* concept of economics, i.e., that the true costs of a certain action are equal to the value of the next-best alternative action on which the same resources could have been spent, but which was not chosen.

the costs and the benefits of the alternatives are taken into account simultaneously and with equal weight.

The purpose of the present report is to give a comprehensive survey of the published economic evaluations in the broad field of cancer in order to describe and assess what is currently known about the relative costs and benefits of the treatment alternatives available. Another purpose has been to assess the state of the art of the methodology commonly employed in the published economic evaluations in cancer and, further, to try to identify the areas in which further research is most obviously needed. The survey is concerned only with cancer treatments and care; thus contributions on prevention and screening have not been included unless they have been judged to provide especially detailed and reliable estimates of the costs of one or more specific treatments. This, however, has not very often been the case. As the number of full economic evaluations in cancer is so far rather limited, the available costing studies, typically concerned with determining the cost of only a single treatment regimen, have also been included, as they may represent a first step in a subsequent full economic evaluation.

Another facet of the economics of cancer has to do with the total drain that it constitutes on the aggregate resources of society. This drain is made up of the direct medical costs, i.e., the medical resources (e.g., personnel, equipment, materials) directly used in diagnosing, staging, and treating cancer, plus the loss of time and production for the patients, their relatives and friends, and society at large due to the morbidity and premature mortality caused by cancer. This way of considering the costs of a disease, the "cost-of-illness" (COI) approach, has previously attracted a considerable amount of interest, and also in cancer a number of studies taking this approach have been published. Therefore, one of the sections in this book has been devoted to a survey of studies concerned with determining the COI of cancer (see "Cost-of-Illness Analysis" in "A Brief Introduction to Economic Evaluation"), although it is questionable whether these studies should rightly be considered as economic analyses, at least if it is claimed, as it is in this report, that it is not so much the absolute amount of resources or costs involved which determines the economic interest of an issue, but rather the existence of alternatives between which a choice may be made. Knowing the total economic burden of cancer is of very limited value in a decision-making context, as it is difficult to imagine the resulting figures (typically very large amounts) playing any role in actual decision making, except perhaps in setting priorities in the allocation of future research efforts. (For a more comprehensive critique of COI analyses, please refer to the above-mentioned section, in which the studies on the economic burden of cancer are discussed.)

The studies reviewed in this survey were identified by means of a computerized search of abstracts on Medline combined with an examination of the reference lists of all the papers thus identified and retrieved. The search term used in the Medline search was "cost analysis – explode all options," which was believed to result in the most comprehensive list of studies, comprising not only proper economic evaluations comparing two or more treatment alternatives but also studies aiming at determining the cost of a single treatment regimen. The drawback of this search strategy was that it resulted in a list with a very large proportion of "misses," in which the terms "costs," "economic evaluation," or the like were only mentioned in passing. The preliminary sorting into "hits" and "misses" was carried out by reading the abstracts of the papers provided by Medline.

The Medline search was not restricted to papers published in any specific language, and papers in English, French, German, Dutch, Italian, Spanish, or any of the Scandinavian languages would be included, if retrievable. However, 95% of the papers identified were in English, and the main exclusions were a certain number of papers in Japanese and Russian. The search comprised papers published between 1985 and the fall of 1996. A minimal requirement for inclusion in the survey was that the studies contain actual attempts at determining the costs of one or more specific treatment regimens. Apart from this, no strict inclusion or exclusion criteria were employed.

As this is the first attempt at providing a comprehensive survey of the economics of cancer treatments, it was considered worthwhile including more or less all published studies of relevance for the subject. Despite a determined effort, however, it has not been possible to retrieve all of the papers identified, so this survey cannot claim to be exhaustive, as even important contributions may not have been included for one reason or another. While regrettable, my inability to provide an exhaustive survey is not a major problem, given that the principal aim of the effort was to provide a survey of state of the art of a particular research area rather than to determine a definitive quantitative result. It is doubtful that even important papers that were not retrieved and included would have changed the overall impression obtained.

In the clinical literature, meta-analysis, defined more or less strictly as a statistical synthesis of a number of similar, but not necessarily completely homogeneous clinical trials, has become a widely recognized and almost indispensable tool if a global overview and quantitative summary of a particular clinical issue is aimed at. It must be clearly stated from the outset that the ambition that guided the following survey is much more modest - largely for no other reason than the very limited number of replications (even if conceived of very broadly) of individual economic evaluations. Very few of the published studies overlap in the clinical issues, so there has been very little occasion for dealing with the potentials and hazards of attempting a quantitative summary of the evidence.[3]

The ambition has rather been to provide a more traditional review of the literature, without any attempt at achieving the kind of objectivity obtained by the tools of formal meta-analysis. In order to limit the subjectivism inherent in the procedure chosen, the individual studies have been described and discussed in sufficient detail that the reader will hopefully obtain a clear impression of the methods and data employed. It is also hoped that the premises

[3] A first attempt at developing a formal methodology for reviewing and summing up evidence from several individual economic evaluations may be found in Jefferson et al. (1996).

of any critical remarks put forward has been stated with sufficient clarity and objectivity that the reader may assess the validity of the criticism.

In most cases, the results of the evaluations described are stated in the form of a cost per outcome measure. Results in anything but US$ have been converted to this currency using the Health Purchasing Power Parities (PPPs) published by the Organization for Economic Cooperation and Development (OECD).[4] Readers are therefore not expected to have immediate recollection of the currency exchange rates as of a particular point of time in the past and require no intuition about the general relation between, for instance, Australian and American dollars. PPPs are only published every 5 years and the latest available are from 1990. Nevertheless, they have been used just as they are (if necessary by interpolation between the figures for 1985 and 1990 or by extrapolating the latter), without any attempts at attaining higher accuracy. This procedure has been chosen deliberately in order to avoid giving any false impressions of precision. Many published papers may be criticized for giving such an unfounded sense of precision, e.g., by presenting results with very "exact" numbers (sometimes even with several decimals), even though the methods and data employed certainly do not warrant such exactness.

A final caveat should also be made clear from the outset. No attempt has been made at establishing anything resembling a so-called *cost-effectiveness league table* for the various treatments based on the results reported in the studies. Such a league table is a ranking of a number of treatments of different diseases according to a single, common criterion, e.g., the incremental costs of saving an additional year of life. It is my contention that, even under the best of circumstances, the establishment of such league tables is a hazardous undertaking with plenty of pitfalls and risks of reaching misleading conclusions. The "best of circumstances" require at the very least a considerable homogeneity in the methods used for the individual studies and even this minimal requirement is certainly not fulfilled by the economic assessments included in the survey, as will become obvious from the detailed descriptions in the following chapters. Any attempt at ranking the studies according to the results of the cost calculations published must therefore be considered as strictly tentative.

---

[4] The most easily accessible mechanism for converting prices between national currencies is to use the official exchange rate prevailing between two currencies at a point in time. However, the official exchange rates are determined by many factors and they usually do not accurately reflect the actual purchasing power of the individual currencies within the respective countries. For instance, it has been demonstrated that the higher the relative income of a country is, the higher its relative price level is. In other words, the internal purchasing power of rich countries compared with the poorer ones is considerably lower than implied by the official exchange rates. In order to make international comparisons of incomes and prices more realistic, it is therefore necessary to calculate PPPs, i.e., artificial exchange rates which make a correction for divergences between the countries in the internal purchasing power. The OECD calculates such sector-specific PPPs (e.g., for the health care sector) by calculating an index for the relative prices in each individual country compared to the average international prices for the same set of goods and services.

In the second chapter ("Epidemiology of Cancer"), an outline of the epidemiology of cancer is given, while the third chapter ("Cancer and Some Basics of the Main Treatment Modalities") contains a short description of the biological and clinical features of the disease and of the main current treatment modalities. The fourth chapter ("A Brief Introduction to Economic Evaluation") briefly discusses some of the methodological issues in economic evaluations and the usefulness of clinical trials as a vehicle for collecting the necessary data for economic evaluations. The fifth chapter ("The Economic Burden of Cancer") describes and summarizes a number of studies that have attempted to determine the economic burden of cancer for society, either by the traditional COI approach or by using other approaches.

From the sixth chapter onward, a survey of economic evaluations of treatment alternatives in cancer is given, with separate chapters devoted to the most common types of cancers, i.e., lung, breast, colorectal, and prostate cancer. There is also a separate chapter on hematological malignancies, which are not the most common but have always attracted a disproportionate amount of research interest, both basic and clinical, and thus have also been the subject of several economic analyses. These types of malignancies are generally considered as good models for oncology in general, inter alia because the disease itself has many points of resemblance with some of the most common and serious side effects of the main treatment modalities for many other tumors, in particular chemotherapy.

Further, there are separate chapters on genitourinary and gynecological tumors and on palliative care and two rather long chapters on supportive care, i.e., prevention or reduction of various adverse effects of the conventional treatment regimens. These toxicities often limit the dose that can be safely administered or may in many patients even prevent administration of the intended normal doses of treatment. Severe toxic side effects are usually considered as a considerable limitation on the potential effectiveness of conventional therapies, and a large part of the research effort in recent years has been focused on reducing or eliminating these restrictions. The aim of this research is not only to ensure that the intended normal dose of treatment may be administered more frequently than currently possible, but also to allow higher doses to be delivered. It is widely believed that an intensification of conventional therapies will lead to appreciable improvements in the outcomes obtained, although the available evidence of a steep dose–response relation is in most cases not very convincing.

In the chapters on the most frequent cancers and on the most important forms of supportive care, an attempt has been made to provide nonmedical readers with a concise summary of the pertinent clinical problems, the state of the art of treatment possibilities, and an indication of the dominating current approaches in clinical research. Such clinical information has been considered to be of superior importance in order to provide a perspective allowing a better assessment of the economic analyses already performed and perhaps to provide some useful suggestions for future research priorities. The main sources of the clinical information given in the various chapters were the two latest editions of the volume by deVita et al. (1993, 1997), which is often referred to as the "bible" of cancer. This was complemented by some other sources, notably the Physician Data Query (PDQ) database provided by the United States National Cancer Institute (updated to the second half of 1996). To a large extent, the PDQ is based on the individual chapters of the volume by deVita et al., but if there has been a divergence between the two sources, the PDQ has generally been preferred. Not every single statement in the text is followed by an exact reference, as this would have made it completely indigestible. However, if sources other than the two already mentioned were used for specific paragraphs, they are cited in the text.

In the final chapter, the body of research contained in the review is considered in its entirety and some indications of the most pertinent issues for future research are given.

Epidemiology of Cancer

This chapter gives some basic facts about the epidemiology of cancer, based on data from the United States and from Western European countries. Internationally, and even regionally, there are large variations in cancer incidence rates[1] and in cancer mortality. However, while the precise incidence rates may differ to varying degrees in many details, the broad picture based on a ranking of the most common cancers is rather similar between the United States and several Western European countries. The following overview of the epidemiology of cancer does not purport to give a detailed picture of the situation in any specific country. It is merely intended to give the reader an idea about the order of magnitude of the problem and has been based on the most readily accessible data, which have not been scrutinized any further.

In Western Europe and in the United States, cancer is the second leading cause of death after cardiovascular diseases, accounting for 20%–25% of the total number of deaths per year. The yearly incidence rate is on the order of 0.5% of the population, and prevalence is about 1%. Although it is an important cause of death in certain younger age-groups, cancer is primarily a disease of the aged. In the United States, the incidence rates per 100,000 in 1987–1991 for all cancer sites combined was 198 for people under 65 and 2145 for those aged 65 or older. In the following, some descriptive epidemiological data will be given to provide the reader with a sense of the magnitude of the problem represented by cancer. In most countries, these data are collected by special cancer registries.

The beginning of continuous registration of new cancer cases in Europe was marked by the setting up of the first population-based registry in Hamburg, Germany, but the first registry covering a whole nation was begun in Denmark in 1942. Today, all of the countries of the European Union (EU), except Luxembourg and Greece, have population-based cancer registries covering all or part of the population, gathering information about the size, nature, and distribution of cancer in the community. The main objective of these registries is to express factual information on cancer incidence and mortality in a standardized way, calculating incidence and mortality rates for

[1] Internationally, 20-fold differences in cancer incidence rates are not unusual, even for the more common cancers such as lung and colon cancers. Even larger variations may be seen, e.g., a 150-fold difference between Australia and Japan in the incidence of melanomas among men in the period 1978–1982.

their population. These rates may be used for comparisons of incidence with other nations or geographical areas, to compare subgroups of the population within the registry area itself, and to study the evolution over time of specific cancers. Incidence rates may also be used to set priorities for various cancer control measures such as prevention and screening programs, in analytical epidemiological studies attempting to improve our understanding of causes, and also in evaluating the effects of control measures.

The following descriptive data are taken from *Facts and Figures of Cancer in the European Community*, a booklet published by the Network of European Cancer Registries, which was launched in 1990 within the Europe Against Cancer program of the European Community (EC). The figures given are from 1990 and are the latest available. In some cases, data are also given for the United States for comparison. It appears that the incidence of cancer is somewhat higher in the United States, around 50% higher for both men and women for all sites combined, while the mortality rate is at the average European level (Table 1).

Within the EU, there is also a difference in incidence of about 50% between the country with the lowest and the highest incidence, respectively, for both men and women. Greece, Portugal, and Spain are low-incidence countries for both sexes, while the highest incidence rates for men are seen in Belgium, Germany, and Luxembourg. For women, by far the highest incidence is seen in Denmark, followed by countries such as Ireland, Belgium, and Germany. In general, the incidence for men is somewhat higher than for

Table 1. Estimated incidence and mortality rate of all cancers in the countries of the European Community (EC) in 1990

Country	Males		Females	
	Incidence	Mortality	Incidence	Mortality
Belgium	310	219	237	122
Denmark	288	190	269	149
France	311	212	208	100
Germany	283	189	234	120
Greece	231	151	174	83
Ireland	257	177	240	133
Italy	276	199	204	107
Luxembourg	307	213	233	120
Netherlands	291	203	235	120
Portugal	229	146	190	184
Spain	248	166	177	86
United Kingdom	252	188	211	137
EC (average)	274	191	209	112
USA (1984–1994 data)	433	212	340	138

Age-standardized rates per 100,000, rounded figures.

Table 2. The most common cancers in newly diagnosed men and women in the EC countries in 1990

Men		Women	
Cancer site	Proportion of all cases (%)	Cancer site	Proportion of all cases (%)
Lung	22	Breast	24
Colorectal	12	Colorectal	14
Prostate	12	Lung	5
Stomach	7	Stomach	5
Bladder	7	Corpus uteri	4
Mouth/pharynx	4	Ovary	4
Larynx	3	Cervix	4
Kidney	3	Pancreas	3
Pancreas	3	Leukemia	2
Leukemia	3	Non-Hodgkin's disease	2
Non-Hodgkin's disease	3	Bladder	2
All others	22	All others	30

women, and it is remarkable that the difference between the yearly incidence and mortality rates is much smaller for men than for women. This is an indication that men are more frequently affected by cancers with very bad survival prospects, especially lung cancer.

For all ages combined, the total number of new cases of cancers in the EC countries in 1990 was estimated to be 647,000 for men and 645,000 for women. The most frequent diagnoses are given in Table 2, which shows that lung cancer is by far the most frequent specific site in men, followed by prostate and colorectal cancer and stomach and bladder cancer. There is a large group of patients in the category "all others," which is very heterogeneous. This is also the largest category for women, where breast cancer and colorectal cancers are the dominant sites.

Age-standardized incidence and mortality rates for the most common cancers for men and women are given in Table 3 below, which includes the average rates for the EC countries in 1990. Particularly large divergences in these rates between the individual countries will be mentioned in the text.

For those of the above cancers that are common for men and women, the incidence is always higher for men, with the smallest difference in colorectal cancer and the largest differences in bladder and lung cancer. For the latter, however, the incidence for women is rapidly rising, while the incidence for men is generally falling. For men, there is generally a difference of a factor 2–3 between the countries with the lowest and highest incidence, respectively, but the ranking of the countries varies greatly according to the site of disease. The smallest difference is seen in leukemia, where the lowest-incidence country is Portugal with 6.9 and the highest-incidence country is Den-

Table 3. Incidence and mortality rates for the most common cancers in men and women (EC averages)

Men			Women		
Site	Incidence	Mortality	Site	Incidence	Mortality
Lung	59	55	Breast	59	23
Colorectal	32	18	Colorectal	26	14
Prostate	28	17	Lung	11	10
Stomach	19	15	Stomach	10	8
Bladder	19	8	Corpus uteri	10	2
Mouth/pharynx	13	7	Ovary	10	6
Larynx	9	5	Cervix	10	4
Kidney	7	4	Pancreas	5	5
Pancreas	7	7	Leukemia	5	4
Leukemia	8	6	Non-Hodgkin's disease	5	3
Non-Hodgkin's disease	7	4	Bladder	4	2

Rates per 100,000 age-standardized persons.

Table 4. Incidence of the most common cancers, according to age-group, in the United States from 1987 to 1991

Site	Age <65 years	Age ≥65 years	All ages
Prostate (men)	27	1002	123
Breast (women)	73	445	110
Lung	28	330	58
Colorectal	18	323	48
All sites	198	2145	390

Rates are given per 100,000 individuals, age-adjusted.

mark with 10.4. The largest difference is seen in mouth/pharynx cancer, for which the incidence is 5.3 in Portugal and 23.3 in France. For women, the differences between high- and low-incidence countries are generally a little smaller than for men, around a factor 1.5–2. The smallest difference is again seen for leukemia, where the range is from 4.8 in Spain to 6.8 in Denmark, and the largest difference is observed in lung cancer, with an incidence of 4.8 in Spain and 23.1 in Denmark.

The age dependency of cancer (Table 4) and some recent developments in incidence and mortality will be illustrated with some data from the United States, as equivalent European data have not been identified. Presumably, the trends are rather similar, although the level of incidence rates differ considerably. The data for the United States are taken from the latest update of the PDQ database.

Table 5. Cancer sites with highest and lowest 5-year survival rates, respectively, for patients diagnosed 1983–1990

Site	5-Year survival rates (%)		
	<65 years	≥65 years	All ages
All sites	58	50	54
Thyroid gland	97	80	95
Testis	93	80	93
Melanoma	86	82	85
Corpus uteri	88	72	84
Breast	79	82	80
Bladder	86	75	80
Hodgkin's disease	83	40	79
...	...	...	...
Chronic myeloid leukemia	33	12	24
Stomach	20	17	19
Lung and bronchus	16	11	13
Acute myeloid leukemia	17	2	10
Esophagus	10	8	9
Liver	9	3	6
Pancreas	5	2	3

Percentages given are rounded values.

There are quite remarkable differences between the United States and the EU countries with respect to the incidence of these cancers, especially for prostate and breast cancer with a four- and twofold difference, respectively. It is also quite clear that cancer is primarily a disease of the elderly, with an incidence in the oldest group which is 11 times higher than in the youngest. The age dependency is especially clear for prostate cancer and colorectal cancer, with a 40-fold and a 20-fold difference, respectively.

Over the period from 1973 to 1991, the greatest increases in incidence for all age-groups combined has been observed for prostate cancer (+126%), melanoma (+94%), non-Hodgkin's lymphoma (+73%), and testis cancer (+43%), followed by increases of about a third in kidney, lung, brain, and breast cancer. Decreases in incidence of around 30% over this period have been observed for cervix uteri and corpus uteri cancers for women and for stomach cancer in general. Over the same period, the mortality rates have increased by 48% for lung cancer, 35% for melanoma, and by around a third for non-Hodgkin's lymphoma and multiple myeloma, while the greatest decreases in mortality have been seen in testis cancer (–67%), Hodgkin's disease (–57%), and cervix uteri cancer (–42%).

Finally, some information on the 5-year survival rates for the various cancers will be given (Table 5), again based on data from the most recent update of the PDQ database. Despite the criticisms that may be directed against their lack of sophistication and potential for inducing misleading conclusions, x-year survival rates are rather popular and widely used as outcome measures for the treatment of various diseases. However, for our purposes, they may be considered as useful summary measures.

In general, the survival rates are higher in the younger age-group, but the differences are not very marked, except for thyroid gland and testis cancer and for Hodgkin's disease at the best end of the scale and acute and chronic myeloid leukemia at the worst end, where the younger age-group seems to fare much better. However, for many of these diseases (thyroid gland, testis, Hodgkin's disease), the incidence in the older group seems to be very small relative to the incidence in the younger group. The only exception with a higher 5-year survival rate for the older age-group is breast cancer, but the difference is not statistically significant.

Cancer and Some Basics of the Main Treatment Modalities

This chapter aims to give a summary overview of some of the clinical aspects of cancer, intended primarily for readers without a medical background. First, a short and extremely simplified description is given of cancer understood as a cellular disease or rather as a large number of cellular diseases, sharing some basic common characteristics. In the subsequent part of the chapter, an introduction to the main treatment modalities in cancer and their possibilities and limitations is given. This should give the interested reader without a medical background the necessary information for a better understanding of the later chapters, in which the published economic evaluations will be reviewed and discussed in the light of short descriptions of the most important clinical issues concerning the various cancer sites.

The main existing treatment modalities are surgical resection, radiotherapy, chemotherapy, and biological therapy, including hormonal therapy. While the new developments within biotechnology seem to offer the potential of quite new treatment modalities[1], such as gene therapy, the following description will be limited to the existing, well-known modalities, as the economic evaluations published to date are concerned with these.

Cancer Understood as a Cellular Disease

Cancer is a group of more than 100 different diseases. The unifying characteristic of these is a disordered proliferation of cells, where cells become abnormal and keep dividing and forming more cells without any control or order. The recognition of cancer as a cellular disease followed the development of the microscope in the nineteenth century, which allowed microscopic examination of tumor tissue, and since then most of the research into its biological properties, etiology, and treatment has been based on this concept.

All organs of the body are made up of cells. Most normal cells are differentiated, i.e., they have developed specific morphology and function, but during this process of differentiation, normal cells tend to lose their ability to proliferate. However, many tissues of the body undergo a process of re-

[1] This includes newer developments which are still being tested in clinical trials, e.g., the use of intensified chemotherapy supported by prophylactic use of hematopoietic growth factors.

newal in which the loss of mature cells is replaced by the proliferation of less mature precursor cells (so-called stem cells), which in turn undergo the differentiation process. Normally, this renewal process is orderly, so that the cells divide to produce more cells only when the body needs them, but if the cells keep dividing even when new cells are not needed, a mass of tissue forms. This mass of extra tissue is called a *tumor*, which may be benign or malignant. Benign tumors are not cancerous, and they can usually be removed without, in most cases, coming back. Most importantly, cells from benign tumors do not spread to other organs or parts of the body.

Malignant tumors are cancerous. In addition to the proliferation of new cells independent of the normal requirement for new cells, cell differentiation is also impaired. An indication of the malignant nature of a cancer and the major property that leads to death of the host is the ability of cancer cells to invade other tissues and to spread to other parts of the body, where they can generate new tumors, referred to as *metastases*. The mechanisms involved in the process of metastasis are still rather poorly understood, but usually the spread occurs through the bloodstream or through the lymphatic system. Tumor invasion and metastasis is the major cause of treatment failure in cancer patients. About 30% of patients with newly diagnosed solid tumors already have clinically detectable metastases at the time of first diagnosis of cancer, and of the remaining 70% that are clinically free of metastases, about half can be cured by local tumor therapy alone. The remaining third of all patients have clinically occult metastases that later become manifest; thus more than 60% of patients have microscopic or clinically evident metastases at the time of primary tumor treatment.

Despite the impairment of cell differentiation in cancer, it is usually possible for the pathologist to recognize the tissue of origin. Most cancers are named after the type of cell or the organ in which they begin. When a cancer spreads, the new tumor has the same kind of abnormal cells and the same name as the original tumor. For instance, if a lung cancer spreads to the liver, the cancer cells in the liver are lung cancer cells and the disease is called metastatic lung cancer and not liver cancer.

Most patients suffer from multiple metastases, where a few large, identifiable metastases in various organs are frequently accompanied by a greater number of micrometastases that were seeded more recently in the continuous process of formation of metastatic colonies. This process commences early in the growth of the primary tumor and increases with time. The size and age variation in metastases, their heterogeneous composition, and their dispersed location in the patient's body are factors that hinder surgical removal and limit the effective concentration of anticancer drugs that can be delivered at the sites of metastatic colonies. Patients with metastatic disease usually die as a result of their compromised anatomy directly caused by the metastases or as a result of the complications associated with antimetastatic therapy.

Despite many years of intensive research directed at finding properties of cancer cells which are consistently different from properties of normal cells, none of the differences so far identified have been shown to be unique. This absence of specific identifiable differences between normal and malignant cells is a major barrier to the development of specific anticancer therapies. Treatment has therefore had to rely on either a spatial separation between tumor and critical normal tissue in local treatment modalities or on minor and empirical differences in the responses of tumors and normal tissue to systemic treatments such as chemotherapy. Not surprisingly, then, almost all types of cancer treatments cause significant damage to normal tissue, and this is often a factor which critically limits the efficacy of treatment.

Tumor cure requires the treatment to cause all tumor stem cells to lose their ability to generate progeny that can cause the tumor to regrow. The most important way of testing cell survival after treatment is therefore to test the cell's ability to form a colony of progeny. Cell survival, thus defined, is frequently found to be exponentially related to the radiation or drug dose over a wide range, implying that repeated identical courses of therapy kill a given fraction of cells rather than a given number. For instance, a clinically detectable tumor weighing 10 g may contain 10^{10} cells. Complete clinical remission, which is a central outcome of many treatment trials and which means that there is no longer evidence of tumor by physical examination or X-rays, may still be consistent with survival of as many as 10^8 cells (tumor weight approximately 0.1 g), so the dose of radiation or radiotherapy required to produce cure may be much larger than the dose required for complete remission.

If a cancer is diagnosed before metastasis has occurred, it is often curable by local treatment with surgery and/or radiotherapy. Surgical removal of a tumor must involve an adequate margin of normal tissue to allow for local spread of tumor cells. Radiation kills both malignant and normal cells, and a major goal of developing new radiation techniques is therefore to simultaneously maximize the killing of tumor cells and to minimize the damage to surrounding normal tissue. If the cancer has metastasized, the only treatment that may influence all sites of metastatic disease is frequently systemic treatment with cell-killing (cytotoxic) drugs. A major limitation to the efficacy of drug treatment is the presence in the tumor of drug-resistant cells. These may either result in initial resistance to treatment or to the subsequent development of resistance after an initial response. Alternative approaches to cancer treatment include the use of hormonal therapy, which may induce remission of some cancers that arise in tissues sensitive to hormones, such as breast and prostate. Various approaches to immunotherapy, i.e., specific killing of tumor cells via immune system-mediated effects, have been tried for many years with minimal success. However, recent developments in biochemical engineering have raised the hopes of major breakthroughs in the treatment possibilities.

The main forms of treatment modalities will be further described below.

The Main Treatment Modalities

Surgical Therapy

Surgery is the oldest treatment for cancer and, until recently, the only treatment modality that could actually cure patients with cancer. However, surgery also plays a role in the prevention of cancer and in the diagnostic work-up of suspected cancers. Advances in surgical techniques and development of alternative treatment strategies have on the one hand allowed surgeons to perform successful resections for an increased number of patients and on the other hand made them reassess the magnitude of surgery necessary.

Direct surgical intervention for the *prevention* of cancer is relevant for a limited number of underlying conditions or congenital or genetic traits that are associated with an extremely high incidence of subsequent cancer. Examples of diseases with a high incidence of cancer that can be prevented by prophylactic surgery are familial colon, breast, and ovarian cancer, where individuals with a family history of such cancers have a substantially higher risk than normal (but far below a risk of 100%) of developing these cancers. In the *diagnosis* of cancer, the main role of the surgeon is to provide the histologist with the appropriate tissue for an exact histologic diagnosis. Various biopsy techniques for obtaining the tissue are used, depending on the site and the natural history of the tumor in question. In the *treatment* of cancer, surgery has a number of different functions:

1. Surgery for primary cancer, which may be subdivided into:
   a) Definite surgical treatment of some localized cancers, which requires accurate identification of patients who can be cured by local treatment alone.
   b) Selection of local treatment that provides the best balance between local cure and morbidity due to treatment.
   c) Application of adjuvant treatments that allow reductions in the magnitude of surgical resection and improve the control of local and distant metastatic disease.
2. Surgery for residual disease in patients in which the extensive local spread of cancer precludes surgical resection of all the involved tissue, but in which surgical resection of the bulk of disease may lead to improvements in the ability to control residual disease that has not been resected by other modalities.
3. Surgery for metastatic disease, which is of primary importance for patients with a single site of metastatic disease, especially for cancers that are more or less refractory to chemotherapy. Many patients with few metastases to lung, liver, or brain can be cured by surgical resection of the metastases and surrounding tissue. In patients with soft tissue and bone sarcomas, the cure rate with surgical resection of metastases in the lung is 30%, and in patients with solitary liver metastases from colorectal cancer, resection can lead to long-term cure in 25% of patients.

4. Surgery for oncologic emergencies, especially because the oncologic patient is often neutropenic or thrombocytopenic with a high risk of sepsis or hemorrhage.
5. Surgery for palliation, primarily required for the relief of pain or of mechanical problems, e.g., intestinal obstruction.
6. Surgery for reconstruction and rehabilitation after definitive therapy, where the reconstruction of anatomic defects may improve both function and cosmetic appearance substantially.

Radiotherapy

In radiotherapy, high-energy rays are used to destroy cancer cells and to stop them from growing and dividing. Radiation may be *external*, where either electromagnetic rays such as X-rays or gamma rays are produced by a machine or electrons or other charged particles are emitted by a particle accelerator, or it may be *internal*, where the radiation comes from an implant of a small container of radioactive material placed directly into or near the tumor. Some patients receive both kinds of radiation therapy.

Radiation can cause damage to any molecule in a cell, but it is generally believed that damage to DNA is the most crucial in relation to the cell-killing potential of radiation. One of the most radiation-sensitive functions of cells is their ability to retain the capacity for continued proliferation, which, as mentioned above, is one important way of defining cell survival. There are no systematic differences between normal and malignant cells in the survival curves that have been observed with various methods. Some of the radiation damage in cells can be repaired (within a few hours), and this repair is the major mechanism explaining the clinical observation that a larger total dose can be tolerated when the dose is fractionated than when given as a single acute dose. Oxygen acts as a radiation sensitizer such that cells treated with a specific type of radiation in the absence of oxygen require a much higher dose than cells irradiated in the presence of oxygen. The presence of hypoxic cells in significant proportions (approximately 10%) in some tumors may limit the efficacy of radiotherapy.

Radiotherapy is usually given on an outpatient basis and involves delivering 25–35 individual dose fractions of about 2 Gy over a period of 5–7 weeks, i.e., one fraction per weekday with a rest during weekends. Four factors likely to influence the response to a fractionated treatment such as this are believed to be (1) repair of radiation damage, (2) repopulation of damaged tissues by proliferation of surviving cells, (3) redistribution of proliferating cells, and (4) reoxygenation of hypoxic cells. Repair and repopulation are the reasons why cells and tissues can tolerate a larger dose when it is fractionated, and they occur both in tumors and in normal tissue. However, repopulation has only a minor effect on the late radiation damage in slowly proliferating normal tissues, which may therefore be a dose-limiting factor, while repopulation during the latter part of conventionally fractionated treatments may cause an increase in the dose required to obtain control of the tumor. Reoxygenation occurs mainly in tumors and may be one of the main reasons for the improved therapeutic efficacy obtained by fractionation compared to single doses.

Different fractionated schedules that give equal levels of tumor control (and normal tissue response) may be expressed in the form of isoeffect relations, i.e., plots between total dose and increasing number of fractions (decreasing fraction size). A difference in isoeffect relationships between early- and late-responding tissues has been observed, and this difference implies that reducing fraction size may reduce the damage to late-responding tissue more than to early-responding. A therapeutic gain may therefore be expected by using hyperfractionation, where treatment with smaller dose fractions are given two or more times a day. Reducing the overall treatment time, and thereby preventing the significant repopulation believed to take place in the latter part of conventional 5- to 7-week treatments, may also imply a therapeutic gain, because the required dose to obtain tumor control may be reduced.

Several other approaches to improve the therapeutic efficacy have been examined, including attempts to reduce the resistance to radiation due to hypoxic cells in tumors. One approach, with very limited success, has been hyperbaric oxygen breathing before and during treatment, and studies using certain drugs capable of specific sensitization of (and toxicity for) hypoxic cells are under way.

Chemotherapy

As opposed to surgery and radiation, which are (normally) local therapies, chemotherapy is usually a *systemic* therapy, meaning that the drugs flow with the bloodstream to nearly every part of the body. The first modern chemotherapeutic drugs, the alkylating agents, were a byproduct of the secret war gas programs during both World Wars, in which an explosion and the exposure of seamen to mustard gas led to the observation that the alkylating agents could cause bone marrow and lymphoid hypoplasia (i.e., incomplete or defective development of an organ, impairing its growth to normal size). Following this, many drugs have been developed and tested for their potential clinical activity, and currently about 35–40 cytotoxic drugs (excluding hormonal agents) are licensed and in general use, while several new agents and new combinations are undergoing clinical trials.

As the aim of tumor treatment is cure or long-term remission, the cell-killing capacity of cytotoxic drugs is measured by their lethality for the stem cells, which have a very large capacity for proliferation, i.e., in the same way that the efficacy of radiotherapy is measured. Other types of damage often also occur, and these effects may lead to toxic side effects or may contribute to remission of the tumor without leading to cure. The toxicity to normal tissue limits both the dose and the frequency of administration of chemotherapy. Many drugs cause toxic side effects precisely because of their preferential activity against rapidly proliferating cells, which in normal tissue are found in the bone marrow, the intestinal mucosa, hair follicles, and the reproductive organs (the gonads). Common side effects of many cytotoxic drugs are loss of hair, nausea, vomiting, and carcinogenesis, while several drugs produce specific side effects in various types of normal tissue.

The use of chemotherapy increased dramatically during the 1960s, when it became clear that, with a few exceptions, single drugs do not cure cancer and that combinations of drugs are necessary to obtain durable clinical responses. By combining two or more drugs, it is possible to achieve several objectives which are not possible if only a single agent is used for the treatment:

- It may provide maximum cell kill within the range of toxicity tolerated by the patient for each drug.
- Tumor cells resistant to specific drugs may be covered by other drugs in the combination.
- It prevents or slows the development of resistance in initially responding cell lines.

New drug combinations are being developed and evaluated according to the following principles:

- Only drugs with single-agent activity, preferably with a fraction of complete remission rather than partial remission, should be included.
- If possible, the toxicities of the drugs in a combination should not overlap.
- The individual drugs should be used in their optimal dose and schedule.
- The therapy should be given at fixed intervals, with the treatment-free period between each cycle being the shortest possible time necessary for recovery of the most sensitive normal tissue, which in most cases is the bone marrow.

Chemotherapy is normally used in one of four principal ways. In *induction therapy*, it is given as the primary treatment for patients who present with advanced cancer for which no alternative treatment exists. Induction therapy in patients who fail after one course of drug treatment and require further chemotherapy is referred to as *salvage therapy*. These patients are particularly difficult to treat because of widespread drug resistance, their poor general health, and often sizable tumors. *Adjuvant chemotherapy* denotes the use of systemic treatment after the primary tumor has been controlled by a form of local treatment such as surgery or radiotherapy. Determination of the suitability of adjuvant therapy for specific types of tumor is based on data concerning their average risk of recurrence after local treatment and on the presence or absence of factors which are known to have a negative influence on prognosis.

If chemotherapy is used as the initial treatment for patients who present with a localized tumor for which there is a possible alternative treatment regimen, it is referred to as *primary* or *neoadjuvant chemotherapy*. In this case, the preservation of the primary tumor makes it possible to use it as a biologic marker of the responsiveness of the cancer to the drugs. Assuming that the response of possible metastases is similar to or greater than the response of the primary tumor, a poor response of the primary tumor to the chemotherapy can be used to indicate a group of patients for whom alternative treatment possibilities, if they exist, should be used as quickly as possible. In some cases, primary chemotherapy may be used to reduce the size of the tumor before operation, thereby allowing less mutilating surgery. In general, in some of the common cancers, where the standard treatments are less than satisfactory, clinical trials examining the possibility of curing selected groups of patients by chemotherapy alone are being performed. If these current trials are successful, this would lead to shorter and more effective treatment regimens that cause less morbidity.

Research in chemotherapy is taking many directions. One is to use our increasing understanding of the biological mechanisms that lead to the development of drug resistance to test new agents that may increase the sensitivity of drug-resistant cells. Another is the investigation of drugs that inhibit metastasis without causing direct toxicity to tumor cells, while others are attempting to increase the delivery of the cytotoxic drugs to the tumor cells by the use of special carriers such as antibodies or liposomes. Already in widespread clinical use, but also under intensive examination, are agents that inhibit or modify drug toxicity, such as growth factors that stimulate the recovery of bone marrow or bone marrow transplantation (BMT), either from the patients themselves or from a close relative, which allows an intensification of the chemotherapy regimen, usually by increasing the doses. A further field of active research is the exploitation of the theoretical benefits of combining chemotherapy with radiotherapy, including use of each modality to treat tumor cells that have developed resistance to the other and use of drugs that are selective for hypoxic cells resistant to radiation.

Hormonal Therapy

For tumors growing in organs under hormonal control (in particular the reproductive organs), manipulation of the hormonal environment may result in regression of the tumors. Hormonal therapy may consist in either surgical resection to remove the source of a normal hormone, the administration of an antihormone, or the administration of other hormonal substances. Generally, hormonal therapy is not curative, but it has the potential advantage of obtaining long-term control with only limited side effects.

Tumors of the breast, prostate, endometrium, and thyroid respond to specific hormones. For instance, prostate cancers respond to surgical resections which remove the source of testosterone, but also to medical treatment with the female hormone estrogen. Hormonal management of breast cancer may comprise the administration of estrogen and the antiestrogen tamoxifen, eradication of the endogenous estrogen production by surgical resection of the ovaries, and various other means.

Biologic Therapy

Biologic treatment is becoming an important new treatment modality in cancer, stimulated by an increasingly better understanding of the basic biologic aspects of host defense mechanisms against cancer and rapid biotechnical developments making the relevant molecules available in the quantities needed for clinical testing etc. The common principle is to produce antitumor effects primarily through the action of natural host defense mechanisms or the administration of substances occurring naturally in mammals. The field is still in its infancy but is considered very promising, and a number of successful applications of biologic therapy for cancer have been observed.

The most frequent approach to biologic therapy of cancer has been to stimulate the immune defense mechanisms of the host, often by trying to make the tumor appear more "foreign" compared to normal tissue or by magnifying relatively weak host immune reactions to growing tumors. Strategies for immunotherapy can be divided into *active approaches*, in which the patient is immunized with materials designed to elicit an immune reaction capable of preventing or retarding tumor growth, and *passive approaches*, which involve the transfer to the patient of immunologic reagents (e.g., cells or antibodies) that have the ability to mediate antitumor responses directly or indirectly. Recent efforts have concentrated on the passive approach, because many studies have shown that patients are immunosuppressed by the growing tumor, which may render attempts at immunotherapy intrinsically disadvantageous. The center of current interest is adoptive immunotherapy, which denotes passive immunotherapy with cells (e.g., lymphocytes or macrophages) that are sensitized with antitumor reactivity (i.e., antibodies).

Examples of *biologic response modifiers* (i.e., substances normally produced in small amounts as part of the body's natural response to cancer and other diseases) that are being evaluated in the treatment of various cancers include the following:

1. *Cytokines* are proteins formed in small amounts by all human cells to help regulate cell processes and which may act directly on cancer cells by inhibiting their growth or promoting their development into more normal cells.
2. *Interleukins* are another type of cytokine produced by lymphocytes (i.e., the white blood cells that fight invading antigens, particularly viruses), carrying regulatory signals between blood-forming cells. Interleukin-2, the most studied, stimulates the growth and activity of white blood cells.
3. *Colony-stimulating factors* (CSFs) are proteins that stimulate bone marrow cells to divide and differentiate into platelets, red blood cells, and various forms of specialized white blood cells. These can be used both to help patients overcome the side effects of high-dose chemotherapy and possibly also to make certain tumor cells more sensitive to antitumor drugs.

Supportive Treatment

With a serious and sometimes immediately life-threatening disease such as cancer, patients and their families and also the treating health care personnel have a much higher tolerance of toxic side effects of the treatments than would be the case for most other less serious diseases. The more or less complete loss of head and body hair (alopecia), which is an almost certain consequence of many chemotherapy regimens, is accepted by most patients as an unavoidable and tolerable, although regrettable, fact of current treatments. It would almost certainly not be accepted to this degree as a side effect of antihypertension therapy of completely asymptomatic "patients" with somewhat elevated blood pressure.

A number of toxic side effects of treatment are different, however, because they (may) directly influence the way planned treatment schedules are carried out in clinical practice and thereby presumably affect also the outcomes of the treatments. Supportive care may be defined as therapy which is intended to enhance the possibilities of delivering anticancer therapy according to the planned schedule, without a reduction in doses or delays in the delivering of doses. Considerable research resources have been devoted to the field of supportive care during the last couple of decades. At least to a certain extent, this is because many researchers and clinicians perceive the often rather disappointing outcomes of new treatment regimens as (partly) a consequence of disturbances to the scheduled administration of the regimens which have been necessitated by the side effects of the treatments. Another consideration behind this particular allocation of research resources may be a belief in a positive dose-response relation, where dose increases would be expected to lead to a larger proportion of cures. However plausible such an hypothesis might appear, it has not received generally convincing corroboration by empirical studies so far.

Several important toxic side effects have attracted particular research attention, and promising new products and methods have resulted from this effort. Understandably, these have also attracted the interest of economists, because many of the new products or treatment methods have high acquisition prices or are expected to be costly to implement in practice. It is therefore important to assess the therapeutic benefits and costs of the new treatments and consider them in relation to the existing alternatives.

One of the important side effects receiving particular attention is *emesis*, i.e., nausea and vomiting, which is associated with many different chemotherapeutic regimens and also appears in some patients receiving radiotherapy. The emetogeneic effects of chemotherapy depend on the specific drugs in the combination and on their doses, with cisplatin being one of the most emetogeneic of the currently available and often used drugs. However, the appearance of the emesis syndrome also depends on subjective factors in the patients, in that it seems clear that psychic conditioning plays a certain role, i.e., patients having experienced emesis in an earlier cycle react much more strongly later on. Great variations are observed in patients' susceptibility to emesis, and this corroborates the hypothesis that an important psychic component is involved.

Emesis may be more than a very unpleasant side effect, endured but tolerated by the patient as an unavoidable consequence of current state-of-the-art treatment. In some patients, the experience or probably more often anticipating the experience of emesis is so troubling and disturbing that scheduled cycles of chemotherapy may have to be postponed or the doses reduced until the patient feels able to face the threat of a renewed emetic episode. Instances in which a patient completely refuses future chemotherapy after having experienced a severe emetic episode are reported with some degree of frequency.

In recent years, research on antiemetic regimens for the management of chemotherapy-induced nausea and vomiting has resulted in the marketing of a new group of interesting products with an important antiemetic effect. The best known of these new chemical entities is called ondansetron. As is frequently the case, this new drug, which seems to have a number of therapeutic benefits compared to the already available antiemetic agents, has a relatively high acquisition price. Accordingly, there is an obvious need to assess the relative costs and benefits of ondansetron and the other new agents compared with the older alternatives.

Another important and pervasive side effect, which is often the cause of delays or modifications of planned treatment schedules, is the *myelosuppressive effect* of most chemotherapy and radiotherapy regimens. In general, chemotherapy and radiotherapy work by affecting cells that are dividing, and they are used to treat cancer because cancer cells divide more often than most other cells. High-dose treatment with chemotherapy or radiotherapy increases their efficacy in killing cancer cells, but at the same time it can severely damage or destroy the patient's bone marrow so that the patient is no longer able to produce the vitally needed blood cells. Destroying the bone marrow may be either an essential part of the treatment (for diseases that affect the bone marrow, such as leukemia) or it may simply be an unfortunate and unavoidable side effect of the treatment of cancers that affect other parts of the body. The most serious effect of myelosuppression is *immunosuppression*, causing the patient's body to be unable to defend itself against infection because of too few white blood cells.[2] However, myelosuppression may also imply an increased risk of anemia (too few red blood cells) and of bleeding that is violent or difficult to stop (because of too few platelets in the blood).

Supportive care for immunosuppression usually includes protective isolation of patients, who stay in a more or less isolated hospital room in an environment kept free of infectious agents. Depending on the institution, the

---

[2] The white blood cells, or leukocytes, constitute the most important part of the human immune system. A reduction in the number of white blood cells is called leukopenia and increases the patient's susceptibility to infections. About 65% of the leukocytes are granulocytes (primarily neutrophils), which fight mainly bacterial infections, and 35% are agranulocytes (primarily lymphocytes), which fight invading antigens, especially viruses.

medical staff and visitors entering the patient's room may be required to go through preventive measures such as thorough hand-washing or putting on masks and gowns. In general, the patients may also often start receiving antimicrobials (e.g., antibacterials, antifungals, and antivirals) just before or soon after chemotherapy or radiotherapy in order to prevent infection. Some centers also use intravenous *immunoglobulin therapy* as a preventive measure against infection.

Despite the various measures taken to prevent infections, these continue to be a major concern in the management of cancer patients, particular those with hematological malignancies. More intensive treatment regimens have produced a larger number of immunosuppressed patients, who suffer an increased risk of infectious complications. In addition to bacterial and fungal infections, parasitic and viral infections are also major primary or secondary complications, and often the same patient develops superinfections or multiple infections, which contribute to making their management a complex matter. Seeking improvements in the management of infections in granulocytopenic patients is a very active research area, where much progress has been achieved. However, overall survival depends mainly on rapid recovery of an adequate leukocyte count as well as remission of the underlying disease.

Rapid initiation of empiric antimicrobial therapy as soon as the patient develops signs or symptoms of infection, e.g., the onset of fever, is mandatory. The standard treatment regimen has been parenteral administration on an inpatient basis of a combination of two or more antibiotics. As no particular combination has been documented to be clearly superior to others, the recommendation has been to let each particular institution make its own choice, taking the local epidemiology of the various bacteria and other pathogens into consideration. Patient response to treatment is evaluated after 3–5 days, and if the patient responds, the regimen should be continued for at least one more week. If the patient remains febrile, the initial regimen should be modified on the basis of culture and sensitivity results and the patient's clinical state.

Newer antibiotics, such as third-generation cephalosporins and carbapenems, offer a single-agent alternative to the standard combination regimens. This alternative seems to offer several advantages in the form of easier administration, lower cost, and a significant reduction in toxicity, which, inter alia, reduces the requirement for close monitoring of the patients. Despite the apparent advantages, there is still considerable controversy regarding the use of single-agent antibiotic therapy, and a number of clinical trials aiming at clarifying the issues are in progress. Another contentious issue is the optimal duration of therapy, which is also the object of several current trials.

In addition, several potent antibacterials have recently been introduced in an oral form, and this has led to a reassessment of the routine use of parenteral antibiotic therapies, which is also the subject of trials. For instance, severely ill patients might be switched to an oral regimen after a few days of receiving parenteral treatment during which the pathogen may be identified, while patients with less severe infections may be able to receive oral antibiotics from the beginning. These oral forms of antibiotics usually have lower acquisition costs, and they reduce or eliminate the costs for preparing and administering the medications. In addition, oral medications seem to offer a number of important advantages, e.g., greater clinical flexibility, possibility of earlier patient discharge or avoidance of hospitalization altogether, reduced need for nursing of hospitalized patients, and a reduction in the risk of nosocomial infections, because of a reduced risk of catheter-related infections and possibly shorter hospital stays. Many ongoing trials aim at assessing and quantifying these apparent advantages of oral antibiotics for cancer patients, also in economic terms.

A number of procedures and products allowing the patients to receive high doses of chemotherapy and, in many cases, radiotherapy as well have been developed during recent years and have attracted the attention of clinicians and economists alike, because of their potential therapeutic benefits and relatively high acquisition prices. These groups of interesting products include the hematopoietic growth factors, i.e., proteins that stimulate the growth and development of cells in the bone marrow. They are produced naturally by the body itself, but they may also be produced in the laboratory in large quantities. The most studied hematopoietic growth factors are the CSFs, which increase the production of white blood cells and therefore help protect against infection. The CSFs are already widely used in cancer treatments to reduce the risk of life-threatening infections, and a fair number of economic evaluations of CSF-supported treatments have been published in recent years.

Another important innovative procedure is BMT or, more recently, peripheral blood stem cell transplantation (PBSCT). These techniques allow stem cells that have been damaged by treatment to be replaced with healthy stem cells that can produce the blood cells that the patient needs. In patients with leukemia, BMT provides bone marrow that is free of disease, either from a donor or from the patients themselves after their own marrow has been treated to remove cancer cells. For certain types of leukemias and lymphomas, BMT is considered the best available treatment option under certain circumstances, but it is also being evaluated in other types of cancer, including cancers of the breast, lung, and ovary. BMT and PBSCT are also being studied for their potential usefulness in the treatment of diseases that have spread and are not responding to other treatment or cannot be removed by surgery (such as some tumors in the head and neck).

BMT is a highly technical procedure requiring extensive hospitalization and follow-up care, and it is therefore also very costly. Advances in BMT treatment methods and the increasing use of PBSCT have reduced the time that many patients spend in hospital by accelerating recovery, but the costs are still considerable and the need for economic evaluations is obvious.

A Brief Introduction to Economic Evaluation

During recent years, a relatively new academic discipline, health economics, has been growing and has gained increased importance and attention, both in the academic world and in business, public administration, intergovernmental organizations, etc. A growing number of universities are offering courses in health economics and establishing chairs or even specific departments dedicated to research and teaching within this field, and the number of scientific journals focusing on health economics is increasing year by year. The number of people employed as health economists has also been rapidly increasing. This is especially true for the pharmaceutical industry (and perhaps also other important suppliers of products used for the production of health care services), which is increasingly often faced with the need to document the economic value for money of new products. Not surprisingly, then, health economics is very often perceived as identical to one of its (important) subdisciplines, economic evaluation, which was very recently dubbed pharmacoeconomics, for obvious reasons.

This is an extremely reductionist view of health economics, which, speaking in very general terms, is concerned with the more or less successful application of the general economist's "tool kit" to questions concerning the demand for and supply of health care services. The beginning of this endeavor dates back to the early 1960s, when a seminal article by the later Nobel prize laureate Kenneth Arrow was published, providing an in-depth and original discussion of the similarities and distinctions between health care services and other economic goods and services. The discipline has since evolved by employing an increasing number of concepts and ideas from general economic theory and from developments in econometrics, i.e., the use of mathematical, statistical models to estimate empirical economic relationships.

Health economics and the ideas evoked and discussed by health economic analyses are very commonly associated with crude cost cutting and with determining whether the treatment of certain groups of patients is worthwhile financially. This is not too surprising, given that the discipline evolved during a period marked by tightening of the health care budgets in all Western societies due to steadily increasing costs, an aging population presumably requiring more care, new and more expensive treatments, and perceived difficulties in financing health care by higher general taxes or increases in compulsory contributions to the national health insurance systems.

However, the popular view is a misconception which fails to appreciate that, even though costs are of central concern for economic analysis, economics is as much about the attributes of what is being purchased as about what it costs. In economic assessments properly conceived, the aspiration is to take both benefits and costs into account simultaneously and on an equal footing, without any of these factors taking precedence over the other. It should also be stressed that economic assessments do not, in and of themselves, have any particular implications with respect to the possible need for containing cost. Just as often as not, the results of an evaluation may be used to argue for a cost increase, justified by the benefits which may be obtained.

In this chapter, a brief introduction to the aims and methods of economic evaluation will be given in order to provide the reader with a minimal theoretical background for understanding the following survey and for appreciating the comments given on a number of the contributions reviewed. The reader should be aware and appreciate, however, that the field is frequently much more complex than it initially appears to be and that there are still many methodological issues which have not been finally settled and on which there are quite divergent opinions. To this may be added that the vast majority of published studies do not adhere to even the methodological rules on which there is general agreement. It will of course be quite impossible to cover these complications adequately in an introductory chapter like this, but a number of references for further reading will be given throughout the chapter.

Before embarking on economic evaluations proper, another type of analysis, the so-called cost-of-illness (COI) analysis, will be dealt with. This type of analysis was very common in the early stages of health economics and may have to take some of the blame for the common misconceptions about analyses in health economics. Today, most health economists are very critical of COI analyses on a number of theoretical grounds, but the approach continues to be used from time to time and new analyses are still appearing, also for cancer.

Cost-of-Illness Analysis

The COI approach to calculating the economic burden of a specific disease or of illness in general is an intuitively reasonable way of determining the costs for society at large. These consist of the resources directly consumed in the treatment processes and of the loss of valuable production which is caused by morbidity and mortality. To this is usually added another category of costs, which is usually given labels such as "intangible costs" and comprises factors such as grief, pain, and anxiety experienced by the patients and their families. However, this type of cost is usually only mentioned in passing, and attempts at actually valuing them in pecuniary terms are very rare indeed.

The *direct costs* of illness are the costs of the resources consumed or used directly in the treatment processes. Examples include the time and knowledge of physicians, nurses, and other medical care personnel, machines and equipment (e.g., operating theaters, high-energy beam generators for radiotherapy, tubes and bags for intravenous administration of drugs), and drugs and other consumables (e.g., cytostatic drugs and blood transfusions). Other examples may be care delivered by primary-care physicians, specialists, and visiting nurses, home help services, and changes in the physical environment of the patient's home required by the disease. Yet another category of direct costs is the transport of the patient to and from the place where care is provided.

The *indirect costs* of illness consist in the value of the loss of production or productive time due to morbidity or premature mortality caused by the illness concerned, and this is the most controversial point of the COI approach. Conventionally, this type of cost has been valued by the Human Capital method, which determines the value, for instance, of premature mortality by the loss of expected production of the person concerned. In practice, this has been accomplished with various levels of detail in the data used, but very often it has been done on a very general level using data for the average wage earner. The mortality cost for a 45-year-old man dying of cancer is then found by estimating his future expected income year by year until expected (normal) retirement age, discounting this figure by a proper discount rate[1], and summing all these yearly figures to an aggregate amount, which is the capitalized present value of his future income. The same principle has been applied, with the appropriate modifications, to value the costs due to morbidity. It has also been widely used in other connections, principally in the methods used for calculating the amount of compensation for damages, which the courts in many different juridical systems are using. This fact may contribute to (or be caused by) the common sense validity attached to the principle, but it is nevertheless extremely problematical from the point of view of economic theory[2].

As a method of measuring the value of a human life, e.g., in considering whether a specific preventive measure is economically worthwhile, the Human Capital model may be criticized on a number of counts. In essence, the notion amounts to regarding medical care as only a means to maximize na-

[1] Discounting is the opposite of the more familiar calculation of the future stream of annual returns on a capital investment made today. The purpose of discounting is to make allowance for the differential timing of costs and benefits, which are made comparable by calculating their present value through discounting. A stream of future incomes (or costs, or whatever) is thus turned into a capital value. The reasoning behind the use of discounting is the hypothetical principle of *time preference*, i.e., that people are assumed to prefer to receive a benefit earlier and incur a cost later, because it gives them more options. The proper rate of discount is a contentious issue, the subject of hundreds of articles in academic economic journals, which will not be dealt with here.

[2] By calculating the amount of compensation in this way, the courts may be claimed to give potential tortfeasors the wrong kind of incentive to exert the proper amount of care in going about their business. The courts' determination of the amount of compensation is based on microdata for the plaintiff, which make the compensation depend on the individual's current income at the time of the accident; thus the compensation payable at the death of a child, for instance, is very limited.

tional income; it ignores essential features of medical care such as the relief of pain, distress, and anxiety and the improvement of physical and psychological well-being, and it leads to fundamental inequity in the setting of priorities. This is because the elderly, children, and generally people outside the normal labor market[3] will be disfavored compared to people active in the labor market and with high incomes. At another level, the method may be criticized for not taking into account fundamental adjustment mechanisms in the labor market, which may attenuate the costs significantly. For instance, the workload of an employee who dies prematurely will probably eventually be taken over by somebody else, perhaps by hiring someone who was previously unemployed. If this is the case, the estimates of indirect cost based on the traditional Human Capital method will be highly exaggerated[4].

COI calculations used to be very popular and were a very widely used method in health economics, also enjoying considerable attention from the political decision makers. However, it is completely uncertain what the resulting figures, usually extremely large amounts, may actually be used for, except perhaps for deliberations about research priorities. In a number of studies, the value of a new treatment has been determined by means of the (potential) avoided costs, i.e., by calculating the COI of the disease with and without this new treatment, respectively. The decision criterion to be used with this kind of analysis has never been made clear, however. What is to be concluded, for instance, if the new treatment actually leads to an increase in the costs? There is no way to take the potential therapeutic gains from such a new treatment into account, and by increasing cost it may appear undesirable. It has also been common to use the Human Capital approach to calculate the treatment benefits in analyses misleadingly given the label "cost-benefit analysis", but it is now more widely recognized that this approach is incompatible with the theoretical welfare foundation of cost-benefit analysis.

The Human Capital approach to valuing human life and suffering has been discarded by most health economists, while the friction cost method is considered as interesting for the purpose of determining the production loss due to disease or premature mortality (but *not* for valuing human life, it should be stressed!). There is disagreement about the proper handling of indirect costs in economic assessments, i.e., whether they should be included or not, and if so, how. In most published studies they are ignored, but this "solution" gives many analysts an uncomfortable feeling, because they con-

[3] It is usually stressed in discussions of principle that the concept of productive activity should be interpreted very broadly in order to reduce this potential for bias and to ensure that household and leisure activities are also considered as having an economic value. However, in practical calculations, this tends not to be done because of lack of data. If such calculations are made, rather low wage rates are generally used for the imputations.

[4] An alternative method of calculating indirect cost, the so-called friction cost method, which tries to take the likely adjustments via the labor market into account, has been developed by researchers at the Institute for Medical Technology Assessment in Rotterdam (see, e.g., Koopmanschap and Rutten 1993; Koopmanschap et al. 1995). Comparative calculations show that the indirect cost calculated by the traditional Human Capital method should be divided by around a factor of 10 in order to approach the results of calculations by the friction cost method.

sider it obvious that loss of productive output and possibilities is an undeniable fact of disease and of many treatments. Alternative treatment regimens may have very different impacts on indirect costs, and ignoring these costs in a comparison of the treatments is equivalent to leaving out important information, according to this viewpoint.

The reader may be referred to Koopmanschap and Rutten (1993) and to Hodgson (1994) for concise accounts of the contentious issues surrounding indirect costs, their measurement, and their inclusion in economic assessments.

The Meaning of the Term "Economic Evaluation"

The term "economic evaluation" refers to a general methodological approach to assessing the relative worth of various activities.[5] In principle, the approach can be used to analyze any type of activities, and it should always be characterized by two conditions:

1. The analysis comprises both advantages (benefits or effects) *and* drawbacks (costs) of the activities.
2. Economic evaluations are concerned with *choices*.

In relation to human beings' desire for satisfaction of needs, the resources in any society, even the richest, are strictly limited. Since most resources cannot be used for several different activities at the same time, it is necessary to *choose* between the possible uses of the resources (see the definition of economics as the science of choice referred to in the "Introduction"). By using a certain amount of resources for one particular activity, one has at the same time chosen not to employ the same resources for other activities and thereby chosen to forgo the satisfaction of needs that could have been obtained by these competing activities. The central cost concept of economic theory follows by implication: The *opportunity cost* of an activity is the utility or satisfaction that could have been obtained by employing the resources used for the activity for other activities or purposes[6].

---

[5] For goods and activities traded in normal markets, this valuing of the relative worth of the various possibilities is performed by the market participants, especially by the buyers when they consider the acquisition of goods. The use of formal economic evaluations as an aid to decision making becomes relevant for goods or activities for which the normal market mechanisms cannot be assumed to function or where their normal function may be assumed to be impaired, for one reason or another. The methods used in economic evaluations were first developed in connection with attempts at determining the economic implications of large public investment projects in the United States in the 1930s, e.g., the Tennessee Valley Authority's building of a dam to generate electrical power.

[6] Every action has a potential opportunity cost, but the size of this cost depends on the viewpoint of the analysis and on the specifics of the situation. This makes the concept rather elusive, and its empirical estimation is very difficult. In most published economic evaluations in health care, the costing problem is "solved" by using whatever data are readily at hand, e.g., charges or prices used in transactions between hospitals and pharmaceutical producers or laboratories. It is only by coincidence that these charges or prices will have anything to do with the actual opportunity costs.

On the basis of the characteristics mentioned, economic evaluation may be defined in general terms as a comparative analysis of alternative lines of action including both their effects and their costs in the appraisal. The basic tasks in any economic evaluation are therefore to identify, measure, value, and compare all the costs and effects of the alternatives under consideration. The purpose is to carry out a structured collection of information regarding each of the alternatives and to ensure that the information about all the alternatives is collected, treated, and assessed according to uniform and consistent criteria.

These two basic characteristics of economic evaluations may be used for classifying a number of types of analyses frequently encountered in health care.

The dimensions of Table 1 are accordingly determined by the answers to the following two questions:
1. Are two or more alternatives compared?
2. Are both the effects and the costs of each alternative taken into account?

Field 1 includes descriptions of the effects of a single treatment (e.g., a case series), while field 2 contains only assessments of the costs and may be termed a cost identification study. Field 3 refers to investigations including both costs and effects, but without a comparison with one or more alternative treatments. Case series of type 1 have been abundant in the medical scientific journals for many years, but the two other types are now seen increasingly often. An early example would be Smith's calculation of the costs of intravesical chemotherapy in bladder cancer (P. Smith 1985).

Studies in fields 4 and 5 may be called partial evaluations, because they entail a comparison of two or more alternatives, but only include *either* effects *or* costs. Field 4 covers the randomized clinical trial comparing the effects of two or more treatment alternatives, while ignoring their costs. Investigations of type 5 are uncommon as formal studies adhering to strict criteria, while they are very common as "back-of-an-envelope" comparisons of the prices of more or less equivalent drugs, based on a postulate of essential

Table 1. Different types of studies in health care categorized according to their inclusion of cost and/or effects and to whether two or more alternatives are compared

	Includes only the effects	Includes only the costs	Includes both the costs and effects
No comparison between alternatives	Field 1: Effect description	Field 2: Cost identification	Field 3: Effect and cost description
Comparison between two or more alternatives	Field 4: e.g., randomized clinical trial	Field 5: Cost comparison, e.g., cost minimization	Field 6: Full economic evaluation (cost-benefit; cost-effectiveness; cost-utility)

Source: Department of Clinical Epidemiology and Biostatistics (1984).

equivalence (ignoring, for instance, differences in types and frequencies of side effects). During recent years, a number of so-called *cost-minimization studies* have been published, trying to identify the least costly among a number of equally effective treatments. However, equivalence of treatments is more often assumed than documented, and in reality treatments are rarely essentially equivalent in all important respects, except for generic drugs. There is, therefore, a tendency in cost-minimization studies to put too much emphasis on the costs at the expense of consideration of (perhaps) relevant differences in treatment effect.

Field 6 contains full economic evaluations comparing two or more alternatives with respect to both their costs and effects. *Cost-benefit analysis* is usually considered the ideal assessment method, but it is very demanding with regard to data collection and therefore seldom used in practice. One of the attractions of cost-benefit analysis proper is that it is firmly grounded in theoretical welfare economics, which is concerned with determining an allocation of society's limited resources so as to maximize social welfare, given individual preferences and the technological possibilities. Another is that only this type of analysis allows a comprehensive comparison of very different activities, i.e., competing uses of society's scarce resources, in order to maximize the net benefits obtained.

In cost-benefit analyses, the costs and effects or benefits of each alternative in the comparison are made comparable by using a common yardstick, i.e., money. In this way, it becomes possible to quantify the net benefits of a program, i.e., the benefits minus the costs, and the net benefits of various programs may then readily be compared. In general, the decision criterion in cost-benefit analysis is that the treatment regimen with the highest positive net benefits will be preferred to a treatment with a lower, but still positive net benefit. Treatments with a negative net benefit, i.e., where the costs exceed the benefits, should not be carried out at all.

In principle, the total benefits of a given treatment should be determined by measuring the sum of the willingness to pay for having (access to) the treatment of all the people affected by the decision about offering the treatment or not. Not surprisingly, the main problem with the practical use of cost-benefit analysis is to obtain a reliable evaluation of the consequences of the alternatives compared. In fact, very few cost-benefit analyses in the strict sense of the term have been carried out in health care, and there has been widespread *misuse* of the term, but there may at present be an increasing interest in using this type of analysis[7] (see, e.g., Johannesson and Jönsson 1991).

Currently, *cost-effectiveness analysis*, with its variant *cost-utility analysis*, may be claimed to be the method of choice for economic evaluations, be-

[7] This may perhaps be a consequence of the continuing methodological developments in the field of economic evaluation, which have revealed hitherto unrecognized or ignored complexities in applying the apparently simpler types of analysis, such as cost-effectiveness analysis.

cause the problems in obtaining pecuniary valuations of the therapeutic effects for cost-benefit analysis are often considered as prohibitive. In cost-effectiveness analyses, there is no attempt at calculating net benefits by using a common yardstick (such as money) for costs and effects. Rather, the effects of the alternatives are measured in terms of "natural units" (e.g., by the number of survivors 5 years after treatment for a certain cancer, by a reduction in morbidity and/or mortality obtained by a new treatment compared to the old treatment or treatments) or in terms of improvements in the patients' utility or quality of life. The final result of the analysis will usually be presented in the form of a ratio, as the costs per "unit" of effect or as the effect per unit of costs. For example, two treatments may save lives with different probabilities and costs, but can be described by their costs per (statistical) live saved, thereby being made comparable.

Generally, the purpose of carrying out a cost-effectiveness or cost-utility analysis of various treatment regimens for a certain indication may be said to be to determine which of the treatment alternatives gives the highest degree of goal attainment within a fixed budget (or a resource constraint expressed in other terms). The dual (inverse) formulation is that the purpose is to determine which alternative minimizes the costs of obtaining a given size of the desired effect.

Cost-effectiveness analysis is concerned with determining to what degree two or more treatment alternatives attain a common type of effect, e.g., an increase in expected survival, and at what costs. However, the outcomes of health care interventions are rarely so simple as to be measurable in only one dimension, and in comparing treatment regimens for most diseases one will generally be interested in more than a single dimension of outcome. For instance, the interesting outcome of many cancer treatments would not only be "mere" survival, but also the types, frequencies, and severity of side effects. Given this, one might choose to carry out a separate cost-effectiveness analysis for each interesting dimension of outcome, with the risk of ending with equivocal results, where no single treatment comes out best in all the dimensions of interest. Other possibilities are to choose one dimension of outcome as the single most important and only carry out the analysis for this or to design a weighting scheme according to which each dimension will be assigned a certain weight in the final assessment of the treatment alternatives. However, these kinds of solutions are usually considered unsatisfactory because of their arbitrariness.

Another drawback of cost-effectiveness analysis is that all effects are assumed to be valued identically. Thus a gain of 20 years of life for one person is considered equal to a gain of 1 year each for 20 people, and possible variations in the quality of life in the years gained are ignored.

The development of cost-utility analysis may to some extent be perceived as an attempt to overcome the unidimensionality and disregard of variations in quality of life found in cost-effectiveness analysis. Physicians, psychologists, and health economists alike have been struggling for more than 20 years to develop outcome measures that would allow comparisons of disease states or treatments with widely varying consequences for the patients' health status and quality of life. A great deal of research effort has been put into the development and validation of various measurement methods that may be used for quantitative assessments of complex outcomes of health care interventions, unfortunately without resulting in a consensus about a preferred index or measurement method. As no "natural" gold standard is conceivable in this area, the only way to reach an agreement on a preferred method will be by trying to reach consensus by decision.

In principle, cost-utility analysis, when suitably developed and applied, should allow an assessment and mutual comparison across all conceivable treatment regimens of every possible disease. The results of the assessment for each treatment would be expressed in a single dimension in the form of a ratio, e.g., as incremental[8] costs per quality-adjusted life year (QALY), and a complete ordering in this dimension would be possible. So far, however, the published studies using a cost-utility approach have used widely differing methods for assessing and quantifying treatment outcomes in terms of utilities, QALYs, or whatever other term has been preferred. Possible comparisons across studies of different illnesses (see the so-called cost-utility league tables, e.g., in T. Smith et al. 1993) must therefore be treated with extreme caution, and usually their value should be considered as limited to giving an indication of orders of magnitude.

A Framework for Economic Evaluations

The framework described below is most directly related to cost-effectiveness analysis, which is the most frequently used method for economic evaluation. With the appropriate modifications, the framework is of equal relevance for the other types of economic evaluation.

Data for an economic evaluation may come from a variety of sources, and these may be combined in various ways. It is generally agreed that data on the relative efficacy of the alternatives should be based on results of adequate randomized clinical trials. It is also widely believed that an ideal way to collect data on resource utilization for the cost calculations is to integrate the data collection into the clinical trial context, either by adding a limited num-

[8] Despite virtual unanimity on this particular methodological issue, *average ratios* (often referred to simply as cost-utility or cost-effectiveness ratios) are frequently used in the presentation of study results instead of the appropriate *incremental ratios*, which assess the addition in therapeutic gain and costs of going from one treatment to another. It is generally inappropriate to investigate any treatment in isolation from alternatives, but this is what is implied by using average ratios. Only if the alternative to a given treatment under investigation is associated with virtually zero costs and zero effects will the incremental be equal to the average. However, even if no active treatment is chosen for a particular disease, it cannot normally be rationally assumed that there are no costs associated with the disease, and a certain number of patients may experience an improvement despite not being actively treated, so the effect will not be zero (see Rittenhouse 1996).

ber of economic questions to an already planned trial (the "piggyback" approach) or by making economic evaluation an integral purpose of the trial from the beginning. It is thus assumed that the prospective collection of cost data will ensure that the necessary data actually are collected and that they can be considered as reliable, thereby avoiding the problems encountered in the much more common approach of collecting the data retrospectively, where data are often missing and generally considered unreliable.

Whether one shares the belief in the value of collecting cost data through clinical trials,[9] it will almost always be necessary to combine these with data from a number of other sources. This is because economic evaluations typically adopt a much longer time span than clinical trials and because an important element in economic evaluations is to analyze what happens to patients who fail to respond to the treatments of the trial, i.e., patients who will not be monitored closely in ordinary clinical trials despite being included in intention to treat analyses. It is imperative that the analysts provide the recipients of the analysis with full and explicit information about the data used, clearly explaining the reasoning behind the choices made and the assumptions used. Unfortunately, it is not common to find a satisfactory description and discussion of the data-generating process, but this may perhaps partly be excused by the space limitations set by most journals.

Formulation of the Objectives of Treatment

In order to assess the relative effectiveness of different treatments, it is necessary to have one or several well-defined and detailed objectives to relate to. Preferably, the objectives should be clinical measures, directly related to the patients' functioning or well-being. Some consider it one of the attractions of cost-effectiveness analysis that it can also be used to assess intermediate outcomes, such as a reduction in blood pressure or changes in laboratory values, but this is a contentious issue (see Johannesson et al. 1996).

Choice of Treatment Alternatives

The choice of treatment alternatives to include in a comparison may have a decisive influence on the results. A common advice is to include all relevant alternatives, i.e., all types of intervention that have a common type of effect on the disease in question. This advice is never adhered to in practice, but it

[9] For an opposing view, see, e.g., Rittenhouse (1995), whose main objection is that the patients recruited into clinical trials can never be considered representative of the general population of the potential users of the treatments, because the proportion of those patients meeting the inclusion criteria of clinical trials that are offered and accept the possibility of treatment choice by randomization is strictly limited. However, the very purpose of cost-effectiveness analysis is to assist in decision making on the general use of the treatments, where the patients will generally differ from those participating in the trials.

is important to make sure that the most commonly used treatment alternatives are actually included in the evaluation if it is to be relevant for decision making. This may give some problems with availability of data on relative effectiveness. Placebo comparisons are rarely relevant for economic evaluations, but many clinical trials are placebo comparisons and many treatments are never directly tested against each other.

Identification and Quantification of Costs and Effects

The relevant costs to include in an economic evaluation depend completely on the viewpoint chosen for the analysis, as what are costs from one point of view may not be so from others. It is therefore imperative that the viewpoint of an analysis is clearly stated from the outset. (This is another instance where published studies only too rarely adhere to a generally agreed upon methodological standard.)

It is usually recommended that a societal viewpoint be adopted for the analysis to ensure that all costs connected with each treatment, no matter who is bearing them, are included. This advice is, however, rarely adhered to in practice, where costs are most often computed from the viewpoint of the hospital or the health care financing system. In this way, significant cost elements may be concealed, and this may lead to important biases when seen from a broader (i.e., societal) viewpoint. A classical example of this is that a policy of diminishing the duration of hospital stays may lead to a large increase in the costs for patients and their families if they have to be taken care of in the home instead. Even if recognized and carefully mentioned in the analysis, this cost element tends to be ignored in the actual decision making, partly because it is rarely quantified as a specific, "tangible" amount and partly because it does not influence the budget constraint of the decision makers.

The total costs of a treatment are determined by the sum of the costs of all the resources committed to the "production process," e.g., doctors' and nurses' time, pharmaceuticals, equipment and materials, ordinary care, and accommodation services. A central part of determining the costs of each treatment is to make an accurate and detailed description of all those activities that are part of the treatment in order to be able to *identify* all the types of resources involved. The subsequent logical step is to *quantify* the amount consumed of each resource, i.e., to count the number of minutes of physician and nurse time, total dose or doses of particular drugs, the number of days of hospitalization etc.

The outcome measures of interest for determining the relative treatment efficacy should be closely related to the ultimate objective of the treatment. If, for instance, a new cancer treatment is primarily expected to reduce the side effects of treatment without significantly improving (or reducing) the expected survival, an outcome measure relating to the patients' quality of life would be of greatest relevance. A second principle is that outcome measures should reflect as closely as possible the patients' own experience of (changes in) their (ill) health and not be based only on laboratory measurements, e.g., neutrophil counts.

Valuation of the Costs

The total costs of the treatments are calculated by multiplying the quantity consumed of each type of resource by a unit cost or price. These also depend on the viewpoint for the analysis. The ideal is to calculate the social cost of the alternatives using social opportunity cost values for the unit costs of the various resources. The usual practical advice given, however, is that, whenever possible, the determination of the unit price of each resource should be based on known market prices (but excluding taxes or subsidies), as these may in general be considered as reasonable approximations to the real opportunity costs (see Gold et al. 1996). Where this is not possible (i.e., where there are obvious market failures such as monopoly), "shadow prices" should be set, either by imputing values (i.e., drawing parallels to known market prices) or by more or less subjective estimates.

Presentation and Interpretation of the Results

From the viewpoint of the final user of an economic assessment, the decisive problem is whether the complexity of the analytical method employed corresponds to the scope of the decision problem posed. As a cost-benefit analysis entails an evaluation of the treatment effects in monetary terms, it is more suited to answering questions of the type "Is the intervention worthwhile? Does it give value for money?" than a cost-effectiveness or cost-utility analysis. Without some additional assumptions, these types of analysis cannot answer this kind of question, while they are well suited to identifying a cost-minimizing way of attaining a given objective.

The results of a cost-benefit analysis will usually be expressed in terms of the net benefits of each alternative, i.e., benefits minus costs. For cost-effectiveness and cost-utility analyses, the most common way to express the result is in a ratio form, usually as the costs per unit of effectiveness or utility. The results of a comparison between the alternatives A and B must logically fit into one of the cells in Table 2, where A may be taken to signify a new treatment and B the standard.

Of crucial importance for a cost-effectiveness analysis is whether the added therapeutic gain when going from one treatment to another is worth the added cost, and it is therefore imperative to use incremental analysis. A proper analysis would not just provide a stand-alone cost-effectiveness ratio, but would incorporate the knowledge and implications of treatments that already exist.

A cell in Table 2 marked by either an A or a B is usually called a *dominant solution.* If, for instance, treatment A is less or at least no more costly

Table 2. Possible outcomes of an economic evaluation of the alternatives A and B and the decision indicated

Costs	Effectiveness		
	A>B	A≈B	A<B
A>B	?	B	B
A≈B	A	A or B	B
A<B	A	A	?

than treatment B and is more or at least as effective, A is the dominant solution, meaning that in going from B to A there is either a gain in effectiveness at no extra cost or a cost saving without any sacrifice in effectiveness. This, however, does not imply anything about the "absolute value for money" of any of the treatments, as cost-effectiveness analysis is only suitable for establishing superiority relative to an alternative and not absolute worth.[10] The decision makers must decide whether the treatment effects obtainable are worth their costs in the first place. In principle, it is important to ensure that the comparator for a new treatment is itself deemed worthwhile, but this is never done in practice (except implicitly, if the comparator is in fact the standard treatment, because, by implication, this must be considered worthwhile by the decision makers).

The most common results of economic evaluations of health care interventions are probably the cells marked by a question mark in Table 2. In these, either a gain in effectiveness can be achieved but only at the expense of an increase in costs, or a cost reduction can be achieved but only at the expense of a loss in effectiveness. In both cases, the incremental cost-effectiveness ratio is positive (whereas this ratio will be negative, zero, or approaching infinity when there is a dominant solution). As before, the analyst will only provide the details and results of the analysis and leave it to the individual decision makers to interpret the results. If their willingness to pay for a particular type of therapeutic gain exceeds the incremental cost-effectiveness ratio for obtaining this gain by going from one treatment to the other, they will probably decide to take this step. One way of helping the decision makers to

[10] For many years, it was regarded as a major advantage of cost-effectiveness analysis compared to cost-benefit analysis that no attempt has to be made to value the effects of the (treatment) alternatives compared in monetary terms. Through the methodological discussions of recent years, it has now become clear, however, that the decision makers cannot avoid this, as they must ultimately decide upon both the absolute and the relative value of the alternatives. By deciding on either treatment alternative, the decision makers will implicitly make an evaluation of the effect in monetary terms, in the same way as they generally do when budgetary decisions are made. In other words, earmarking a budget for particular activities is equivalent to carrying out an implicit evaluation of the effects of these activities. In contrast, in cost-benefit analysis, it is not the decision makers but the (potential) users of the treatments who decide upon their pecuniary value.

determine their own willingness to pay and to make such choices is to provide them with the results of economic evaluations of other treatment alternatives using the same methodology.

It should be stressed once again that these economic assessment methods should be considered exclusively as instruments for critical thinking, a systematic approach to a structured and consistent analysis of decision problems, intended to ensure that the collection of information relevant for each decision alternative is performed according to homogeneous and explicit criteria. The assumptions of the calculations should therefore be clearly stated, and their implications for the interpretation of the results must be made clear, inter alia by *sensitivity analysis* examining the robustness of the results of the analysis with respect to "reasonable" variations in the data and assumptions.[11]

Lastly, it is also necessary to emphasize the importance of making a distinction between the objective of cost containment and that of ensuring value for money. The purpose of performing economic evaluations is to aid decision makers in a particular field to ensure better value for money of their activities. The ultimate value of such analyses must therefore be assessed according to whether they induce the decision makers concerned to make better decisions than they would do in the absence of this kind of information. In practice, this will be rather difficult to assess one way or the other.

---

[11] Sensitivity analysis has been the traditional way of treating uncertainty in the data for an economic evaluation. With the increasingly widespread use of clinical trials as a "vehicle" for collection of the data for economic evaluations in health care, the proper statistical methodology for handling these stochastic data has become an issue in recent years. O'Brien et al. (1994) set out a number of the pertinent considerations on this question.

The Economic Burden of Cancer

Illness creates a burden for the patient and for his or her family, relatives, and friends as well as for society at large. The social and economic implications of disease for the direct victims and for society at large are pain, suffering, disability, and death. Vast amounts of human and technical resources are devoted to detection, diagnosis, and treatment of diseases, but despite this effort, millions of years of life are lost or spent in a state of less than full health. Because of morbidity and premature mortality, large amounts of production, voluntary work in organizations, household activities, and leisure time are forgone by the patients and their families and friends.

There is general agreement that the economic burden of disease for society at large should be measured by the value of goods, services, and productive activities diverted from other uses to provide medical services plus the loss in productive output (defined very broadly) due to morbidity or premature mortality.

Methodological Considerations

The dominating approach to measuring the economic burden for society of illness is called the cost-of-illness (COI) analysis, a method which has already been briefly described and discussed in the previous chapter. The purpose of such a calculation is to provide an estimate of the aggregate economic burden at the social level of a specific disease or group of diseases or of illness in general. The data for COI analyses are usually collected on an aggregate level rather than on the micro level typical for economic evaluations of different treatment or management strategies. It is not uncommon to find no or only very limited primary data collection for a COI analysis, and most frequently such analyses are only based on readily available secondary data, e.g., administrative data registries.

The COI may be calculated using either an *incidence* approach or a *prevalence* approach. With the incidence approach, a longitudinal perspective is chosen and the idea is to calculate the costs of a certain disease (or of illness in general) from its time of diagnosis (or first symptoms) until the patient is cured or until he or she dies of the disease or for any other reason. In the prevalence approach, which is the most commonly used, the time perspective chosen is short and a cross-section analysis is performed. The estimation concerns a given point in time or rather a short time period such as 1 year and summarizes the costs during that year for all the patients suffering from the disease in question during that period. Using a cross-sectional approach, the prevalent patient population may be considered to contain patients in every conceivable state of the disease and thus provide a picture of the expected future course for a patient suffering from it. Data collected in this way may accordingly be used to obtain an estimate of the incidence costs, which otherwise may be difficult to measure, at least for chronic diseases or diseases with a prolonged course.

The COI may be calculated as the losses, pecuniary or otherwise, originating from a certain disease or group of diseases or from all illness taken together. It is common to distinguish between the following three types of cost:

1. *Direct costs* result from the use of resources to prevent, diagnose, and treat the disease in question and from the continuing care, rehabilitation, and terminal care of patients. *Direct medical costs* include costs for the hospitalization, outpatient clinical care, services of primary-care physicians, specialists, nurses and other health care practitioners, drugs, drug sundries, and other materials, etc. *Direct nonmedical costs* include costs borne by patients and their relatives and friends, including costs of transportation to health care providers, extra expenditure for household help for cleaning, laundering, and cooking, help provided by family and friends, special diets and clothing, alterations of property to accommodate the needs of the patient, expenditures for retraining and rehabilitation, and certain financial costs (e.g., interest lost when treatments are paid by patients themselves out of savings or loans).
2. *Indirect costs* are the time and production lost by the patients, family, friends, and others from employment, housekeeping, volunteer activities, and leisure. The patients suffer a reduction or cessation of productive or other activities because of the morbidity, disability, or mortality associated with the disease, while family and friends may incur indirect costs from the time spent caring for the patient or perhaps from loss of opportunities or unwanted job changes necessitated by the patient's illness. The indirect costs also include the time patients and sometimes family members spend visiting physicians and other health care professionals.
3. *Psychosocial* or *intangible costs* are (some of the) terms used to refer to a variety of vaguely defined effects of the disease. It is usually assumed that disease has a negative impact on the quality of life of the patients and the people around them. The patients may lose a part of body or speech and may become disabled and dependent on others for practical help; they may be in pain and grief and be deeply troubled by the prospective of the possible progression of the disease and further deterioration of their state of health. They and their family may become socially isolated and economically dependent, and the "psycho-social environment" created by the disease may induce anxiety, diminished self-esteem, and reduced feelings of well-being. It may also lead to severe emotional problems, personality changes, and disrupted personal relationships.

Most COI calculations focus on the direct medical costs and sometimes on some of the major components of indirect costs such as the loss of production due to premature death and morbidity of the patients. Indirect costs are often measured in a very rough and ready fashion, using aggregate data on average incomes in various age-groups up to retirement age. As data are lacking for most of the nonproducing, but nevertheless valuable and useful activities that patients and their relatives would spend their time on if they were not (pre)occupied by the illness and its treatment, such indirect costs are rarely valued or included in the estimations. The same applies for the intangible, psychosocial costs, which are, practically speaking, *never* valued for inclusion in the total cost estimate.

Conceptual and methodological critiques of the COI approach abound, as already alluded to in the previous chapter. They often focus on the *inappropriate interpretation* of the results of an COI analysis as an input for cost-benefit analyses, as it has been quite common to regard the result as an estimate of the benefit of a treatment in a cost-benefit analysis. Another critique focuses on the way of calculating indirect costs and on a common interpretation of the estimated value. This has often been considered as a form of rough and provisional minimum estimate of the value of human life. The standard way of calculating the indirect cost for an individual, e.g., a man who dies prematurely at the age of 47 of non-Hodgkin's lymphoma, is to estimate his expected future income for each year until expected retirement, say at age 67, to discount the figure for each year by an appropriate discount rate to take care of the time preference problem, and to sum the discounted annual figures to a single total. This total is then the capitalized value of the expected future stream of income, also called the net present value of future income. This is then aggregated over all the individuals concerned to obtain total indirect costs. If the disease in question leads to morbidity rather than premature mortality, the principles of calculations are modified correspondingly.

Calculation of indirect costs by this so-called Human Capital approach is habitually criticized for focusing too much on the productive capacity of the patients and their relatives, while ignoring other and more essential aspects of health care provision, such as generating freedom from pain, anxiety, and suffering. It is claimed that the Human Capital approach implies that the ultimate objective of providing health care is to maximize the productive capacity or the gross national product of the country. Furthermore, the use of the method leads logically to a discrimination against people no longer or not yet in the workforce, i.e., the elderly and children,[1] in favor of people active in the labor market and in particular those with high incomes.

Notwithstanding the legitimacy of these criticisms, it seems undeniable that an important consequence of disease, whether it results in morbidity or premature mortality, is a loss of productive possibilities (in the widest sense, includ-

[1] For children, the net present value of their expected future earnings will become so small, because of the effect of discounting, that they will not carry much weight in the calculations.

ing the leisure activities freely pursued by individuals in their spare time) and thereby a loss of output seen from the social perspective. This important consequence of disease should arguably not be ignored, but the question then is how to obtain a realistic estimate of the real size of the loss of output and, finally, how to interpret and make use of the results. These questions will not be considered further here, but a possible solution would be to carry out the calculations, e.g., using the friction cost method mentioned in the previous chapter, and present them alongside the calculations of the direct costs, without any attempt at aggregating the two types of cost. Presented with this information, the decision makers would then have to decide what weight they want to attach to the indirect costs compared to the direct ones.

Despite the widespread agreement among economists about the problems with and limitations of the traditional Human Capital approach to COI calculations, studies of this kind continue to be produced in large numbers. An important reason for this is probably that the data collection effort required is modest, because COI calculations are traditionally based on easily available secondary data. Another reason for their popularity may be that the estimates seem to generate an intuitively appealing measure of the overall magnitude of a particular problem in terms that are comparable to budgetary items and decisions and therefore familiar to decision makers (see Brown 1990). One may, for instance, come across statements such as the following: "The total societal costs of non-Hodgkin's lymphomas in country X in 1993 was almost exactly the same as the societal costs for lung cancer, even though the latter was four times as frequent measured by the number of new cases." This is certainly an interesting piece of information, but it is not immediately apparent for what purposes it might be of any practical use. It is sometimes claimed that COI calculations for various diseases might be used for prioritizing future research efforts, but if this is the case, it should at least be ensured that all the COI calculations made for such a purpose are fully comparable in the methods and quality of data sources used. This is hardly the case at present.

Nevertheless, considering the importance of cancer as the second major killer in all Western societies, surprisingly few studies of the COI of cancer have been identified through the literature search performed for this overview. This may have to do with the widespread perception of cancer as a terrifying disease which must be fought by any means whatever the costs, making any considerations of the costs be considered as unethical per se. It may also have to do with a realization that cancer is primarily a disease of the elderly, which makes the indirect costs as calculated by the traditional Human Capital approach relatively small. Accordingly, the potential reduction in indirect costs obtainable by improved treatment regimens will also seem small. This hypothesis would be a variant of the common criticism of the Human Capital approach of discriminating against the elderly.

Calculations

Most of the published papers originate in and concern the United States. Brown and Fintor (1994) have given a chronological overview over this work, which will be briefly summarized in the following. Additional sources have been Baker et al. (1989, 1991). The emphasis will be on the methods used rather than on the precise results obtained.

In the Third National Cancer Survey (1969–1970; Scotto and Chiazze 1976), a sample of 10,000 cancer patients newly diagnosed in 1969 or 1970 were followed for up to 2 years from the date of diagnosis, and information was collected on their use of hospital-based care services and the costs of these. Data are available, by cancer site and stage at diagnosis, about the number of hospital admissions per patient, the average length of stay, and the average dollar payment per stay. Combined with data on the costs of outpatient services obtained from patient surveys, these data have also been used to obtain estimates of the lifetime costs of treatment per cancer site. It is estimated that hospital costs are 60% of the total direct medical costs.

The Cancer Care Inc. Study (1973) was carried out by a private organization providing social services to cancer patients and their families in the New York area. A total of 275 families of cancer patients who died in 1971 or 1972 were contacted, and 115 completed the questionnaire about the duration of illness from onset to death, total costs of illness, sources of funds, annual family income, and family hardships related to the illness. There was no identification of the site of disease. The patients were atypically young, with a median age at death of only 60 years. The total costs were related to the duration of the illness, not to the family's income. Hospital and physician costs plus burial expenses accounted for 71% of all costs, and more than half of the families reported cutbacks in planned consumption and loss of income. Sources of payments other than medical insurance included financial assistance, savings, and salary and wages.

The annual economic cost of cancer to the nation was estimated as one major category in the National Center for Health Statistics' estimation of the total cost of illness for 1963, 1972, 1975, and 1980 (Rice and Hodgson 1981). These estimates, recently updated for 1985 and 1990, include direct medical costs, morbidity costs, and mortality costs and are based on national estimates of health expenditures by type of service and nationally representative surveys of service use. This means, for instance, that the cancer-related expenditure for hospital care is obtained by multiplying total national expenditure for hospital care as reported by one government institution by the proportion of days spent in hospital by cancer patients according to another government agency. For 1990, the total costs are reported to be $ 90,000 million (unfortunately, the total COI is not given), of which 29% are direct medical costs and 71% indirect costs. Two thirds of the direct medical costs are due to hospital care, 24% to physicians services (both in primary care and physicians' services in hospitals).

A Blue Cross/Blue Shield study (1978–1979; Gibbs and Newman 1982) was based on claim records from three different federal states to assess the costs in the last 6 months of life for 1054 cancer patients, all under the age of 65, who died in 1978 or 1979. All insurance-covered inpatient, outpatient, and physician expenditure was included. The distribution of costs was strongly skewed toward the last month of life, and there were only minor differences by age, sex, and cancer sites, while there were some large geographical variations, many of them due to longer hospital stays in one of the states (after controlling for diagnoses and service mix).

A variety of studies have used claims records from Medicare (a government program of medical care in the United States for the elderly), which means that they are limited to patients over 65 years. They comprise an analysis of the monthly costs during the last year of life for patients dying of cancer, a comparison of cancer patients dying in hospice and nonhospice settings, and a study of treatment costs during the last year of life for patients dying of cancer compared to patients dying of other diseases. Average costs for the cancer patients were 50% higher than for the other deceased.

The Continuous Medicare History Sample File (CMHSF), a 5% longitudinal sample of Medicare beneficiaries with a retrospective tracking of medical expenses from 1974 to 1979 and cancer deaths identified from death certificates, has been used for several studies, inter alia to estimate lifetime treatment costs per cancer site. The costs are based on charges to Medicare, adjusted to reflect patient copayments and deductibles and divided into three phases, i.e., initial care (the first 3 months following diagnosis), terminal care (the last 6 months before death), and continuing care (the period in between). There is very little variation in the terminal phase between cancer sites, but some variation in the initial phase, i.e., a factor of 2.2 between stomach cancer (expensive) and melanoma (cheap). The same data have been used to construct estimates of annual aggregate medical expenditure per cancer site by combining the data on the expenditure in the three phases with data on cancer incidence and survival. The estimate given for the total expenditure per year is over $ 40 billion (dollar value of 1990).

The CMHSF data found no significant differences according to cancer site in the average expenses during the last year of life, while there was a marked age variation with a rapid decline for patients over 79 years old. Higher total expenditures were found for patients with a longer survival. The costs attributable to some cancers were found by summing the average expenditure found for patients in the initial, continuing, and terminal phases and comparing them with age-matched control groups that did not have a cancer diagnosis. In 1990 dollars, the attributable costs for lung and breast cancer were calculated as $ 18,000 and $ 52,000, respectively.

At the beginning of the 1990s, a link was established between the SEER project (Surveillance, Epidemiology and End Results, a database containing information on cancer cases diagnosed and reported in nine geographically distinct population-based tumor registries covering 10% of the United States population) and Medicare (billing information on the health care of the disabled and more than 95% of the population aged 65 and over). Thus data has become available for all patients diagnosed with cancer in SEER between 1973 and 1989 (and of course also for the period from 1990 onwards), although the Medicare data from before 1984 are not very detailed. This database has made it possible to construct reliable estimates of the lifetime costs of cancer treatment by cancer site and stage at diagnosis and to analyze these costs in terms of treatment regimens and utilization of health care services by demographic characteristics and by geographical location (see Potosky and Riley 1992; Potosky et al. 1993). However, the Medicare data are obviously still limited because they only cover patients aged 65 years and older and health care services actually covered by Medicare. An example of the publications made possible by the SEER/Medicare link will be described later.

Another possible, but little used approach is based on ideas used in modeling for decision analyses, e.g., by constructing a series of treatment scenarios for a typical patient or by more rigorously constructing a probabilistic decision tree for a hypothetical patient population. The medical procedures and services consumed can then be costed by using a set of unit costs or prices, e.g., by using any desired health care accounting system. This approach can mainly be recommended for a form of informal cross-validation check for data obtained by other means. It may, for instance, be used to check estimates based on retrospectively collected data, or it may be used to indicate major gaps in other registry-based files, such as Medicare.

In addition to these, a number of studies based on convenience samples and focusing on aspects of costs other than the direct medical costs have been published, but they are of course of limited generalizability due to the nature of the samples. The economic impact of childhood cancer, with parents in their prime age for earnings becoming primary caregivers, has been well studied, and the average weekly out-of-pocket expenses plus lost wages have been estimated to be around 40% of family income. For adults in chemotherapy (for breast, colon, or lung cancer), another study estimated the sum of total expenses and loss of pay to be more than 25% of family income.

Brown (1990) provides an example of calculating the national economic burden of cancer by compiling and combining data from several administrative data registries. It is an update of a study performed in 1985 by Dorothy Rice, one of the pioneers of the COI methodology, and her coworkers (Rice et al. 1985). The revised calculation takes into account the rising cancer incidence since then and the inflation in health care costs. Rice et al. (1985) found that the direct costs for cancer care comprised 10.7% of all medical care costs in 1985. The new estimate uses data on hospital discharges, health care expenditures, disability, mortality, and earnings for 1985 and adjusts them by the above-mentioned factors.

Direct medical costs were obtained starting from the estimates of national health care expenditure by each type of service (e.g., hospital care and physician services) produced by the federal agency administering Medicare and

Medicaid (a program of medical aid designed for those unable to afford regular medical service and financed by the state and federal governments). The share attributable to cancer was then derived from other sources, e.g., the share of all expenditures attributable to cancer was obtained by using the number of days of hospital care identified as being cancer related in a National Hospital Discharge Survey. Mortality costs were estimated by calculating the number of lost person-years due to premature cancer-induced deaths by age and sex, using data from the National Center for Health Statistics. The number of lost years in each age–sex category was then multiplied by expected earnings for each group, including imputed values for housekeeping services. Morbidity costs were estimated by using work-loss data due to illness (by diagnoses) from a National Health Interview Study and finding the economic value of these lost days for various population groups, such as full-time employees, housekeepers, and those normally unable to work.

Finally, these estimates were adjusted to take into account a 14% increase in cancer incidence from 1985 to 1990 and a 42% rise in the health care price index. The final results, in 1990 dollars, are total direct costs of $ 35 billion and indirect costs of $ 69 billion, comprising $ 12 billion in morbidity costs and $ 57 billion in mortality costs. In other words, only one third of the total costs thus calculated are accounted for by the direct costs, while more than 80% of the indirect costs are caused by premature mortality.

Riley et al. (1995) presented the first analysis of data from the combined SEER/Medicare database mentioned above and gave estimates of total Medicare payments from diagnosis to death by stage of disease at diagnosis for the five most common cancer types in the elderly, i.e., lung, breast, prostate, colorectal, and bladder cancer. Costs were estimated by the actual Medicare payments rather than by the billed charges, which are usually higher. Excluded from the analysis were health care services not covered by Medicare, such as nursing home services and self-administered prescription drugs. At diagnosis, all patients were 65 years old or older, which is the criterion for becoming eligible for Medicare. Costs were allocated to the various phases of illness defined by the date of provision of the service.

For all the cancer types, a U-shaped cost curve was found, regardless of how long the individual patients survive: expenses are very high in the initial phase (1 month before to 6 months after diagnosis) and again in the final phase (the last 6 months of life), while they are rather low in the continuing phase (between the initial and the final phases). For some purposes, a fourth phase is distinguished, the prefinal phase, i.e., the 12 months immediately preceding the final phase. Within the initial phase and the continuing care phase, there were substantial differences between the five cancer sites, while there was little variation in the final and prefinal phases. This may mean that terminal cancer may be rather similar regardless of the site of origin, but it should also be kept in mind that many patients in the sample died of causes other than cancer, which may also tend to diminish the variations. Except for lung cancer, expenditure in the final phase was largest for those patients for whom cancer was registered as the cause of death. For all cancer sites and in all phases of disease, inpatient hospital care causes the largest proportion of expenditure. This proportion is always higher than 50%, and in the final phase the share of inhospital care was about two thirds of total expenditure for all tumor sites.

On average, lung cancer patients were the most expensive in the initial phase, with costs about the double of those of breast cancer patients, who were the least expensive. There are also appreciable cost differences in the initial phase by stage of disease at diagnosis, where the treatment decisions are often determined by the assessment of the stage and grade of disease. In breast cancer, for instance, the average costs in the initial phase were $ 7000 for carcinoma in situ and about $ 12,000 for distant disease. The expenses in the continuing and prefinal phases were generally also higher for patients diagnosed with distant disease than for those diagnosed earlier, while no such differences were found for the final phase. A direct relationship between the extent of staging and expenditure is seen, because extensive staging requires a number of expensive procedures to be performed.

The lowest total expenditure from diagnosis to death is seen for lung cancer patients (about $ 29,000), who also have the shortest average survival (only 1.7 years), while the highest expenses are seen for bladder cancer (around $ 58,000). The total expenses for the three other sites are slightly lower than the latter figure, and the longest average survival is seen for women with breast cancer. Clearly, the total expenditure between diagnosis and death is positively related to survival time, and the expenditure is substantially higher for patients diagnosed at an early stage than for patients diagnosed with distant disease.

A rather similar exercise was performed by Koopmanschap et al. (1994) for the Netherlands, supplemented by a prediction of future costs determined by a combination of the cost calculations and a model for determining (changes in) the incidence of cancer. Again, the five most common cancer types are distinguished, with stomach cancer included instead of bladder cancer as in the American study. The cancer model used is a Markov model, i.e., a deterministic state transition model, which divides the population into subpopulations defined by states. Transitions from one state to the next are governed by probabilities extracted from cancer registries and from the clinical literature. Again, three phases of the disease are defined, i.e., initial (first year following diagnosis), final (the last year before death for people dying of cancer), and the intermediate phase between these. The number of patients in each disease phase per cancer type, age, and sex is calculated by the incidence model described above. Values for the prevalence of disease are calculated from incidence figures, disease-specific mortality rates, and all-other-causes mortality rates (assumed to be independent of cancer mortality). This model is used to determine the anticipated future costs of cancer.

The calculation of costs per tumor site and phase of disease is based on a top-down approach, taking as the point of departure an estimation of the total health care costs of the Netherlands, based on national registers (for inhospital and nursing home care) and data from recent surveys (for general practitioners, physical therapy, and district nursing). These total costs are allocated to cancer and 42 other disease categories by means of data on the utilization of services or the number of patients in order to calculate the costs of inpatient care and nonhospital care for cancer patients. Costs for outpatient hospital care are determined as follows: Radiotherapy costs are determined by assigning the costs of the Dutch radiotherapy centers to cancer types on the basis of new patients receiving radiotherapy by type of cancer; the total costs of cytotoxics are assigned to cancer types in proportion to the distribution of the costs of in-hospital care.

For breast cancer, the costs of the intermediate phase are determined on the basis of a detailed follow-up study, while for the other sites, costs are assigned by extrapolation from United States data, where the relative follow-up costs have been estimated from data for 87,000 patients. Hospital costs in the initial phase are calculated by data on length of stay from a 1988 nationwide Dutch hospital register for the various types of cancer, age, and sex. Results are stated in 1988 Dutch guilder.

The total health care costs of cancers in 1988 are estimated as 1894 million guilder,[2] or as 4.8% of the total health care costs. In-hospital care accounted for 60% of this sum, outpatient hospital costs for 29% (chemotherapy and radiotherapy for about 11% each, follow-up visits for about 7% of the total), and nonhospital care for 11%. Lung cancer accounted for 16% of the total, breast and colorectal cancer for 13% each, prostate cancer for 6%, and stomach cancer for 5%, while the category "all other sites" accounted for 47% of the total direct health costs of cancer.

For all the six cancer types described (including the category "all other sites"), the general pattern of consumption of health care services coincides remarkably well: the costs peak in the initial phase and again in the terminal phase, while they are very modest in the intermediate phase. The total costs related to the prevalence of cancer only become important if the intermediate phase is very long (say, 15 years), as the costs of the intermediate phase are primarily dependent on the length of disease-free survival. For all six cancer types, the length of hospital stay increases uniformly with age, especially for women, while the admission rate falls with age. For patients older than 75, the second factor dominates, resulting in lower costs.

In order to examine the importance of demographic developments and of changes in incidence and in treatment effectiveness, four different scenarios for the development of the future costs (for the year 2005) of colorectal cancer are analyzed by means of the model. An improved survival is assumed in these simulations, based on a true decrease in mortality due to anticipated improvements in treatment effectiveness and on a spurious increase of survival due to earlier diagnosis (lead time) and increased detection of slow-

[2] About US$1150 million according to the authors' own conversion to US$, for which they do not mention the source of the exchange rate used. Approximately the same result is obtained by using an estimated value for PPP of US$1 = 1.65 guilder, found by interpolation between the relative PPPs of 1985 and 1990.

growing tumors. If only the demographic evolution from 1988 to 2005 is taken into account, the costs will rise by 23%. If the prevalence of disease is assumed to rise due to treatment improvements, prolonging the period of disease-free survival, the costs will rise by 20%. If the same increase is due instead to an actual increase in incidence (separate from the demographic evolution), the costs will rise by 58%, while if all three factors are assumed to be active simultaneously, the increase will be 67%. The last assumption is considered to be the most likely.

Finally, a Swedish study by Lindgren (1990) should be briefly described for the sake of completeness. The year of the study is 1983, and it is based exclusively on secondary data, published, for instance, by the Swedish National Social Insurance Board and the Swedish National Bureau of Statistics, as collection of primary data tailored to the measurement of COI was deemed to be too resource consuming. The total COI in Sweden in 1983 is estimated to have been SKr 162 billion (about US$ 435 billion if converted by the relative purchasing power parity (PPP) between SKr and US$ for 1985), of which 61% were indirect costs (morbidity 46% and mortality 15%). Of this total, the share for cancer is estimated as 6.9%, of which 71% is estimated as being due to indirect costs. The share of cancer in the total direct medical costs is estimated as only 5.1% (SKr 3.2 billion), and of this about 92% is for treatment of in-hospital patients, 5% for outpatient treatment, and 3% for pharmaceuticals.

Concluding Remarks

If one momentarily ignores the legitimate criticisms of the methodology and data employed that may be raised against the studies summarized above, and they are taken at face value, they seem to converge in two respects, both of which appear to make intuitive sense and are not surprising. One is the typical U-shaped curve for the development of costs over time for the average individual cancer patient, with high costs in the phase of diagnosis, initial work-up, and staging and in the terminal phase and with usually moderate costs in the period in between, whatever its length. The other result which seeks to impose itself as an established fact is that the economic burden of cancer on society appears to be disproportionately low compared to the proportion of all deaths attributed to cancer and to the associated grief and dread. Arguably, if a good estimate of the intangible costs of cancer could somehow be produced (instead of this cost item always just being noted in passing with an excuse for not attempting to estimate it, however approximately) and included in the calculation of the overall costs, this picture of the overall economic burden of cancer might change drastically.

Whatever speculations one may come up with about the anticipated impact of including an estimate of the value of the intangible costs, the whole COI approach to obtain an estimate of the societal costs of cancer is rather flawed, as argued above and in the previous chapter. According to welfare economic theory,[3] a much more relevant measure of the economic burden of cancer would be found by estimating the willingness of people concerned to sacrifice something else in order to obtain a reduction of the risks associated with cancer. This beneficial effect might, for example, be a reduction of a certain size in the risk of contracting cancer or of dying of cancer. The currently preferred method of obtaining such estimates is called the *contingent valuation method*, which has largely been developed in environmental economics in response to the need for valuing environmental "goods" or "bads," for which there are generally no markets where a value (price) might be determined through the interplay of demand and supply. The general idea of this approach to evaluation is to ask a sample of the population concerned about their willingness to pay for a certain "good" or for avoiding a certain "bad." Alternatively, one may ask about the population's willingness to accept, i.e., the amount of money that people will claim as compensation in order to accept having to forgo a certain "good" or to suffer a certain "bad."[4]

It is clear that there is a fundamental conceptual difference between these two approaches to evaluating the costs of cancer, even if an estimate of intangible costs were to be included in a COI analysis. Only by mere coincidence will the resulting estimates have any resemblance, and it seems very likely that a cost estimate based on the willingness to pay approach will be very much higher than a COI estimate.[5]

[3] Welfare economics is the branch of *normative* economic theory which is concerned with determining conditions for the optimal allocation of resources given the technological possibilities and individual preferences.

[4] The pros and cons of contingent valuation methods will not be discussed any further here, but it should be mentioned that all the obvious and many (or even all) of the sophisticated objections against the validity of this evaluation method have been dealt with, although not necessarily (satisfactorily) solved, in the literature on environmental economics.

[5] As briefly alluded to above, the continued use of COI methods is often justified by their feasibility (data are easily available) and by the argument that the result of the calculations may at least be considered as a minimum value of the benefits that would be found in a proper cost-benefit analysis. Thus, according to this line of argument, if the minimum value of benefits is higher than the costs, net benefits are at least positive, and the minimum value of net benefits may be compared with other interventions. This line of reasoning is very pragmatic, but not very convincing from a more theoretical viewpoint.

Breast Cancer

Breast cancer is the most common cancer in women, and its incidence has been steadily increasing over the past couple of decades. According to the American Cancer Society, the estimated risk of a woman developing breast cancer at some time in her life is now 1:9, almost double the risk observed in 1940, and breast cancer is the most common cause of cancer death among women in most Western countries. For many cancers, a patient surviving 5 years after primary treatment is considered cured. This is not so for breast cancer, where the risk of recurrence persists after 5 years of survival, although it is decreased.

Breast cancer is highly treatable by surgery, radiotherapy, chemotherapy, and hormonal therapy, and it is usually curable when detected in early stages. About 90% of the women presenting for the first time have disease clinically limited to the breast and axillary lymph nodes. Mammography is the most important screening modality for the early detection of breast cancer.

Prognosis and selection of therapy are influenced by a number of factors. Among these are the age of the patient, stage of the disease, pathologic characteristics of the primary tumor (including the presence of tumor necrosis, estrogen receptor (ER), and progesterone receptor (PR) in the tumor tissue), measures of proliferative capacity, and the patient's menopausal status and general health. Age greater than 50 is often substituted for a definition of postmenopausal status, as the criteria of menopausal status vary widely. Breast cancer is classified into a variety of cell types, but only a few of these affect prognosis or selection of treatment.

Patient management after initial diagnosis generally includes confirmation of diagnosis, determination of stage, and choice of treatment. Diagnosis may be confirmed by aspiration cytology or by some type of biopsy, and part of the removed tissue should be used to determine ER and PR levels. Apart from anatomic stage (size of primary tumor and axillary node involvement), which is an important prognostic factor, other histologic and biologic characteristics are currently being examined for their possible predictive value, but often with inconsistent results between the studies.

Staging of breast cancer is done according to the TNM classification system. Stage 0, carcinoma in situ, now constitutes about 15%–20% of all breast cancers. The increasing use of screening mammography means that such noninvasive cancers, of which there are various types which may be difficult to distinguish from each other, are more frequently diagnosed. Stage I refers to small, invasive tumors with no spread to local lymph nodes. Stage II includes small to moderately sized tumors (≤5 cm) but with spread to the axillary lymph nodes plus larger tumors without spread. Stage III include large tumors with spread to the axillary lymph nodes and tumors of all sizes with spread to lymph nodes inside the chest wall or to the skin of the breast. Inflammatory carcinoma, a rare and special entity which tends to spread quickly, is categorized as stage IIIB. Usually there is no underlying palpable mass, but the skin of the breast appears inflamed due to tumor embolization of dermal lymphatics or to capillary congestion. Stage IV includes tumors of any size and degree of node involvement, but with distant metastases or with local spread to homolateral supraclavicular nodes. The most common sites of metastases are the bones, lungs, the liver, or the brain.

Treatment Options

The current standard treatments for breast cancer, according to the stage of the disease, are described below.

The standard treatments for intraductal carcinoma in situ are either total mastectomy or excisional biopsy with radiotherapy. Different types of breast-conserving techniques for partial resection are under clinical evaluation. For lobular carcinoma in situ, which is considered a marker for the subsequent development of invasive disease (with a risk of around 25% of developing invasive cancer in either breast within the next 25 years) rather than a premalignant lesion, the standard treatment alternatives differ radically: either bilateral total mastectomy (with/without low axillary dissection) or long-term periodic examinations and follow-up after biopsy, but without any further therapy until indicated by the examinations.

Stage I disease, i.e., early or node-negative breast cancer, is often curable by a variety of surgical techniques, but 10–20 years of follow-up of patients managed by surgery alone have shown an ultimate relapse of around 20% for this group. The surgical options include total mastectomy (with or without reconstruction) or conservative surgery with radiotherapy. Both local tumor control and survival are equal with any of these options, as documented in a large number of prospective randomized trials. As the clinical staging is inadequate (about one third of patients with clinically negative nodes have histologic node involvement and are candidates for additional treatment as node-positive stage II patients), there is a need for an axillary node dissection. However, there is controversy as to the extent of the required extension of lymph nodes because of the long-term morbidity associated with axillary node dissection, mainly arm discomfort and swelling.

Because of the significant number of ultimate relapses in patients with node-negative breast cancer, adjuvant chemotherapy or hormonal therapy has been studied in several prospective randomized trials. However, as up to 80% of these patients are cured by surgery alone, it has been suggested that it would be highly desirable if adjuvant therapy could be limited to those patients with the highest risk of relapse, as adjuvant treatment is costly and the regimens can cause toxicities which may ultimately also require treatment. Ideas about the optimal management of these patients diverge, but some clinicians advocate the use of multiple prognostic factors in order to identify patients with a high risk of recurrence and offer them adjuvant treatment. The problem then is to identify the relevant risk factors.

The standard treatment for stage I disease may therefore be said to be either total mastectomy or breast-conserving surgery with or without radiation therapy plus adjuvant systemic therapy depending on the patient's tumor characteristics (ER status, size, and grade). Under clinical evaluation are various other regimens for adjuvant chemotherapy or hormonal therapy and no adjuvant therapy for selected subsets of patients with favorable prognostic factors. Likewise, it is argued that irradiation after breast-conserving surgery may be considered unnecessary overtreatment in a large number of patients, so several trials in which low-risk patients are not given any adjuvant radiation therapy after limited surgery are under way.

Stage II or local breast cancer is curable using various accepted surgical procedures, namely conservative surgery with separate axillary node dissection and radiation to the breast, or modified radical mastectomy with axillary dissection. Long-term, prospective, randomized trials indicate that survival is equivalent with either of these types of surgery. Local recurrence is seen for about 20% of the patients treated with conservative surgery, so careful monitoring for this occurrence is mandatory. In most of the patients with recurrence, a subsequent mastectomy will succeed in controlling the disease.

Several randomized trials comparing conservative surgery with or without radiation therapy have shown a high rate of local recurrence in patients that have not received irradiation, and these trials have not been able to determine a subset of patients that do not benefit from radiation therapy. However, even if postoperative radiation markedly reduces the risk of locoregional recurrence, its effect on survival remains uncertain. An overview of several trials shows postoperative irradiation to be detrimental to survival, primarily due to an increase in late cardiac deaths, evident in patients treated for left-sided breast cancer in trials that gave large doses of radiation to the heart. A clear positive relation between cardiac dose and cardiac death has been established. However, newer trials suggest that the radiotherapy can be given safely and is associated with a modest benefit in survival of node-positive patients. Nevertheless, there is still controversy about the need for delivering a boost dose to the primary site, and there is also no consensus about the advisability of treating nodal areas with irradiation.

The recommendations with regard to adjuvant treatment following the treatment used to control the local disease depend on the patient's hormonal and menopausal status. The best evidence concerning the use of adjuvant systemic therapy comes from a large meta-analysis performed by the Early Breast Cancer Trialists' Collaborative Group, which comprised 75,000 women with stage I or II carcinoma who were enrolled in randomized trials of hormonal, cytotoxic, and biologic systemic therapy. Current treatment recommendations are to a large extent based on this comprehensive meta-analysis, supplemented with a number of other studies performed by various collaborative groups, e.g., comparing various combinations of cytotoxic drugs in chemotherapy.

For women with positive nodes, adjuvant combination chemotherapy has been found to prolong the disease-free interval and overall survival for all patients, no matter what their menopausal status. The standard duration of administration of this chemotherapy is 4–6 months, and several different regimens seem to produce similar results in terms of disease-free survival, while there are differences in toxicity which may influence the choice of regimen. For women with positive nodes and hormone receptor-positive (ER^+) tumors, hormonal therapy with the antiestrogen tamoxifen prolongs disease-free interval and perhaps also overall survival. Some studies have shown a benefit in terms of the disease-free interval and overall survival when a combination of tamoxifen and chemotherapy is used compared to tamoxifen alone. Tamoxifen is relatively nontoxic, but it has nevertheless been associated with certain toxicities. The most important of these is the development of endometrial cancer, which in some large clinical trials has been shown to occur at a rate that is two to seven times higher than in untreated women.

Patients with stage II node-negative breast cancer generally have a lower risk of recurrence than patients with positive node involvement. The risk of relapse may be related to a number of factors, including tumor size, as shown by an analysis of patients with no nodal involvement. At 20 years, there was a 33% risk of relapse for tumors between 2 and 3 cm, compared to a relapse risk of 44% for tumors between 3 and 5 cm. The current recommendation is to give ER^- patients adjuvant chemotherapy with one of the regimens of proven efficacy and to give ER^+ patients tamoxifen according to an established schedule.

Currently under clinical evaluation are protocols evaluating new types of chemotherapy and/or hormonal therapy and others aiming at determining optimal adjuvant therapy regimens for various subsets of patients, including no adjuvant therapy for subsets of patients with favorable prognostic factors. Other (preliminary) data indicate that chemotherapy given before the operation (neoadjuvantly) may allow breast-conserving therapy in a number of patients whose lesion or breast size would otherwise not have allowed this option. There are also some ongoing clinical trials in which women with more than ten positive lymph nodes are treated with high-dose chemotherapy supported by bone marrow transplantation (BMT). This approach remains investigational, however.

A total of 10%–20% of women with breast cancer present with stage III or locally advanced disease at first diagnosis. This is a heterogeneous group of tumors, ranging from neglected, relatively slowly growing, large primary tumors to small breast tumors with extensive nodal metastases. The biologic diversity of these tumors makes the comparison of various treatment results and the formulation of treatment recommendations difficult, but it is useful to subdivide them into operable (IIIA) and inoperable (IIIB) disease. Usually, inflammatory breast cancers are classified with IIIB disease, as the treatment options are the same.

For operable, locally advanced breast cancer, it is usual to treat the patients with a combined-modality treatment consisting of induction or primary chemotherapy (with or without hormones) and a combination of mastectomy (radical or modified radical) and radiotherapy. The potential benefit of induction chemotherapy before undertaking local treatment is the prompt treatment of presumed systemic disease, the reduction of tumor burden before definitive local therapy, and the use of the response of the primary tumor as an in vivo chemosensitivity assay. After maximal tumor shrinkage has been obtained by the induction chemotherapy, it is still uncertain whether the next step should be surgery followed by radiation therapy or the opposite sequence.

Currently under clinical evaluation is the usefulness of maintenance chemotherapy after induction chemotherapy and surgery and of giving tamoxifen as postoperative adjuvant hormonal therapy for postmenopausal ER^+ patients. Clinical trials of these questions are under way, as are studies of the potential for neoadjuvant chemotherapy to allow breast-conserving therapy in selected patients. Another area of study is the use of high-dose chemotherapy with hematopoietic stem cell support.

In stage IIIB cancers and in inflammatory breast cancers, surgery is usually limited to the initial biopsy aiming at staging and determination of ER status. If followed by neoadjuvant chemotherapy prior to local therapy by irradiation to the primary tumor and regional lymph nodes, it may result in tumor shrinkage and early systemic control. Surgical removal of residual tumor may be performed if a good response is achieved with the other therapies employed. If the response is poor, a mastectomy may be performed, if technically feasible. The local treatment is often followed by either combination chemotherapy or, if this is contraindicated, by hormonal therapy for patients whose tumors are ER^+.

Under clinical evaluation are studies using combination chemotherapy initially, followed by surgery and/or radiation, and maintenance chemotherapy. Other ongoing trials are examining the potential of high-dose chemotherapy with hematopoietic stem cell support.

Stage IV or clinically overt metastatic disease is often responsive to treatment with lasting complete remission obtainable in 10%–20% of patients, although long disease-free survival indicative of cure is rare. The clinical situation is somewhat complicated by the fact that many patients with metastatic disease have relapsed after prior adjuvant chemotherapy, and their tumors may be resistant to most effective drugs. The current treatment of this patient subset is largely palliative, particularly using radiotherapy for palliation of pain caused by bone metastases. Radiotherapy may also be used to control local disease, or a hygienic mastectomy may be performed. Hormonal therapy or combination chemotherapy is used, depending upon the patient's ER status and upon whether visceral disease is present or absent.

The treatment possibilities for overt metastatic disease are perceived to be in a rather static phase, with no consistent and substantial improvement in survival in the last decade, despite numerous clinical trials using the available cytotoxic drugs, hormonal agents, biologic response modifiers, and various combinations of these modalities. Second-line treatment is mainly empirical, and clinicians are in the process of testing new drugs in phase II and phase III trials, either alone or in multiple combinations and/or doses. The current recommendation is to enroll patients into one of the many ongoing trials. The taxoids (paclitaxel and docetaxel) are often perceived to be some of the most promising new drugs in this field, and in some countries (e.g., the United States) they have been approved for second-line treatment of patients with recurrence after an anthracycline (doxorubicin) chemotherapy regimen (alone or in combination considered the most active single agents against advanced breast cancer). Other treatment possibilities under clinical evaluation are various forms of high-dose chemotherapy regimens with hematopoietic stem cell support.

Local recurrence after breast-conserving therapy is defined as recurrence in the breast parenchyma, skin of the breast, or nodal areas. Mastectomy is the treatment of choice, and the use of systemic therapy after recurrence is controversial. Local recurrence is usually the first sign of widespread disease, but in a subset of patients it may be the only site of recurrence. For patients in this subset, surgery and/or radiotherapy may be curative and the 5-year disease-free survival may be around 25%, with a 10-year survival rate of 15%. Some other sources cite a much higher 10-year survival rate after salvage mastectomy, however. Apart from local treatment consisting of surgery and/or radiotherapy, the current treatment options are various hormonal therapies or combination chemotherapies. The choice between these possibilities for systemic treatment should be governed by the patient's menopausal status, ER status, and the presence/absence of visceral disease (any metastases to any inside organs).

Current clinical evaluations are centered around determination of the optimal hormonal therapy - including oophorectomy or castration with luteinizing hormone-releasing hormone (LHRH) agonists - or chemotherapy - including the taxoids - for various subsets of patients. For recurrent patients with metastatic disease, there is an ongoing National Cancer Institute (NCI)-sponsored trial comparing high-dose chemotherapy supported by autologous BMT with standard maintenance chemotherapy for patients not refractory to standard chemotherapy.

Diagnostic work-up procedures are intended to determine the clinical stage of disease and to identify disease sites that may modify or completely alter the treatment plan. The following staging procedures are recommended as essential: complete history taking and physical examination of the patient, chest X-rays, complete blood counts, liver chemistry, and bilateral mammography. The following types of diagnostic procedures are not generally recommended: bone scans (large numbers of false-positive and false-negative results), liver scans, and evaluation of serum tumor markers (e.g., carcinoembryonic antigen, CEA). In most cases, however, histologic staging will be performed based on an excisional or aspirational biopsy.

The intensity of follow-up and the appropriateness of screening tests after the completion of primary treatment for stage I–III breast cancer is controversial. There is convincing evidence from randomized trials that periodic screenings with bone scans, liver sonography, chest X-rays, and blood tests of liver function do not improve survival when compared to routine physical examinations. While these tests permit earlier detection of recurrence, patient survival and quality of life are unaffected, so an acceptable follow-up scheme for asymptomatic patients after completion of primary treatment for stage I–III disease may be claimed to be physical examination along with annual mammography.

Economic Evaluations

The economic studies which have been published in breast cancer cover quite a wide range of aspects of the treatment of the disease, from an analysis of the costs of the various diagnostic procedures in common use to studies of the costs of palliative care of terminal patients in their own home compared to institutional care. A number of the more controversial issues in breast cancer treatment, such as the use of adjuvant systemic therapy in local disease, are also addressed. The two first studies to be discussed are both concerned with establishing a sort of cost function for progressive diseases, with the aim of determining whether the treatment costs vary by the stage of disease at diagnosis. The functions established are intended to be general, but are exemplified with data from breast cancer patients. A determination of the relationship between stage of disease at diagnosis and treatment costs is of interest in its own right, but the implications of a finding of such variations would be of particular interest in the evaluation of the costs and benefits of screening programs, which aim at diagnosing cancers at an earlier stage.

Taplin et al. (1995) use a kind of case-control design with retrospective data collection to analyze whether cancer treatment costs vary by stage at diagnosis, age-group, or level of comorbidity. The analysis is based on data for the more than 380,000 members of a health maintenance organization (HMO) in Puget Sound, Washington. All incident and prevalent cases of breast, prostate, and colorectal cancer during 1990 and 1991 were identified (by means of the NCI's SEER program), and the presence of comorbidity was determined by examining the members' use of pharmaceuticals in 1988, using a scoring system reflecting use of pharmaceuticals associated with more serious conditions.

The costs included are for materials and disposable goods, physician and other personnel salaries, and administrative overheads. It is claimed that the cost-accounting system of the HMO ensures that the cost per unit of service reflects the actual costs of medical personnel and supplies to provide the service plus overhead costs. For services not delivered directly by the HMO (but contracted out to other provider organizations), the unit price used is the charge in the contract plus overhead costs to manage billing and payments. Actual longitudinal data (incidence costs) are not available, so the analysis is based on a pooling of cross-section and time series data for the "observational window" of 2 years. The costs are calculated for 3-month periods.

The "attributable cost" of cancer is determined as the average cost per cancer case minus the average medical cost per control case, i.e., the difference between the two is attributed to cancer. Control subjects are members of the HMO who did not have a diagnosis with one of the relevant cancers. Controls were matched to each individual case subject on the basis of sex, age (5-year groups), and level of comorbidity. It is hoped that the resulting net costs of care per stage at diagnosis will reflect the net effect of cancer diagnosis and all the related changes in care of other conditions. The separate effects of stage, age, and comorbidity on the total costs of cancer and of the various phases of disease (initial care, >6 months after diagnosis; continuing therapy, ≤6 months after diagnosis; terminal care, >6 months prior to death) are determined by an analysis with a multivariate regression model, with a correction for the likely autocorrelation of the quarterly cost data.

The most detailed results given are for the average total cost (including cost of care for comorbidities) for the cancer patients, while the results given concerning net attributable costs are more selective. For the breast cancer group, average total costs in the initial phase were about $ 10,800, rising with stage at diagnosis, falling with age, and unaffected by comorbidity. For the continuing phase, average total costs were about $ 1100, rising with stage at diagnosis and level of comorbidity. For patients in terminal care, the average total costs were $ 17,700, falling with rising age and unaffected by stage and level of comorbidity. When controlling for age, the net cost of breast cancer was $ 9400 in the initial phase (about 90% of the total costs), rising with stage at diagnosis. In continuing care, the average net cost is only about $ 270, a fourth of the total, but rising sharply with stage. The net costs in these two phases were not related to age or comorbidity, while the net costs in the terminal phase were not estimated.

Butler et al. (1995) developed a treatment cost function for a progressive disease on the basis of a multiproduct-firm theory (i.e., an economic theory assuming that a firm produces two or more products) and applied it to empirical data for a group of 300 breast cancer patients from one Australian hospital, randomly selected among all breast cancer patients treated at this hospital from 1983 to 1989. It is assumed that the disease without treatment will progress through a number of exclusive and exhaustive successive stages of progression. The general form of the cost function for the treatment of such a disease can then be written as a function of the number of patients treated within each stage category and a vector of input prices. The cost functions are assumed to be restricted to exhibit nonjointness in inputs; in effect, therefore, the disease stages are to be seen as distinct outputs, each with a separate cost function, which is furthermore restricted to have constant returns to scale, meaning that the relative costs between the various output classes are only determined by the stage at detection and not by the number of patients treated within each category. It is further assumed that input prices are constant across stages at detection.

Given this formulation of the cost function, the question of whether the cost of treatment varies by stage can be examined empirically by testing whether the estimated parameters for the various stage categories in an econometric model differ significantly from each other. The estimation is made more complicated by the fact that variations in the cost of treatments are not only due to differences in stage at detection, but may also be caused by other factors which cause the exact nature and course of the disease and the prognosis to differ between patients during the follow-up period. In addition, the empirical estimation may be complicated by differing follow-up times or otherwise incomplete data.

The empirical analysis is based on a retrospective extraction from the patient records of 300 breast cancer patients treated in one Australian hospital. Any treatment given outside this hospital is not recorded, while the data extracted include the following: total number of days hospitalized, stage at diagnosis (five stages according to the TNM classification), primary and secondary treatment or treatments given, number of follow-up visits etc.. The data from the patients' charts provide information on the number of the various types of resources used, which must then be multiplied by a unit price. Most of these are based on running expenses for the hospital for the year 1987–1988. The data do not include any capital costs, as the authors have not been able to obtain any meaningful estimates of such costs.

A number of different calculations are presented, but the most interesting is based on the detailed data extracted from each patient's record, discounted at 5%. It shows the cost estimates rising steadily from about AUS $ 3800 for a stage 0 patient to around AUS $ 14300 for a stage IV patient[1], with the largest increase seen from stage I to II, and with very large standard deviations around the mean. A multivariate analysis shows that, even after allowing for the effects of age, status at latest hospital discharge, and duration of follow-up (to allow for different follow-up times in the sample), stage at detection exerts a statistically significant influence on treatment cost, i.e., the mean treatment costs are generally higher the more advanced the disease at presentation. However, the factors included in the model explain no more than 35% of the variation in treatment costs between patients in the sample, so there is still a large amount of heterogeneity within each stage category.

A number of cost identification studies, dealing separately with the various disease stages, have been published. Hillner (1993) determined the financial costs of treating women with low-risk local disease (node-negative, ER^-) with or without adjuvant chemotherapy. The calculation is based on a

[1] The purchasing power parities (PPPs) between AUS $ and US$ were US $ 1 = AUS $ 1.09 in 1985 and AUS $ 1.27 in 1990, so by interpolation an exchange factor of 1.2 might be used.

Markov state transition model, which is used to simulate a clinical trial of a large number of patients over several decades. The model is used to calculate the cumulative outcomes when a cohort of women is followed until the age of 90 or death. Central assumptions of the model are that (a) the annual probability of the first recurrence of breast cancer is constant, (b) chemotherapy alters only the probability of first recurrence, and (c) chemotherapy is equally effective or ineffective for high- and low-risk cancers (justified by the findings of the Early Breast Cancer Trialists' Collaborative Group's meta-analysis of adjuvant systemic treatment of local disease).

The initial estimated annual risk of recurrence for the untreated is 4%. The reduction in risk from combination chemotherapy (not specified) is assumed to be 30%, so the annual risk of recurrence for the treated women is 2.8%. The primary cost data used are based on estimates of the typical charges for physician, laboratory, office, and hospital services for a typical patient not enrolled in a clinical trial. The costs of care for recurrence and terminal care are estimated from Medicare data and the author's own "best guess" estimates. Both costs and health benefits are discounted by 5%. A quality adjustment of the various health states of interest was performed, based on a survey of the local oncology staff at the author's institution.

The paper gives baseline results for 45- and 60-year-old women. For a 45-year-old woman, the average gain in overall survival from adjuvant chemotherapy is 0.92 years (median benefit, 1.0 year). When quality of life is considered, the gain from therapy is considerably less, i.e., 0.43 quality-adjusted life-years (QALYs), resulting in a cost per QALY of $ 15,400. For a 60-year-old woman, the benefit is even less, i.e., 0.34 QALY, resulting in an incremental cost of $ 18,800 per QALY.

Richards et al. (1993) performed a cost identification study for advanced disease, concentrating on the hospital cost, without, however, clearly stating the perspective of the analysis. The calculation is based on a retrospective analysis of the hospital records for 50 patients with advanced disease who were primarily managed in one specific institution and who died within a specified period. For each patient, information on the duration of inpatient admission, number of visits to outpatient clinics, all treatments administered, all laboratory and radiologic investigations, and whether a hospice or a home care team were involved was registered. From the patient records, fairly reliable information on the quantities of the various resources consumed is available (at least within the hospital or its outpatient clinics), and, as usual, the most difficult problem is to find the right unit prices for these resources.

Although the costing methodology used is described at some length by giving a number of sources of data and calculation methods for the unit prices used, the information provided is rather inadequate, and this makes it difficult to judge the quality and consistency of the set of prices used. For instance, it is stated that both direct and indirect overheads were included, but nothing is explained about how this is accomplished. Examples given of direct overheads are portering and domestic services, while administration is an example of what they mean by indirect overheads. Likewise, an amount of 19% is added to the calculated costs in order to cover capital costs, without any explanation or justification for this figure being given.

The mean duration of advanced disease (from diagnosis of metastases in patients initially presenting with operable disease or from the date of presentation for patients initially presenting with inoperable locally advanced disease or overt metastases) was 27 months (range, 7 days to 12 years), with a mean duration of inpatient stay of 32 days and mean treatment costs of around £ 7600.[2] The distribution of costs were as follows: inpatient care, 57%; outpatient clinic visits, 12%; surgical treatment, 2%; tamoxifen, 2%; drugs for chemotherapy, 8%; radiotherapy, 7%; radiologic investigations, 9%; and laboratory investigations, 3%. Further information is provided on the number of radiologic and laboratory investigations per patient and their cost. The most common radiologic tests were bone and chest radiographs (eight and six per patient, respectively), but the most expensive item is the radionuclide scan (2.9 performed per patient, accounting for 41% of the cost of radiology). The most common laboratory tests were hematology (16.6 per patient and 28% of the cost) and biochemistry (14.6 per patient and 44% of the costs).

A similar cost identification study focusing on breast cancer recurrence has been published by Hurley et al. (1992), who determined the costs of hospital-based health services, although without explicitly stating the perspective of the analysis. Resources consumed were identified by a retrospective analysis of the patient records of two consecutive series of patients from two major Australian cancer hospitals, from first diagnosis of recurrence until the patient died or no further data were available. If necessary, information from other institutions (e.g., hospices) were included. An episode of recurrence was defined as a period during which metastatic disease was known to involve a specific set of anatomic sites, with anatomical sites grouped into five classifications (e.g., visceral, comprising the lungs, liver, pleura, abdomen, and bone marrow) for which the treatments a priori were expected to be the same. Each episode was categorized in a hierarchical manner to one of the five groups and was considered finished when involvement from another group was diagnosed (which is the beginning of a new episode) or the patient died (or history abstraction ceased). Resource utilization was recorded in relation to the episodes thus defined and the sites involved.

The costs of three types of hospital visits were calculated, i.e., an inpatient day, day-patient attendance (no admission, but chemotherapy administered or a procedure performed, e.g., a blood transfusion or bone marrow biopsy), and an outpatient visit (no chemotherapy administered, no procedures performed). Costs for these types of visits were calculated by apportioning oncology unit and ward nursing staff costs to each type on the basis of nursing dependency data and an activity study of the oncology unit. "Hotel costs"

[2] Costs are calculated using 1991 prices, but with the PPP of 1990 (US$ 1 = £ 0.419), this amounts to about $ 18,000.

(e.g., administration, food, cleaning) were allocated on a per diem basis equally for all hospital patients within the three types of visit. The costs of investigations were calculated by means of a special clinical costing system, while drugs and consumables were priced according to their actual costs for the hospital.

The primary measure of central tendency reported is the median, as resource usage, costs, and duration of the recurrence episodes all had skewed distributions. Each patient had on average slightly more than two recurrence episodes, with a median duration of total recurrence of 18 months (16 months for those who died and 30 months for the patients with censored data). The number of inpatient visits, inpatient bed days, and day-patient visits, but not the number of outpatient visits, differed significantly between the five categories of recurrence distinguished. The median cost per episode of recurrence was AUS$ 4300, and the median cost per recurrence was AUS$ 11,300 (by using the PPP of 1990 between US$ and AUS$ of 1.27, this amounts to about US$ 14,300). The total monthly costs for recurrence episodes in the visceral and central nervous system (CNS) groups were substantially higher than for the bone, local, and other groups. For each group, hospital visits and investigations were the major cost items, accounting for 54% and 24%, respectively, of the mean total costs for all episodes combined. Fatal recurrences were more costly than nonfatal ones, and with increasing duration of the episodes the costs followed a cubic pattern, with costs rising initially as the duration increased and flattening off as duration increased further.

As already mentioned, the intensity of follow-up after primary treatment and of screening for recurrence is a controversial subject among clinicians. Schapira (1993) set up a study with the declared aim of examining the possible evidence in favor of an intensive surveillance program for breast cancer recurrence. Such intensive programs include a patient history and physical examination, complete blood cell count, chemistry profile, and tumor markers (either CEA or CA-15-3) plus other procedures such as chest X-rays and bone scans. The assessment is based on findings from the literature on the effectiveness of each type of procedure in first diagnosing breast cancer recurrence. These are coupled with some cost estimates for the various surveillance procedures and with data on the incidence of breast cancer recurrence in order to produce a figure for the potential annual saving on a national basis by sticking to minimal intervention follow-up instead of following a program of intensive surveillance.

The quality of the study does not merit much further discussion, as there is no explanation at all of the sources used for the estimation of costs, and as there is no adequate discussion of the case series used for assessing the "effectiveness" of the various procedures for identifying breast cancer recurrences. The series show on average that 70% of recurrences are detected by the patients themselves, while another 15% are detected by a simple physical examination by the patient's general practitioner. However, case series such as these can hardly be used as an assessment of the relative effectiveness of the various procedures. Not surprisingly, by combining these data with data on the yearly national incidence of breast cancer recurrence, the author can point to a large "potential saving" (in the order of $ 1 billion) by using minimal intervention follow-up instead of intensive surveillance.

The procedures used for diagnosing and staging primary breast cancer have also been examined in some studies, but again with far from optimal methods and rather dubious data. Leivonen (1987) examined the diagnostic procedures commonly used in breast cancer and their costs with the aim of analyzing the possibilities of reducing the costs without impairing the diagnostic quality, i.e., performing a cost-minimization analysis. Leivonen conducted a retrospective analysis of data from 456 patients with operatively verified breast cancer treated between 1978 and 1985 at the University Hospital of Helsinki and judged the effectiveness of the diagnostic procedures used by assessing their sensitivity, i.e., the number of true-positive findings (a finding of possible malignancy by the test is considered positive in this assessment of sensitivities). The costs of the procedures were assessed by using the tariffs of the public health insurance as of April 1986 (and translated into US$ by the author using the exchange rate of that year).

The procedures studied and their average sensitivity[3] was as follows: clinical examination, 88%; mammography, 82%; fine-needle aspiration (FNA) biopsy, 79%; ultrasound, 85%; biopsy, 98%; and frozen section, 94%. As a mirror image of this, the rates of false-negative results vary between 2% and 21%. The sensitivity of most of these procedures is age dependent, with a much higher sensitivity for patients older than 65 than for patients younger than 50. The costs of the procedures vary between $ 21 for FNA biopsy and $ 23 for biopsy to $ 75 for physical examination and $ 68 for ultrasound.

If two diagnostic procedures are combined, the rate of false-negative results varies between 4% and 7%, while it varies between 2% and 4% if three procedures are used. Combining four or more methods does not improve on this result. As a criterion for the "reasonability" of including a specific diagnostic method, the author chooses the cost of false-negative findings per 100 examinations, because "the more false negative results are obtained, the more unnecessary are the costs." The combination of clinical examination, mammography, and FNA is found to be the most accurate, with a sensitivity of 97.5% and "reasonable" costs for false-negative findings of $ 438. Although the reasoning follows common sense and is straightforward, the study fails to be convincing because of a number of errors in the text and tables and because of selectivity in the case series (the patients were referred to the university hospital with an established diagnosis). Accordingly, it should not be considered as anything more than a first and very tentative attempt at addressing the important problem of determining the optimal set of diagnostic and staging procedures.

---

[3] Sensitivity or the true-positive rate is the proportion of patients with the target disease who have a positive test result.

Going into even greater detail, Lannin et al. (1986) compared the costs and effects of FNA biopsy with excisional biopsy on an in- or outpatient basis. Many surgeons will require a (definitive) excisional biopsy in all cases, so the two procedures should not be considered as substitutes. The idea, however, is to analyze a staging procedure in which FNA is used to decide whether the excisional biopsy should be performed on an in- or outpatient basis, which presumably would have consequences for the costs. The data come from a cost analysis for breast biopsies performed at the authors' local institution during the 2 years before publication and based on a review of patient charts. The assessment of the efficacy of FNA comes from a review of the results of the last 100 FNAs performed at the institution and a comparison of these with the results of the definitive biopsy. The costs analyzed include all hospital, operating room, recovery room, laboratory, radiology, pathology and anesthesia *charges*, but not the surgeon's professional fee.

The actual costs of FNA are not considered, while the result of the FNA is used to determine whether the definitive excisional biopsy should be performed on an in- or outpatient basis. The possible cost savings are therefore determined as the difference between routine use of either in- or outpatient biopsy compared to a selective procedure, where positive and suspicious FNA tests are followed by an inpatient excisional biopsy, while negative and insufficient FNAs are followed by an outpatient excisional biopsy. Average costs are calculated for 100 patients with each of these approaches, and on this basis FNA is calculated to save $ 39,000 (per 100 patients) compared to routine use of inpatient excision and around $ 10,000 compared to routine use of outpatient excision. For any sensitivity of the FNA test higher than 37%, the test saves more than it costs to perform, and for any specificity[4] of the test higher than 80%, the same is true. The last 100 FNAs performed by the department showed a sensitivity of 87% and a specificity of 100%. The economic consequences of the FNA strategy also depend on the prevalence of breast cancer in the test population, just as they depend on the costs of routine in- or outpatient excisional biopsies. If the prevalence rate of disease in the population tested is at least 13%, the FNA test "pays for itself" by saving more on other procedures than it costs to perform.

A number of papers have been published by the team of Desch, Hillner, Smith, and colleagues on various aspects of breast cancer treatment, based on decision analytic modeling of hypothetical cohorts of patients with effectiveness and cost data collected from diverse (and sometimes perhaps disparate) sources. Hillner et al. (1993) summarized some earlier studies on the question of giving adjuvant chemotherapy or hormonal therapy to women with early breast cancer, according to the women's age or menopausal status, ER status, and presence or absence of nodal involvement. These studies are all based on efficacy data from the large meta-analysis performed by the Early Breast Cancer Trialists' Collaborative Group (1990) involving 75,000 women. These

[4] Specificity is the true-negative rate, i.e., the proportion of patients without the disease for whom the test result is negative.

are combined with cost data from various sources, e.g., charges from the authors' own medical institution in Virginia, USA, and from Medicare.

Smith and Hillner (1993) assessed the efficacy and cost-effectiveness of adjuvant therapy in premenopausal women with early breast cancer, where surgery is the primary treatment. A societal viewpoint was chosen, and four different strategies were considered: (1) no adjuvant therapy, (2) hormonal therapy (tamoxifen) for 2–5 years, (3) standard combination chemotherapy (cyclophosphamide+methotrexate+fluorouracil, CMF) for 6 months, and (4) tamoxifen+chemotherapy. These treatment strategies were all examined in four different clinical settings, dependent on the presence (N^+) or absence (N^-) of nodal involvement and on the patient's ER status, i.e., whether the patient's tumor was responsive to hormonal treatment (ER^+) or not (ER^-). The incremental benefit and cost-effectiveness ratio for each strategy was calculated for each of the clinical settings. The detailed results will not be reported here, but their general tendency is as follows:

- For tumors responsive to hormonal therapy (N^-, ER^+ and N^+, ER^+), the clinical benefit of either tamoxifen or chemotherapy compared with no adjuvant therapy is about equal, a gain in survival of around 3.5 months for node-negative and about 5.5 months for node-positive patients. The incremental cost-effectiveness ratios for tamoxifen and chemotherapy, respectively, are about the same for node-negative patients, around $ 11,400, while for the node-positive patients tamoxifen is the most cost-effective, with a cost-effectiveness ratio of about $ 5000, while the ratio for chemotherapy is $ 9200.
- Even for tumors unresponsive to hormonal treatment, the meta-analysis has shown a statistically significant clinical benefit of tamoxifen, although naturally very small, about 0.2 months. This results in large cost-effectiveness ratios ($ 58,000–214,000). The clinical benefit of chemotherapy in terms of increased survival is much higher, around 10 months, with an associated cost-effectiveness ratio of around $ 5000.
- No matter what the patient's nodal and ER status, the clinical benefit of a combined modality treatment with tamoxifen+chemotherapy was rather limited (from 0.2 to 2.1 months), with the resulting cost-effectiveness ratios varying between $ 14,700 and 80,700. For the patients not responsive to hormonal treatment, this ratio is always above $ 80,000, while for the hormonally responsive patients the combined-modality treatment adds benefits at a cost-effectiveness ratio within accepted limits, according to the authors.[5]

In Desch et al. (1993), the model is applied to a hypothetical cohort of postmenopausal women, aged 60–80, with a diagnosis of primary breast cancer, no nodal involvement, and not responsive to hormonal therapy, and the ques-

[5] The authors do not explicitly state a threshold for acceptability. Originally based on estimates of the cost-effectiveness ratios of widely accepted procedures such as renal transplantations, a limit of around $ 35,000 seems to be gradually gaining acceptability, perhaps just by being mentioned very often.

tion posed is whether they should receive adjuvant chemotherapy. The assignment of probabilities is based on different sources, mostly (but not exclusively) randomized clinical trials. The risk of breast cancer recurrence is set at 5% per year, and the relative reduction in risk of recurrence obtained by adjuvant chemotherapy (standard regimen of CMF, as in the model described above) is estimated at 20%. The model assumes that chemotherapy alters the risk of first recurrence only, that the patients receive six cycles of chemotherapy, and that its protective effect lasts for 5 years, equally divided over all the 5 years, while the potential toxic side effects of the therapy last only for the year when treatment is given. Probabilities for toxic side effects are taken from a number of different sources. Major toxicities require hospitalization, while minor toxicities require only unscheduled visits to a family doctor.

A distinction between life expectancy and active life expectancy is made. The loss in active life expectancy is defined by the annual rate of decline in health status derived from a health care panel study which studied changes in health status in relation to the panelists' dependence or independence in activities of daily living. For instance, for individuals between 65 and 69 years old, there is a 7% annual loss in independence or active life expectancy, while the annual loss is 34% after the age of 84. Quality-of-life adjustments are performed based on statements from consensus panels of physicians, and the gains in expected survival are discounted by 5%.

The unadjusted survival benefit of chemotherapy declines steadily with age, from 5.5 months for a 60-year-old to 2.5 months for an 80-year-old patient. After discounting and quality adjustments, these gains are reduced to 2.8 months and 1.4 months, respectively. The impact of using active life expectancy can be illustrated with the example of a 75-year-old patient, who gains almost 2 months of quality-adjusted survival when conventional life tables are used. The gain is reduced to 3 weeks when active life expectancy is used as the outcome event, and the resulting cost per QALY is of course more than double the estimated cost-effectiveness ratio with survival as the end point. In general, the cost-effectiveness ratio is increasingly unfavorable with age, rising from $ 28,200 per QALY for a 60-year-old to $ 57,100 per QALY for an 80-year-old patient. The total costs of treatment fall with age, due to a reduction in follow-up costs, fewer late recurrences, and death from other causes, but this fall is more than balanced by the fact that the clinical benefit of adjuvant chemotherapy decreases with age. The results of the analysis of the model are stable, as major changes of the variables (by 30%–50%) did not have any considerable impact, i.e., did not change the direction of the results.

Finally, Hillner et al. (1992) used an equivalent modeling approach to assess the efficacy and cost-effectiveness of standard chemotherapy versus high-dose chemotherapy with autologous BMT in metastatic breast cancer (stage IV). A hypothetical cohort of 45-year-old women was examined in a Markov transition model, with transitions every 3 months and constant transition probabilities over these intervals. Transition probabilities are calculated by using the "best available evidence," which is, however, marked by serious shortcomings. Thus the majority of the data used on standard therapy and all data on high-dose chemotherapy with autologous BMT support consist of case series with no concurrent controls and probably plagued by selection bias.

The standard regimen of chemotherapy used was cyclophosphamide+doxorubicin+flourouracil, while the high-dose strategy used intensive doses of doxorubicin+methotrexate+flourouracil during the induction period. On completion of the first 3-month cycle, the responders to induction therapy were given high-dose alkylating chemotherapy (cyclophosphamide+cisplatin+carmustine) with autologous BMT support. In the baseline analysis, no granulocyte colony-stimulating factor (G-CSF) was used, and the treatment-associated mortality rate and complicated hospital stay rate were assumed to be 7% and 20%, respectively. Quality-of-life adjustments were performed, based on the consensus of a focus group of physicians and nursing staff. Applying institution-specific cost-to-charge ratios, the costs of induction therapy and of autologous BMT were determined by studying a limited number of "typical" patients, while the costs of standard chemotherapy were determined by using typical outpatient charges. Costs for progressive disease and for terminal care were taken from adjusted Medicare data. A discount rate of 5% was used for all future costs and clinical benefits.

With a 5-year time span, the women undergoing autologous BMT had an average survival gain of 6 months (27 vs. 21 months with standard chemotherapy). After quality adjustment, the gain increases to 6.3 months, resulting in an incremental cost-effectiveness ratio of $ 96,600 per QALY. However, limiting the time span to 5 years underestimates the benefits obtained by women in complete remission after these 5 years. If these women are assumed to have normal life expectancy thereafter, the therapeutic gain from autologous BMT becomes 18 months for an incremental cost per year gained of $ 28,600. Sensitivity analyses show that the analysis is driven by the assumptions concerning the effectiveness of the therapy and not by its toxicity or costs. Thus the results are very sensitive to changes in the risk of recurrence with autologous BMT and to changes in the treatment-associated mortality rate with autologous BMT, while an analysis with addition of G-CSF to reduce toxicity and the number of very costly days of hospitalization did not have any appreciable impact on the results.

Dranitsaris and Tran (1995) reported a cost-minimization analysis of two equally effective chemotherapy regimens in advanced breast cancer which differ with respect to the incidence and severity of cardiotoxicity and severe myelosuppression leading to febrile neutropenic episodes (FNE). Epirubicin is an analogue to doxorubicin, which is reported to have the same efficacy (response rate and survival), while being much less toxic. The analysis concerns a comparison of two chemotherapy regimens, consisting of 5-fluorouracil and cyclophosphamide plus either doxorubicin or epirubicin (in equal doses).

An economic analysis from the hospital perspective was performed to determine the budgetary impact of managing cardiotoxicity and FNEs after chemotherapy with either the doxorubicin- or epirubicin-containing regimen. The analysis focuses only upon these side effects and includes the costs of hospitalization, pharmaceutical support (including the pharmacy's preparation of the drugs and administration by a nurse), monitoring of therapeutic drug, laboratory tests, and specialist consultations. The data come from a retrospective review of patient charts from the author's institution, where the standard treatment protocol for breast cancer patients has been changed in the period 1985 to 1994 from the doxorubicin- to the epirubicin-containing regimen. A total of 100 patients were randomly selected from the two groups of patients having received either of the two regimens in the institution.

Sources for the cost data used for the various types of resources are reported in detail along with many of the amounts used, but there is no discussion of how these figures were derived in the first place or of their overall compatibility with the perspective chosen for the analysis. Despite the details provided, it is therefore not possible to evaluate the adequacy of the data used and the ensuing calculations. The acquisition costs of the cytotoxics are left out of the calculations, because the prices of doxorubicin and epirubicin were equal at the time of the analysis. Based on resource utilization data from the retrospective patient chart review, the total costs of each hospital admission caused by cardiac failure or FNE after the administration of chemotherapy were calculated, and the costs per cycle of chemotherapy were determined and compared.

The patients in the two groups were judged to be similar with respect to physical characteristics, diagnosis, metastatic sites, and previous therapy. In the doxorubicin group, there was an incidence of hospitalization for cardiac failure of 5%, compared with 2% in the epirubicin group. The cost per episode was more than 50% higher in the doxorubicin-induced cardiac failures, and combined with the difference in incidence, the authors calculated a potential institutional cost saving on this account if epirubicin is preferred to doxorubicin. Per 100 patients, the potential saving amounts to almost CAN$ 13,000. The incidence of hospitalizations due to FNE was found to be 25% in the doxorubicin group compared with 14% in the epirubicin group, while the costs per episode of hospitalization were almost the same. Per 100 patients, the potential institutional saving by using epirubicin instead of doxorubicin is thus calculated to be around CAN$ 60,000.

Combining the two types of toxicities examined, the potential institutional cost saving per 100 metastatic breast cancer patients amounts to CAN$ 72,000. The potential institutional saving should be balanced against a likely increase in the acquisition cost of cytotoxics, even though the protocols used had identical doses for epirubicin and doxorubicin, which were assumed to have the same price in the calculations. The retrospective chart review revealed that the median cumulative dose of epirubicin received was 25% higher than that of doxorubicin. There is evidence of a positive dose–response relation to epirubicin for metastatic breast cancer patients, so presumably the dose intensification made possible by the reduced toxicity may also lead to better outcomes. However, this remains speculative.

Another study concerning metastatic breast cancer has been published by Launois et al. (1996). This is a cost-utility analysis of three different chemotherapy regimens used as second-line treatment in metastatic breast cancer. All three regimens are single-drug therapies, and the idea of the study was to compare the taxoids docetaxel and paclitaxel with each other and with a standard regimen, although this may be difficult to define, as many different regimens are in common use around the world. Vinorelbine was chosen as the standard comparator, as it is used (alone or in combination) in more than half of the second-line protocols in France. In the absence of data from randomized phase III trials directly comparing these three drugs, the analysis was performed using a Markov state transition model, combining various types of data and evidence.

The model analyses the period from start of second-line treatment until death. The possible health states, which are assumed to last 3 weeks each (corresponding to the duration of each cycle of chemotherapy) until transition to the next state, are defined by using three different criteria, i.e., response to treatment, the nature of toxicities, and complications of the disease. Thus the model comprises 53 different health states, subdivided into 20 for docetaxel, 19 for paclitaxel, and 14 for vinorelbine, corresponding to the clinical criteria mentioned. A maximum limit of six cycles of chemotherapy was assumed for the taxoids, whereas vinorelbine was assumed to be continued until disease progression. The clinical data were taken from pooled phase II trial results (docetaxel), a randomized phase III trial comparing different dosages (paclitaxel), and a case series of patients (vinorelbine). As no relation between response to treatment and survival has been demonstrated, the three regimens were assumed to be associated with identical median survival, i.e., 12 months.

The cost calculations were made from the viewpoint of the third-party payer and patient, comprising all direct medical costs (including, e.g., the patient's transportation costs). Data for the amounts of resources used were taken from a retrospective analysis of case records for 146 patients (those that could be evaluated for response, i.e., having received at least two cycles of chemotherapy) out of a series of 153 patients receiving second-line therapy for metastatic breast cancer. For inpatient hospital care, the services provided were categorized according to the French diagnosis-related group (DRG) classification, and the corresponding unit prices were used for the cost calculation. For outpatient services, the relevant scales of charges were used, while primary care services were costed using tariffs or reimbursement amounts as unit prices. It was assumed that the acquisition price for docetaxel is the same as that for paclitaxel.

The major outcome focused upon in the analysis was quality-adjusted survival, given the postulate of equal survival in the three groups. Measures of utility were obtained by surveying oncology nurses, using an elaborate system of health state descriptions and standard gamble techniques for elicitation.

Total expected medical costs for each regimen, defined as the overall cost for each state multiplied by the likelihood of being in that state, were calculated and should reflect the expected value of all expenditure from the start of second-line treatment until death. The total costs are almost identical for the three regimens, i.e., around FF 250,000,[6] but the lowest figure is found for docetaxel and the highest for vinorelbine. The difference is very small, less than FF 7000 (i.e., less than 3% of the total), but the composition of the total cost figures differs considerably when subdivided in three categories. Treatment and follow-up costs for docetaxel are more than double the amount for vinorelbine, which reflects both a higher acquisition price for the drug and the fact that more patients respond and remain in treatment for a longer time. The costs of treatment-related complications are similar, while the costs of disease-related complications (overall the largest cost category, accounting for 67%–80% of the total costs) are about 20% lower for docetaxel. For all three cost categories, the figures for paclitaxel are very close to those for docetaxel, but the total is slightly higher.

The utility values elicited from the oncology nurses vary according to the patients' response to treatment, degree of toxicities from treatment, and state of progression (i.e., early progression scoring a lower utility value than later progression). As docetaxel reduces the time spent in progression without improving survival compared to vinorelbine, it results in a larger number of progression-free days of survival. When multiplied with the utility values elicited, this implies a gain in quality-adjusted survival, almost double compared to vinorelbine and rather marginal compared to paclitaxel. Combining this gain in utility with the lower expected total costs, the authors claim docetaxel to be a dominant solution. Sensitivity analyses show that the relation between docetaxel and vinorelbine is stable toward changes in the assumptions, while the cost-utility relation between the two taxoids changes under certain configurations of assumptions, although docetaxel appears to be (slightly) more effective in all cases.

Bierman et al. (1991) reported an evaluation of the potential clinical benefits and cost reductions from using clodronate in the management of bone metastases in advanced breast cancer. The agent is not expected to have any impact on survival, while it is expected to reduce the incidence of pathologic fractures and hypercalcemia and the intensity of bone pain. In this way, it is expected to improve the patients' ability to function and their quality of life. It is also presumed that the use of clodronate in these patients may reduce the costs related to patient disability, pain management, and radiotherapy.

Based on a retrospective review of charts of 120 patients with metastatic breast cancer to the bone treated in the authors' university hospital in the late 1980s, an attempt to estimate the costs of managing these patients was made, including an estimate of the costs directly related to the bone metastases. Only costs of hospital-based treatments, but excluding physician fees, were included, and costs were calculated by using a particular cost-to-charge ratio for the institution (55%). The possible impact of clodronate was then

[6] The date of the analysis refers to 1993 values, but as mentioned above, the latest health care-specific PPP values available are from 1990. Using general PPPs for 1993, total costs amount to about $38,000.

examined through a series of so-called "if–then scenarios," i.e., possible cost reductions if clodronate is assumed to have a specific "clinical efficacy" varying from 20% to 50%. The actual meaning of this is that clodronate is supposed to reduce the calculated costs by these rates due to its anticipated effect of reducing the intensity of bone pain and the incidence of pathologic fractures and hypercalcemia requiring hospitalization.

Concluding Remarks

The main characteristics, methods, and results of the economic assessments described and briefly discussed in this chapter are summarized in Table 1. As stated at the beginning of the previous section, the economic assessments in breast cancer cover a wide range of clinical aspects of the disease, but none of these are dealt with by more than one paper. This precluded the possibility of a simple comparison of the results taken at face value, which would be an initial step in assessing their validity. The only exceptions to this are the two studies investigating the total costs of patient management according to stage at diagnosis (inter alia), which both find that management costs are higher for patients diagnosed at a later stage than for patients with early-stage disease. This finding could be interpreted as lending some support to a policy of screening, but this conclusion would of course need corroboration from studies with a design more specifically directed at this issue, in particular taking outcomes into account.

The studies on diagnostic procedures, in connection with primary treatment and in following up patients after this to observe for recurrence, all have a weak design and are therefore not convincing. Concerning the issue of adjuvant treatment of patients with early disease, the cost-effectiveness of standard chemotherapy and tamoxifen seems almost equal in patients responsive to hormonal therapy. The exact value of the cost-effectiveness ratios depends on the question of whether there is nodal involvement. Combining tamoxifen and chemotherapy adds very little benefit at a high cost, implying a very high cost-effectiveness ratio. The quality of life of patients receiving adjuvant therapy is assessed to be quite low, so the cost-outcome ratios calculated are very much influenced by whether quality of life is included or not.

For patients with advanced disease, it seems clear that, from a provider perspective, epirubicin offers a less costly alternative to doxorubicin because of a lower incidence of cardiotoxicity and FNEs. The study comparing the new taxoids (paclitaxel and taxotere) with vinorelbine has equivocal results, and there is no evidence that either of these newer agents are more cost-effective than standard agents such as doxorubicin or epirubicin already are. This underlines the importance of using appropriate comparators if a particular study is to have value for practical decision making.

Table 1. Main characteristics of economic assessments dealing with breast cancer

Reference	Disease category	Treatments examined	Main characteristics of the study
Taplin et al. (1995)	All stages	All treatments given (i.e., those covered by Medicare)	Do treatment costs vary with stage at diagnosis? Third-party perspective (Medicare) Retrospective data for patients enrolled in HMO to find costs attributable to cancer; pooled time series and cross-section analysis to simulate longitudinal (incidence) cost data Costs rise with stage at diagnosis for the initial and the continuing care phase (until 6 months prior to death), no relation in terminal care
Butler et al. (1995)	All stages	All hospital treatments given	Do treatment costs vary with stage at diagnosis? Hospital perspective Retrospective data for 300 random patients from one Australian hospital; resource utilization taken from patient charts Treatment cost estimates rise steadily with stage at diagnosis, largest increase from stage I to II, very large standard deviations around the mean
Hillner (1993)	Local disease, ER^- stage II primarily	Health care services covered by Medicare	Financial costs of treating patients in this group Medicare perspective Markov state transition model, estimates of typical charges for typical patient, some data from Medicare, author's guesstimates
Richards et al. (1993)	Locally advanced and metastatic disease	All hospital treatments given	Costs of hospital care for patients with locally advanced and metastatic disease Perspective not clearly stated, primarily hospital Retrospective analysis of records for 50 patients, deceased within a given period; quantitative data on resource consumption from patient charts Mean duration of advanced disease 27 months, mean duration of inpatient stay 32 days, costs of inpatient care 57% of all treatment cost
Hurley et al. (1992)	Patients with recurrent disease	All hospital-based health care services	Cost-identification study Hospital perspective, though not directly stated Retrospective analysis of patient records for two consecutive series of patients; costing partly based on a top-down approach, with weights derived from activity studies and estimations of nursing dependency Total costs of recurrence episodes vary according to anatomical site of recurrence, highest in CNS and visceral sites; most important cost items hospital stays (54%) and examinations (24%)
Schapira (1993)	All patients after primary treatment	Follow-up and screening for recurrence after primary treatment	Determine the possible national cost savings by using minimal intervention follow-up instead of intensive surveillance Perspective not explicitly stated Effectiveness data for the various follow-up procedures from the literature

Table 1 (continued)

Reference	Disease category	Treatments examined	Main characteristics of the study
			Very large potential cost saving on national basis by using minimal intervention follow-up
Leivonen (1987)	All patients with primary breast cancer	Diagnostic and staging procedures	Cost-minimization analysis Third-party payer perspective Retrospective analysis of records for 456 patients treated in hospital; effectiveness of procedures judged by their sensitivity A combination of clinical examination, mammography, and FNA most accurate (sensitivity, 97.5%) and the costs are "reasonable"
Lannin et al. (1986)	All patients with primary breast cancer	Excisional biopsy on inpatient/outpatient basis and FNA	Cost-minimization analysis Hospital perspective Efficacy assessed by retrospective comparison of test result with definitive biopsies; procedure costs calculated by review of patient charts, using the official charges Results depend on sensitivity and specificity of the test and on the prevalence of disease in the test population; for most reasonable values of these, the use of FNA is cost saving
Smith and Hillner (1993)	Patients with early disease (stage I/II)	Adjuvant therapy with chemotherapy or hormones (tamoxifen)	Cost-effectiveness analysis Social perspective (claimed; in reality more of a third-party payer perspective) Decision analysis Markov model; efficacy data from large meta-analysis, cost data from hospital charges and Medicare unit prices For tumors responsive to hormonal therapy, the cost-effectiveness ratios are about equal, ranging from $ 5000 to 11,000; a combined-modality therapy is in most cases much less cost-effective
Desch et al. (1993)	Early disease (stage I/II), elderly, postmenopausal, ER^-	Adjuvant standard chemotherapy or not	Cost-utility analysis Third-party payer perspective Decision analysis Markov model, efficacy data from randomized clinical trials; quality-of-life adjustments based on consensus panel of physicians; hospital charges and Medicare data used for cost calculation Adjusting survival for quality of life leads to more than a doubling of the estimated cost-outcome ratios; these ratios increase considerably with age; the results are very stable
Hillner et al. (1992)	Metastatic disease, stage IV	Intensive chemotherapy with ABMT vs. standard chemotherapy	Cost-utility analysis Hospital perspective Decision-making Markov model; efficacy data mostly from case series; quality-of-life-adjustments based on consensus of treatment personnel; charges for "typical" patient, transformed into cost by cost-to-charge ratios

Table 1 (continued)

Reference	Disease category	Treatments examined	Main characteristics of the study
			With a 5-year time span, the cost-utility ratio is rather high, $ 96,000; assuming normal life expectancy after this, it falls to a quarter; results are sensitive to efficacy assumptions, not to costs or toxicities
Dranitsaris and Tran (1995)	Advanced breast cancer	Two different chemotherapy regimens, epirubicin vs. doxorubicin	Cost-minimization analysis, determining the budgetary impact of using each regimen Hospital perspective Retrospective review of patient charts for patients randomly selected among those receiving one or the other regimen in the institution (policy change from one regimen to the other); focus on cardiotoxicities and FNE; costs of hospital admission for cardiac failure or FNE based on resource utilization data from chart review; unit cost data from analyses performed in the authors' institution Incidence of hospital admissions for both cardiac failures and FNEs was lower in the epirubicin than in the doxorubicin group and some of these hospitalizations were shorter; as acquisition prices of the two drugs and the costs of administering them are the same, there is a saving with epirubicin
Launois et al. (1996)	Metastatic breast cancer	Three different chemotherapy regimens as second-line treatment, docetaxel vs. paclitaxel vs. vinorelbine	Cost-utility analysis Third-party payer plus patient perspective Markov state transition model; no direct randomized comparison of the three drugs, so efficacy data from various sources, e.g., phase II trials and case series; identical survival assumed; resource utilization data from retrospective review of charts for case series of patients in second-line chemotherapy; unit prices from the French DRG system, tariffs and reimbursements for outpatient services; utility values for quality-of-life adjustment elicited from oncology nurses Docetaxel claimed to be a dominant solution with a gain in quality-adjusted survival and smaller expected total costs of treatment; compared to vinorelbine, this result is stable in sensitivity analysis, while the comparison with paclitaxel is more equivocal
Bierman et al. (1991)	Metastatic breast cancer	Using clodronate to manage bone metastases	Analyzes the impact on costs of using clodronate Hospital perspective Analysis of hypothetical scenarios based on assumptions about the efficacy of clodronate; costs of managing breast cancer patients with bone metastases based on retrospective review of charts for case series of patients; only costs of hospital-based treatments included, not including physician fees; unit costs from charges based on cost-to-charge ratio

Table 1 (continued)

Reference	Disease category	Treatments examined	Main characteristics of the study
			Possible cost reductions if clodronate is assumed to have a specific "clinical efficacy" are calculated, varying the efficacy assumed

ER^-, estrogen receptor negative; ABMT, autologous bone marrow transplantation; CNS, central nervous system; FNA, fine-needle aspiration; HMO, health maintenance organization; FNE, febrile neutropenic episode; DRG, diagnosis-related groups.

Lung Cancer

Introduction

In the United States and many other Western, industrialized countries, lung cancer is one of the most common cancers and the leading cause of cancer death in both men and women. For women, this is a relatively new phenomenon dating back to the late 1980s, while for men it has been so for decades. The incidence in men (presently about 70 per 100,000 men) is falling and has been for some time, while the incidence in women is rapidly rising. This is believed to reflect the fact that women took up the habit of smoking some decades later than men and seem to give up smoking to a lesser extent than men. The prognosis for patients with lung cancer is invariably very poor, as only 13% of patients with the diagnosis will survive 5 years.

The principles of clinical management of lung cancer differ significantly according to the cell type. The major histologic distinction is between small cell lung cancer (SCLC) and non-small-cell lung cancer (NSCLC). The latter is a heterogeneous aggregate of at least three distinct histologies of lung cancer, including squamous carcinoma, adenocarcinoma, and large cell carcinoma. These NSCLC histologies are usually classified together because, when localized, they all have the potential for cure with surgical resection. Compared with other cell types of lung cancer, SCLC has a greater tendency to be widely disseminated at diagnosis, but it is much more responsive to chemotherapy and irradiation. Without treatment, SCLC has the most aggressive clinical course of any pulmonary tumor, with median survival from diagnosis of only 2–4 months.

The proportion of lung cancers diagnosed as SCLC varies with the method for obtaining the data because of the propensity of SCLC to develop early and distant metastases. The proportion ranges from 3% to 12% in surgically resected neoplasms to between 17% and 29% in biopsy and cytology diagnostic specimens. In the large epidemiological surveillance program SEER, run by the National Cancer Institute (NCI) in the United States, SCLC accounts for 18% of all primary lung cancers, and this cell type seems to be the most rapidly increasing type of lung cancer, especially in women.

Small Cell Lung Cancer

By the time of diagnosis, almost 70% of SCLC patients have metastatic disease, and 90% of these have distant metastases. SCLC is therefore often considered to be a systemic disease from the onset, and all patients are treated with initial chemotherapy, regardless of the extent of tumor dissemination. Because metastatic disease is present at diagnosis in most patients, the detailed TNM staging system is not commonly used in SCLC, as survival is usually not affected by small differences in the amount of locoregional tumor involvement. Instead, patients are classified as having either *limited-stage disease*, where the tumor is confined to one hemothorax and the regional lymph nodes, or *extensive-stage disease*, defined as disease beyond these bounds. There is no universally accepted definition of the terms used for delimiting these stages from each other, and different clinical groups are using diverging delimitations.

Performing a larger number of more sensitive staging tests does not influence the prognosis, but the survival of both limited- and extensive-stage disease patients is improved, because patients with minimal metastases outside the thorax are moved from the limited- to the extensive-stage disease group.[1] In some clinical situations, the choice of treatment may be affected by stage, especially when chest irradiation or surgical excision is added to chemotherapy alone for patients with limited disease. Favorable prognostic factors are limited-stage disease, female gender, and good performance status. In general, patients who are confined to bed tolerate aggressive forms of treatment poorly, have increased morbidity, and rarely attain 2-year disease-free survival, but they can often derive significant palliative benefit and prolongation of survival from treatment.

The efficacy of many different combination chemotherapy regimens including two to four different drugs appears to be rather similar, and many different combinations are commonly used. The results of combination chemotherapy are clearly superior to the results of single-drug treatment, and moderately intensive doses are superior to doses that produce only minimal or mild hematologic toxicity. The optimal duration of chemotherapy has not been clearly defined, but there is no significant improvement in survival when the duration of drug administration exceeds 4–6 months, and there is no evidence from randomized trials of any benefit of maintenance chemotherapy. In limited disease, optimal regimens should produce a median survival of 12–16 months and a 2-year disease-free survival rate of 15%–25%. For patients with extensive disease, the corresponding results should be a median survival of 7–11 months, while 2-year disease-free survival is rare.

[1] This phenomenon, whereby improved survival (or other outcomes) is achieved simply by more refined staging at diagnosis, is well described in some malignancies and should always be taken into account as a possibility in historical comparisons. By refining the staging, the average severity is reduced in all the stage categories, and, even when using unaltered treatment regimens in the various stages, the average outcome would be expected to improve for all stage groups.

Combined-modality treatment comprising chemotherapy and radiotherapy has been shown to produce a modest, but statistically significant improvement in survival compared with chemotherapy alone. Two meta-analyses have shown an improvement in 3-year survival rates of 5% from combined-modality treatment, but the trials differed, e.g., with respect to the temporal relation between chemotherapy and irradiation and the dose and schedule of irradiation. Accordingly, the question of whether variations in the relation of the radiation and chemotherapy components of combined-modality treatment influences its antitumor effects is far from resolved. However, several trials report increased morbidity and sometimes also mortality from combined-modality treatments.

Prophylactic cranial irradiation (PCI) has been used by many physicians during the last 10–15 years in order to curtail the development of brain metastases, which is very frequent in SCLC patients. This is especially so for patients with prolonged survival and may be the sole site of clinical relapse from complete remission. Although a beneficial effect of PCI has been shown in several prospective trials, especially in patients with complete response to chemotherapy, it is not recommended as a prophylactic measure for routine administration. This is because of an increasing number of reports of significant side effects in the central nervous system (CNS) and because there is no evidence of an effect of PCI on survival. On the other hand, radiotherapy is the treatment of choice when brain metastases have developed, but the effectiveness of treatment of brain metastases has little influence on survival for most patients, since for them SCLC is a widely disseminated disease. Chemotherapy may also obtain responses in brain metastases from SCLC.

Despite the good response rates of initial chemotherapy at diagnosis, most patients eventually develop tumor recurrence. The prognosis for these patients is poor, with a median survival from disease progression of 2–3 months and infrequent objective responses to salvage therapy. The best response to salvage regimens is seen in patients whose tumors progress after a long period off chemotherapy compared with patients who relapse early. Relapses of SCLC continue to occur between 2 and 5 years, while only rarely 5–10 years after initial therapy, so 5 years of follow-up is considered an appropriate time period for assessment of the curative potential of a treatment. The overall 5-year survival rate based on six studies is only 4% (7% for limited disease, 1% for extended), but even for the long-term survivors the risk of death from other causes is far higher than in the age-matched population. Most notable is a significant risk of developing additional, smoking-related malignancies, especially NSCLC, but the long-term survivors also have a sixfold increased risk of death from other causes, principally from cardiovascular and other pulmonary diseases.

Currently under clinical evaluation are new combination-drug regimens composed of standard and new agents and variation of the doses of the current regimens. The possible benefits of adding surgical resection of the primary tumor or radiotherapy to the chest and other sites are also being studied. There is some controversy about the possibility of improving survival by increasing the dose rate of commonly used front-line regimens over the level that produces modest toxicity. Retrospective studies of this issue, plagued by methodological difficulties as they are, show inconsistent results, while a prospective randomized study in extensive disease does not document any advantage of increasing the standard doses of etoposide+cisplatin. Moreover, intensified chemotherapy with bone marrow transplantation support has not been shown to improve survival in SCLC either.

Non-Small-Cell Lung Cancer

NSCLC is a heterogeneous aggregate of at least the following types of tumor cells: adenocarcinomas (40% of all lung cancers and increasing), squamous cell carcinomas (approximately 30% of all lung cancers), and large cell carcinomas (up to 15% of all lung cancers but decreasing). Staging of NSCLC patients is based on a combination of clinical (physical examination, radiologic, and laboratory studies) and histologic (e.g., biopsy of lymph nodes, bronchoscopy, and mediastinoscopy) staging procedures, and stage plays a critical role in the selection of therapy. The TNM classification system is commonly used.

The results of the existing standard treatments in NSCLC are generally poor, except for the most localized cancers, where the 5-year survival rate exceeds 70% (in completely resected T1N0 tumors). At diagnosis, the patients may be divided into three groups, reflecting the extent of disease and the approach to treatment:

1. Patients with resectable tumors, generally stage I and II; some of these patients will have medical contraindications to surgery, but for about one fifth of these patients, radiotherapy may be curative.
2. Patients with locally (T3–T4) or regionally (N1–N2) advanced disease who are primarily treated with radiotherapy, alone or in combination with other modalities. Highly selected patients in this group may be treated effectively by surgery alone. The overall 5-year survival rate for the group is no higher than 10%, and the median survival is less than 1 year.
3. The final group has distant metastases (M1) at the time of diagnosis and may be given palliative treatment with chemotherapy or radiotherapy. The median survival is less than 6 months, and 5-year survival is extremely rare.

Localized NSCLC, stages I and II, denotes disease limited to one hemithorax with tumor extension no further than the visceral pleural peripherally (T2) or bilar nodes proximally (N1). In these cases, surgery is the treatment of choice, and in most cases lobectomy (resection of part of the lung) is the procedure required. In some cases with greater tumor involvement, pneumonectomy (resection of the whole lung) is necessary. Studies comparing lobectomy with techniques using even more limited resection show significantly higher rates of local recurrence with limited resection, while the overall survival in the two groups is equivalent. In T1N0 tumors, the 5-year survival rate exceeds 70% after complete resection, or perhaps even more than 80%, since about one fourth of the patients not surviving are found to be tumor-free at autopsy.

It is strongly debated whether mediastinal lymphadenectomy should be a routine part of the surgical procedure. By removing all lymph nodes, which can then be analyzed pathologically, this resection provides the best possible surgical staging procedure. The proponents of the method claim that it also improves survival, but a recently completed randomized trial has not corroborated this claim. The trial compared mediastinal lymphadenectomy with intraoperative lymph node sampling and found no differences in survival, local recurrence, or staging accuracy.

Inoperable patients with stage I or II disease and sufficient pulmonary reserve may be given radiotherapy with curative intent, where doses greater than 60 Gy but no more than about 69 Gy are associated with improved disease-free survival. The largest retrospective series to date report an overall 5-year survival rate of 10% for a group of 152 patients treated this way, with a rate of 60% for patients with T1 disease.

Currently, clinical trials are evaluating the effects of combined-modality treatment for inoperable patients, where chemotherapy is combined with standard-dose or hyperfractionated radiotherapy. Another area of current research is the use of adjuvant chemotherapy or radiotherapy following surgery, which is indicated by the fact that many patients treated surgically subsequently develop regional or distant metastases. One randomized trial of postoperative irradiation failed to show any benefit in overall survival, while there was a significant reduction in local recurrences. Adjuvant chemotherapy appears more promising, as two controlled trials of adjuvant combination chemotherapy with cisplatin, doxorubicin, and cyclophosphamide have shown modest increases in disease-free survival and a trend toward improved overall survival.

Locally advanced, stage IIIA disease includes T3 tumor or N2 nodal spread or both, but there is a significant difference in prognosis between patients with T3N0 and those with N2 disease. The goal of surgery will in each case be to perform a complete resection, but once lymph nodes are involved, the prognosis is much worse. After complete resection, a 5-year survival rate of only 20% has been observed in patients with lymphatic metastases. Surgery for patients with mediastinal lymph node involvement (N2 disease) is the most controversial question in the surgical management of patients with lung cancer, the disagreement concerning the optimal degree of nodal resection.

For patients with advanced N2 disease, the use of various forms of induction therapies before curative surgery, such as "neoadjuvant" chemotherapy, radiotherapy, or chemoradiotherapy, have been studied extensively. So far, induction therapy with various forms of cisplatin-based combination chemotherapy regimens seems to be the most promising, with median survival clustering around 20 months. According to the trials reported, the addition of radiotherapy concomitantly or sequentially, while adding to toxicity, does not seem to add significantly to either resection rates or survival compared with chemotherapy alone.

Patients with locally advanced, stage IIIB disease (T4 or N3) are considered inoperable, and radiotherapy is the standard treatment. Most of the patients do not obtain a complete response to radiotherapy, but occasionally a patient will be completely cured, and some patients will survive 3 years. The addition of chemotherapy to radiotherapy has been reported to improve long-term survival in some, but not all prospective studies. There is some doubt about the cause of the variation in results, which may for instance be due to different drug administration schedules. A meta-analysis of data from 54 randomized clinical trials showed that the addition of cisplatin-based chemotherapy to radiotherapy resulted in an absolute survival benefit of 4% at 2 years, and the optimal sequencing of the treatment modalities is under study in ongoing clinical trials.

For patients with metastatic disease, stage IV (M1), systemic treatment is indicated if any prolongation of survival is hoped for. The efficacies of all of the current treatment programs are so low that no specific regimen can be considered standard treatment, but meta-analyses have shown that chemotherapy produces modest benefits in short-term survival compared to supportive care alone. Some cisplatin- or carboplatin-based regimens have recently been shown to result in objective response rates, including a few complete responses, that are better than the results obtained with single-agent regimens, and the outcomes of varying cisplatin-containing regimens are similar, although the toxicities may vary. A higher dose intensity of cisplatin failed to produce improved survival in a randomized trial. A number of new drugs – the taxoids (paclitaxel and docetaxel), gemcitabine, vinorelbine – have shown significant activity in advanced NSCLC.

The poor survival of patients with locally advanced and metastatic NSCLC makes effective palliation an important objective, and a "watch and wait" policy is considered inappropriate for most of these patients because of the risk of development of serious local complications, which are difficult to palliate. Several randomized trials have shown radiotherapy in standard fractionation and doses of around 30–40 Gy to produce palliative benefits, measurable as symptomatic improvements and increases in performance scale measures. In other cases, surgical resection combined with postoperative radiation is recommended for single metastases.

Economic Evaluations

Rosenthal et al. (1992) performed a retrospective calculation of the costs of treating a cohort of SCLC patients in one institution during 1 year. All diagnostic investigations, treatments given, and follow-up examinations performed were recorded retrospectively by examination of each patient's medical and radiotherapy chart. The calculation is based on 31 unselected patients with SCLS treated during 1987 at one institution who received all their treatment at the same institution (out of 39 patients referred to the institution). Survival is measured from the first day of treatment to death or the last day of follow-up, which lasted for 3 years; no patients were lost to follow-up.

Routine diagnostic investigations performed by other physicians before referral are included in the total costs, while the costs of terminal care for the patients are excluded, with the argument that these costs are unavoidable and not dependent on the initial treatment. Costs of paramedical services and what the authors term "infrastructure costs within the hospital departments" are not included, as it is not very clear what is understood by these terms. The unit prices used for costing the various resources consumed are usually semiofficial rates fixed by branches of government or other public bodies such as the Australian Medicare Schedule Benefit for all diagnostic investigations and tests, fees set in this schedule for the costs of radiotherapy, pharmacy purchase price for pharmaceuticals, a standard government rate per day of hospitalization, etc. Quality of life for the patients is considered by first using the TWiST method developed by Gelber and colleagues (see, e.g., Gelber et al. 1991) to divide the overall survival time for each patient into time with toxicity from treatment (tox), time without symptoms of disease or toxicity of treatment (TWiST), and time after relapse to death (rel). Subsequently, the various periods of survival are given arbitrary utility coefficients in order to perform a threshold analysis. The purpose of this is to determine for which constellation of utility values for tox and rel one treatment will be preferred to the other.

The costs were calculated in 1990 AUS$, and the median cost per patient was found to be approximately AUS$ 14,400, with a range from about AUS$ 1200 to 40,000 (the median corresponds to around US$ 11,300 when converted by the PPP of 1990). The median costs for patients with limited disease were almost 50% higher than for patients with extensive disease (AUS$ 18,200 vs. 13,200), while the difference in overall survival was less than 1 month (8.7 vs. 7.9 months). Hospitalization (including outpatient visits) accounted for 42% of the total costs, while initial chemotherapy and radiotherapy accounted for 18% and 11%, respectively, follow-up examinations for 8%, and management of relapse (including second-line chemotherapy or radiotherapy) for 12%. If utility coefficients of 0.75 for tox, 0.25 for rel, and 1 for TWiST are assumed,[2] the difference between absolute survival and quality-adjusted (Q)-TWiST is rather small for patients with limited disease (12.6 vs. 10.2 months), while it is more substantial for patients with extensive disease (9.1 vs. 5.1 months).

The only other identified economic assessment related to SCLC was made by Goodwin et al. (1988), a retrospective cost-effectiveness analysis based on

[2] The authors claim these values to be the clinically most reasonable, but they should of course only be perceived as attempts at approximating the relative "badness" of tox and rel without pretending to be exact measures of their relative utility.

a clinical trial of standard chemotherapy, cyclophosphamide+doxorubicin+vincristine (CAV), versus a new and more aggressive regimen, where CAV is alternated with etoposide+cisplatin. Each regimen was given for six cycles, and responding patients received prophylactic cranial radiation after three cycles. The effectiveness of the treatments was measured as survival after randomization. The costs of treatment were calculated from time of randomization to death, and all costs were identified retrospectively for one of the institutions participating in the trial, treating about half of all the patients (144 patients on the standard arm, 145 on the new arm). Prospectively collected information, such as frequency of hospital visits during chemotherapy and details of the chemotherapies (doses, number of courses) and radiation administered, was taken directly from the trial records, while other information was obtained retrospectively (e.g., the rates of hospitalization, which were taken from a provincial cancer registry).

The authors try to assess costs from a societal viewpoint, inter alia by including costs of patient transport and accommodation, but these are based exclusively on assumptions and not observations. The determination of unit costs for the various types of resources consumed is described in rather great detail, but the distinction between charges and costs is not always upheld. The costs per patient are presented from various viewpoints, i.e., those of the treating hospital, other agencies, the patients, and society, and in all cases the costs are higher for the new treatment. Utility measurement was accomplished by using category scaling and standard gamble techniques with two different proxy groups: (1) patients undergoing similar treatments and (2) a group of health professionals familiar with the treatments. No significant differences in these quality assessments were found either between the two proxy groups or between the two measurement methods.

Compared to the standard regimen, the new, alternating regimen gave a statistically significant gain in response rates and in overall survival (9.7 vs. 8.1 months). The quality-adjusted survival advantage was 1.2 months. The incremental costs from the societal viewpoint were CAN$ 450 (in 1984 CAN$), which translated into an incremental societal cost per quality-adjusted life-year (QALY) of CAN$ 4500 (equal to US$ 3900 if converted by 1985 PPPs). The major cost item in both cases was hospitalization (65% of total costs for the standard treatment, 59% for the new), while the second major cost item was chemotherapy (16% for the standard, 20% for the new regimen). The results are fairly unstable, as sensitivity analyses show that both the magnitude and direction of the cost-effectiveness ratio change if the hospitalization rates are varied by ±20% and also by variations in other variables. The most unfavorable result for the new regimen of these sensitivity analyses was CAN$ 35,000 per year of life gained.

In NSCLC, two studies are concerned with the cost-effectiveness of various preoperative procedures used for clinical staging of the patients, while several other studies are concerned with the controversial issue of using chemotherapy for patients with advanced disease and widespread metastases. Black et al. (1988) analyzed when to perform a chest computed tomography (CT) scan in patients with T1N0M0 NSCLC by means of a decision analysis, based on a decision tree with two arms as starting point, CT staging and no CT staging. CT staging can lead to biopsy (if lymph nodes are greater than a chosen threshold) to examine whether there is mediastinal involvement. If this is confirmed, no surgery will be performed and the patient will only receive palliative care. If involvement is not confirmed or if the CT scan is negative to begin with, the patient undergoes surgery, which is the basis of a new subtree. If no CT staging is performed, the patient goes directly to the surgery subtree, in which there is a small probability that the patient will not survive. Given survival, there are two possible outcomes based on the presence or absence of mediastinal involvement, the probability of which depends on how the patient arrives in the surgical subtree.

The data for the decision tree are derived from a survey of the medical literature, and the study is quite remarkable by giving a thorough description of the available literature, a discussion of the findings, and explicit reasons for the actual choice of values for the variables. On the other hand, the cost estimates for the procedures used in the calculations are given only very summarily and without any details of the methods employed for estimation, only claiming that the cost estimates for chest CT, biopsy, and curative surgery are consistent with figures reported from other institutions.

With the baseline values of the analysis, CT staging is demonstrated to be a dominant solution, because it simultaneously results in an improvement in expected survival and lower expected costs. Threshold sensitivity analyses show that, over the range of most variables, CT staging provides a better life expectancy at lower costs than no CT scanning, so there is no trade-off between life expectancy and costs, as the CT strategy is clearly preferable to the alternative on all counts. The desirability of CT scanning may be stated as a function of the prevalence of mediastinal metastases, when baseline values are used for the other variables. With a prevalence of less than 6%, no CT is preferred. With a prevalence of 15% (which is the baseline value chosen based on the literature review) or higher, CT scanning is dominant. With a prevalence of between 6% and 15%, there is a trade-off, varying from US$ 2.1 million per year of expected lifetime gained when the prevalence is 7% to US$ 13,600 per year when the prevalence is 12%.

Eddy (1989) examined the costs and consequences of assessing mediastinal metastases in operable NSCLC patients by two alternative methods, CT scanning and mediastinoscopy. By the latter method, the lymph nodes can be directly visualized to see whether the tumor has spread to them. If the lymph nodes are not involved, the tumor is resectable, while surgery will normally not be performed if there is nodal involvement. It is expected that 25% of the patients presenting have nodal involvement, and these will be spared the risks and costs of unnecessary surgery if preoperative mediastinoscopy is used. However, the procedure has a false-negative rate of 10%. By the alternative staging method, CT scanning of the mediastinal nodes, the patient will be sent directly to surgery if the scan shows no enlargement of the nodes, while in case of enlarged nodes, the patient will undergo further examinations, primarily mediastinoscopy. The effectiveness of CT scans is less well established, but it is believed that the rate of false-negative results is somewhat lower than 10%, and that the rate of attempted resections is the same as when mediastinoscopy is used alone.

The two staging strategies have not been compared in a randomized controlled fashion, so the analysis proceeds as a decision analysis of a hypothetical cohort of 1000 patients, where the available data on costs, effectiveness, and complications are combined in a decision tree. The perspective chosen for the analysis is that of the Ministry of Health. Probabilities for effectiveness and complications are derived from a number of large published case series of patients undergoing the two procedures, while unit prices to be used for the calculation of the costs of the alternatives are gathered from one specific institution. It is claimed that the unit costs used are fully allocated in the sense that overhead costs and support services (e.g., housekeeping) have been allocated to a number of cost centers and then assigned to patients based on services actually used. It is assumed that the resource consumption prior to and after the staging procedures performed is the same, no matter what staging strategy is used, and that the same number of patients will either undergo surgery for presumably resectable disease or will be denied surgery, regardless of the staging procedure used. In effect, then, the analysis performed is a cost-minimization analysis.

The decision analysis is highly dependent upon the assumed rate of positive CT scans, i.e., scans that lead to further examination by mediastinoscopy, and there is no agreed threshold for the size of lymph nodes that will be considered normal or enlarged. The analysis is performed for assumed rates of positive CT scans between 40% and 80%, but whatever the rate used, the costs of a primary mediastinoscopy of all patients is always higher than the costs of a strategy in which CT scans are followed by mediastinoscopy for only those patients who have a positive CT scan. The conclusion is that, assuming equal pretest and post-test resource use, the CT scan strategy (within the range of rates of positive CT scans examined) always results in smaller costs and fewer days of hospitalization due to complications than the mediastinoscopy strategy. The higher the rate of positive CT scans assumed, the more similar the costs and the number of hospitalization days of the two strategies are, and for a rate of 80%, the difference in expected cost and expected number of days of hospitalization is only about $ 35,000 and 16 days, respectively (for a cohort of 1000 patients).

For patients with inoperable or metastatic NSCLC, the first study by Jaakkimainen et al. (1990) is a retrospective economic evaluation of a randomized clinical trial (performed by the Canadian NCI) of two chemotherapeutic regimens compared with each other and with a strategy of best supportive care (BSC). The chemotherapeutic regimens are vindecine+cisplatin (VP) and cyclophosphamide+doxorubicin+cisplatin (CAP), and the study's measures of the relative effectiveness of the treatments are taken directly from the trial. The costs considered are the costs of all hospital-based services determined from the viewpoint of two public health care plans, while other costs incurred by the public health care plans, by private health insurance plans, and by the patients themselves are excluded. All costs are determined in CAN$ 1984 prices, one of the years of patient recruitment for the clinical trial, and there is no discounting, because mean and median survival in all three arms was less than 1 year. The results are calculated for the outcome mean survival, which in all three arms was some 5–7 weeks higher than the median survival time.[3]

It was not feasible to identify retrospectively the costs for all individual patients in the trial, because these data are not routinely collected in the Canadian health care system. Instead, a detailed costing study was performed based on the resource utilization in two of the centers, which are claimed to be representative for all oncology centers in the country (even though both are university-affiliated tertiary-care institutions.). The costs determined at the two institutions were combined by averaging. Even for these institutions, not all the data on resource utilization could be retrieved from the trial data, so on a number of occasions assumptions have been used. The methods used for determining unit cost are reported in some detail, but, nevertheless, the estimation procedures used are not always very transparent.

No chemotherapy was administered in the BSC arm, while palliative radiation could be given to any patient in the trial. The mean survival and mean costs in the three arms were as follows: BSC. 24 weeks and CAN$ 8600[4]; CAP, 32 weeks and CAN$ 7600; VP, 37 weeks and CAN$ 12,200. Compared to BSC, both chemotherapy regimens gave a statistically significant increase in survival. The cost-effectiveness ratio (i.e., the cost per year of life gained by moving from one treatment to the other) of CAP compared to BSC is *minus* CAN$ 6200 (i.e., a saving per year of life gained), while the ratios were CAN$ 14,800 for VP compared to BSC and CAN$ 49,700 for VP compared to CAP. The direction of these cost-effectiveness ratios is not changed by any of the sensitivity analyses performed, in which the estimates of resource consumption and the unit costs are varied by ±25%. The authors themselves emphasize that one of the important findings of the study is that a policy of BSC for patients with advanced NSCLC was associated with substantial costs, because these patients had higher hospitalization rates and received more palliative radiotherapy than the patients receiving either form of chemotherapy. The favorable results of chemotherapy compared to BSC would be further improved by a recalculation with 1989 prices, because lower-priced generic drug products (cisplatin) have become available on the market since then.

Kennedy et al. (1995) used clinical data from the same clinical trial as that used by Jaakkimainen et al. (1990) for a cost-utility analysis of the choice between chemotherapy and BSC in patients with advanced NSCLC. Interest-

---

[3] This may not sound of much, but for the BSC strategy, for instance, the difference between mean and median (7 weeks) amounts to more than 40% of the median value (17 weeks).

[4] With the 1985 PPPs, CAN$ 8600 is equal to about US$ 6900

ingly, their cost calculations differ from the ones reported by Jaakkimainen et al. (1990) and their results are much more in favor of BSC. The discrepancies in the cost calculations may be explained by several factors, and they underline the difficulties in transferring the results of a cost-effectiveness analysis carried out in one setting to another setting. Important factors are that the two studies were carried out in different provinces of Canada, between which there are discrepancies in treatment patterns (e.g., hospitalization rates) and unit prices and the fact that the two studies include different cost items.

Kennedy et al. (1995) performed a retrospective analysis on 70 patients from two hospitals in the Quebec province (out of the total of 232 patients included in the complete clinical trial), so the study is plagued by large variances of the estimates and low power. All patients had died at the time of data collection. The health services used for these 70 patients were identified and enumerated from the time of randomization into the study until death. For all patients, a complete registration of the services used was performed, except for medications other than chemotherapy due to the considerable workload such a registration would imply. However, a detailed analysis of medication provided was performed for a random sample of 12 patients in order to estimate a mean medication cost, which was then imputed to all the patients.

The costs were calculated from the viewpoint of the healthcare system, with most unit cost figures taken from the reimbursement schedule of the provincial health plan as of 1990. Prices of procedures performed consist of the medical component to which a technical component is added. No capital costs are included, and neither are the costs incurred by the patient and his or her family. Because of the short time period involved (mean survival time for all treatment arms was less than 1 year), neither the costs nor the effects of treatment have been discounted.

Utility values for the different management strategies were obtained from a panel of nine oncologists with extensive experience in treating NSCLC patients. The time trade-off technique was used for eliciting the utility values, and the number of QALYs was then calculated by multiplying the survival time in days with the utility value and dividing by 365. Two health states used for elicitation of utility values, one associated with combination chemotherapy[5] and the other with BSC, were presented by developing two scenarios describing the anticipated beneficial and adverse effects of the treatment alternatives. These scenarios were based mainly on the information provided to the patients in the trial on the form with which they gave their consent to participating in the trial, supplemented with information about the adverse effects actually observed in the trial.

[5] The same state was considered applicable to both, as each contain cisplatin, which causes the most important adverse effects associated with these regimens, and as the incidence in the trial of other important adverse effects differed very little between them.

The average utility value attributed to combination chemotherapy was 0.34 compared with 0.61 for BSC. This difference was found to be statistically significant, and the values were used for weighing the median survival time observed in the trial for the three options in order to estimate median QALYs. This results in median QALYs of 0.19, 0.15, and 0.19 for BSC, CAP, and VP, respectively, i.e., there are no statistically significant differences between them in the quality-adjusted survival. The average total costs for the treatment arms, in CAN$, are 6400 for BSC, 7800 for CAP, and 9800 for VP.

The gain in survival time from giving chemotherapy compared to BSC[6] is thus achieved at an increase in costs, while at the same time there is no gain in QALYs because of the significant reduction in quality of life caused by the adverse effects of chemotherapy. These results were found to be stable after comprehensive sensitivity analyses, varying the costs (±50%), the survival time (using the survival from the complete clinical trial), and the utility values used for determining QALYs (±20%).

Smith et al. (1995) added to the controversies regarding the use of chemotherapy in metastatic NSCLC by a cost-effectiveness analysis of three different regimens of chemotherapy. The evaluation is retrospective, combining efficacy data from a European trial of the three regimens with cost data from an university-affiliated cancer center in Virginia, USA. The randomized trial compared the new cytotoxic agent vinorelbine alone with vinorelbine + cisplatin and with vindesine + cisplatin, which is a very common regimen in Europe. A total of 612 patients were randomized between these three regimens, and all patients were treated until disease progression, unacceptable toxicity, stable disease for 18 weeks, or patient refusal. The objective response rates and mean survival times, respectively, were 14% and 41.6 weeks for vinorelbine alone, 28% and 49.6 weeks for vinorelbine + cisplatin and 19% and 44.3 weeks for vindesine + cisplatin. Major treatment-related toxicities were very limited (only 20 episodes of febrile neutropenia requiring hospitalization and two or three deaths on each arm), while minor toxicities, including nausea, were more frequent on the arms containing cisplatin.

The trial enrolled patients from eight European countries at 45 different sites, so it was decided to use cost data from an American academic cancer center instead of trying to determine average prices for the centers in the trial. All patients received similar supportive care, and they were assumed to have similar costs for palliative radiation therapy, hospice care, and terminal care. Neither the efficacy nor the costs of second-line chemotherapy or supportive terminal care were estimated. Inpatient and outpatient charge data for similar NSCLC patients enrolled in clinical trials (including vinorelbine)

---

[6] In the subgroup of 70 patients, the differences in median survival were not statistically significant due to the small sample size and low power, although median survival was 112 days in the BSC arm, 165 in the CAP arm, and 214 in the VP arm. In the complete trial, survival times in each arm were a little longer, and the difference between BSC and each of the chemotherapy regimens was statistically significant.

were used to calculate charges for treatment and toxicities. Following this, the costs were estimated by using local charge-to-cost ratios. No actual resource utilization data were used, but the charges/costs were determined by multiplying the incidence or frequencies (e.g., of various types of toxicities) observed in the trial with some assumed standard charges/costs per such event. The origin of these standard cost figures and the methods of determining them are not explained. Purportedly, the analysis was performed from a societal viewpoint, but the meaning of this statement is not clear, because only direct hospital costs seem to be included, and the unit cost data used are impenetrable.

After ordering the regimens in terms of efficacy, the incremental cost-effectiveness ratios are determined as $ 17,700 per year of life gained with vinorelbine+cisplatin compared to vinorelbine alone, $ 22,100 per year of life gained with vindesine+cisplatin compared to vinorelbine alone, and $ 15,500 with vinorelbine+cisplatin compared to vindesine+cisplatin. The treatment costs consisted almost entirely of chemotherapy, supportive drug, and laboratory costs, with the costs of chemotherapy alone accounting for around 45% of the total. Using average estimates from 14 oncology physicians and nurses, quality adjustments of the survival gains are made with the values 1 for the state "well," 0.7 for vinorelbine alone, and 0.6 for the cisplatin-based regimens. After this quality adjustment, the costs per gain in quality-adjusted survival are calculated.[7] Vinorelbine alone dominates over vindesine+cisplatin by giving a gain of 18 days at a saving of $ 29,000, while vinorelbine+cisplatin compared with vindesine+cisplatin results in a cost-effectiveness ratio of $ 25,800. The gain with vinorelbine+cisplatin compared to vinorelbine alone is 0.6 weeks, resulting in an incremental cost-effectiveness ratio of $ 241,300.

Evans and Le Chevalier (1996) used data from the same clinical trial as Smith et al. (1995) to examine the relative cost-effectiveness of various chemotherapy regimens in the management of NSCLC patients with metastatic disease. In addition to the three regimens included in the trial (vinorelbine, vinorelbine + cisplatin, and vindesine + cisplatin), the analysis comprises two other chemotherapy regimens often used for NSCLC patients with metastatic disease (VP-16 + cisplatin and vinblastine+cisplatin) and a policy of BSC. Moreover, a regimen of outpatient vinorelbine + cisplatin (but much less cisplatin intensive than the inpatient regimen), under current investigation in an NCI trial in Canada, is included in the analysis.

Survival data and details about the doses administered from the European trial are combined with data from a number of other sources in order to determine the possible therapeutic gains and the incremental costs of obtaining them. Thus survival data and some economic data used for the cost calculation (hospitalization) for the two standard chemotherapy regimens and BSC

[7] In this recent paper, the "accepted benchmark for medical interventions" is revised to about $ 50,000 per year of life gained. Whether the gain is quality adjusted or not is not made clear.

are taken from the Canadian trial from the mid-1980s, upon which the above-mentioned economic evaluation by Jaakkimainen et al. (1990) was based. For the outpatient regimen of vinorelbine+cisplatin, it is assumed that survival is the same as for the corresponding inpatient regimen.

The total expected costs of managing NSCLC patients with the various regimens are found by adding chemotherapy-specific costs to a standard cost model for lung cancer patients. This takes the perspective of the third-party payer (the government) and includes data on diagnostic methods, treatment and its outcomes, health care utilization, and direct costs. The chemotherapy-specific costs are partly based on time and motion studies and workload measures. The costs of BSC and terminal care are obtained by taking the data from the Jaakkimainen study and adjusting them to 1993 figures. It is assumed (as was observed in that trial) that chemotherapy-treated patients use fewer hospital days during terminal care and receive less palliative radiotherapy.

Compared to the BSC policy, four of the six chemotherapy regimens offer a modest gain in survival for a reduction in total expected cost. For the other two regimens, the survival gain is accompanied by increasing costs, resulting in cost-effectiveness ratios of about CAN$ 5500 for vinorelbine+cisplatin (inpatient) and CAN$ 12,000 for vindesine + cisplatin. The standard regimen of vinblastine + cisplatin offers the greatest cost reduction of about $ 3200 compared to the BSC policy. Using this regimen as a standard comparator, the cost-effectiveness ratios of the vinorelbine-containing regimens, which all lead to a survival gain (in no case more than 2 months), vary between $ 16,400 per year gained for vinorelbine + cisplatin (outpatient) and $ 140,000 per year gained for vinorelbine alone. The results are very sensitive to changes in the assumptions about days of hospitalizations for patients in terminal care, while major changes in the assumed survival gain have less of an impact.

Concluding Remarks

Table 1 summarizes the main characteristics of the economic assessments of lung cancer treatments which have been described and briefly discussed in this chapter. A study worth mentioning, which has not been included because it does not deal with a calculation of the costs of treatment for a particular group of patients or comparison of specific treatment alternatives, is the one by Coy et al. (1994). This paper describes a promising method for cost calculations at a very detailed level, i.e., the costs of various activities performed by a radiotherapy unit, exemplified with a standard protocol for lung cancer patients.

In accordance with the relative incidence of the two major forms of lung cancer, the main focus of economic evaluations of the management of lung cancer has been on NSCLC. A survey of the cost and quality-of-life issues involved in SCLC, complementing the description of the published studies giv-

Table 1. Main characteristics of economic assessments dealing with lung cancer

Reference	Disease category	Treatments examined	Main characteristics of the study
Rosenthal et al. (1992)	SCLC, all patients	Complete management, i.e., all diagnostic investigations, treatments given, and all follow-up examinations	Cost-identification study Perspective not clear, mostly third-party payer Retrospective analysis of charts of 31 unselected patients from one institution; unit prices used are semiofficial rates, fee schedules etc.; quality of life is considered by means of Q-TWiST Cost distribution highly skewed; median costs for limited disease much higher than for extensive disease, survival only 1 month longer; small difference in absolute and quality-adjusted survival for limited disease, larger for extended
Goodwin et al. (1988)	SCLC, all patients	New chemotherapy regimen vs. standard	Retrospective cost-effectiveness analysis Social perspective, including direct costs for patients Clinical and some economic data from randomized controlled trial, supplemented with information obtained retrospectively, e.g., rate of hospitalization; utility adjustment of survival using proxy group evaluations Baseline analysis results in moderate cost-outcome ratios for gain in overall and quality-adjusted survival; results are not stable
Black et al. (1988)	NSCLC, local disease	Clinical staging with CT scan or not	Cost-effectiveness analysis Hospital perspective Clinical efficacy data from literature review; cost data from calculations for other institutions Baseline result is that CT scan is a dominant solution, i.e., resulting in survival gain at reduced cost; the result is very sensitive to assumptions about the prevalence of metastases in this group
Eddy (1989)	NSCLC patients, operable	CT scan vs. mediastinoscopy for assessing metastases	Cost-minimization analysis Third-party payer perspective Decision tree analysis; data for effectiveness and complications from published case series; cost data from single institution Results highly dependent upon assumed rate of positive CT scans leading to secondary mediastinoscopy; primary mediastinoscopy almost always the most costly strategy
Jaakkimainen et al. (1990)	NSCLC, advanced disease	Two chemotherapeutic regimens vs. BSC	Cost-effectiveness analysis Third-party payer Effectiveness data from randomized clinical trial; resource utilization data from trial combined with assumptions; unit cost estimated from charges and fee schedules Compared to BSC, both chemotherapy regimens result in significant increase in survival, for one with a cost saving, for the other with a modest cost-effectiveness ratio; the results are stable

Table 1 (continued)

Reference	Disease category	Treatments examined	Main characteristics of the study
Kennedy et al. (1995)	NSCLC advanced disease	Two chemotherapeutic regimens vs. BSC	Cost-utility analysis Third-party payer Effectiveness (survival) data from randomized clinical trial; resource utilization data from retrospective analysis of charts for patients in the trial; unit cost data from public reimbursement plan; utility values elicited from oncologists Costs of both chemotherapy regimens are higher than the costs of BSC, while the quality of life of patients in chemotherapy is much lower than that of patients receiving BSC; adjusting the survival gain of chemotherapy for the reduced quality of life, there is no gain in QALYs of chemotherapy, while the costs are higher
Smith et al (1995)	Metastatic NSCLC	Three chemotherapy regimens, with new agents such as vinorelbine and vindesine	Cost-effectiveness and cost-utility analysis Perspective claimed to be social, in reality hospital perspective Efficacy and toxicity data from a European randomized controlled trial; only first-line treatment costs considered, all other costs assumed to be identical; cost calculated from examination of charges from a single cancer center for similar patients enrolled in similar randomized controlled trials and then converted by local cost-to-charge ratios; no actual resource utilization data used, incidence of events multiplied by assumed standard cost/charge for type of event; quality adjustment of survival based on expert opinion Lowest incremental cost per year of life gained is found for vinorelbine+cisplatin compared with vindesine+cisplatin; after quality-of-life adjustment, vinorelbine alone dominates over vindesine+cisplatin; compared to vinorelbine alone, the addition of cisplatin adds very little to the outcome at very high incremental costs
Evans and Le Chevalier (1996)	Metastatic NSCLC	Six different chemotherapy regimens compared with BSC	Cost-effectiveness analysis Third-party payer (government) perspective Survival data from various randomized controlled trials and, in certain cases, assumptions; chemotherapy-specific cost data, partly based on time and motion studies and workload measures, added to standard cost model for lung cancer patients; BSC and terminal care cost based on adjustment of previous study Compared to BSC, four of the chemotherapy regimens offer a dominant solution, while for two of them a survival gain leads to increased costs; the results are sensitive to assumptions about days of hospital for terminal care, less so to variations in the size of survival gain

SCLC, small cell lung cancer; NSCLC, non-small-cell lung cancer; CT, computed tomography; BSC, best supportive care; QALY, quality-adjusted life-year; Q-TWiST, quality-adjusted time without symptoms of disease or toxicity of treatment.

en here, may be found in Graham and Boyages (1993). Despite being of a comparatively high technical standard, the four studies concerned with the controversial issue of treating patients with advanced NSCLC do not make an unequivocal contribution to finding a definite solution to the controversy, which is also informally discussed by Ruckdeschel (1990). The cost-effectiveness studies (Jaakkimainen et al. 1990; Evans and Le Chevalier 1996) show that several regimens of chemotherapy may be a dominant solution compared to BSC (i.e., giving a survival gain while being less costly). With other chemotherapy regimens there is a trade-off, i.e., a gain in survival is achieved but only at higher costs than for BSC, but the cost-effectiveness ratios reported are quite low.

However, when the survival gain is adjusted to take patient's quality of life into account, as done by Kennedy et al. (1995), BSC becomes the dominant solution, as they find that chemotherapy is more costly than BSC, while there is no gain in QALYs. The panel of oncologists used for eliciting utility values attributed a much lower utility value to patients in chemotherapy compared to BSC. The last paper, by Smith et al. (1995), does not contribute directly to the controversy, because it only compares three chemotherapy regimens with each other without including BSC as an option. However, it is interesting to compare the utility values used in this study, which were also elicited from a panel of oncology clinicians and nurses, with the ones used in Kennedy et al. (1995). Smith et al. (1995) state that the average values given for the chemotherapy regimens were 0.7 and 0.6 for the vinorelbine- and cisplatin-based regimens, respectively, while Kennedy et al. (1990) found mean values of 0.34 for chemotherapy (cisplatin-based) and 0.61 for BSC.

This substantial divergence in utility values attributed is remarkable and certainly one of the factors explaining the opposite results. The usual recommended "solution" would be to elicit utility values from (potential) patients and their relatives, but there is no certainty that such a procedure would not result in just as divergent values if repeated with various groups of responders. In addition, there is considerable discussion about whose (utility) values should be used for decision making. Another methodologically interesting result of comparing these economic evaluations is the divergence in cost calculations between two studies (even performed in the same country) based on the same randomized controlled trial. This underlines the complexity of transferring results from one setting to another and the need for separate reporting of resource utilization data and the unit prices used instead of just reporting total costs.

Colorectal Cancer

Introduction

Colorectal cancer is the second most common cancer after lung cancer. Worldwide the incidence rates vary widely, but in most westernized countries about 5% of the population will be affected during their lifetime. Cancer of the colon is about three times as common as rectal cancer. It is predominantly a disease of the elderly, as about 40% of the patients are over 75 and only 5% are under 50. The age distribution of the population will affect the overall incidence, which is expected to grow by about 10% from the late 1980s to 2005, while the mortality rate is expected to rise by 3%. The 5-year survival rate for both types of cancers have increased by about 10 percentage points since the mid 1950s and is now a little more than 50% for each.

The main treatment option and the only one that can be curative for colorectal cancer is surgery, and between 70% and 90% of the presenting patients are considered suitable for surgical intervention. The most important independent prognostic factor for survival or recurrence after potentially curative surgery is the stage of cancer, which is determined by the degree of penetration through the bowel wall and the presence and number of positive lymph nodes. Other independent prognostic factors include age (the younger the patient, the poorer the prognosis), gender (women have a more favorable prognosis), symptoms (there are several reports of high survival rates in asymptomatic patients in whom the cancer is detected by screening), duration of symptoms (better survival with longer duration, perhaps indicating slow growth of the tumor), and several others. In contrast to most other tumors, there does not seem to be a negative relation between the size of the primary tumor and survival.

Several coexisting systems for the pathologic staging of colorectal cancers have been evolving since the 1930s. The issue of which of these staging systems to use has not yet been definitely resolved, but in this report the common TNM staging system will be used. Stage 0 signifies carcinoma in situ, and stage I indicates that the tumor is limited to the bowel wall, whereas in stage II the tumor has spread to extramural tissue. In stage III, regional lymph nodes are involved, and stage IV is defined by the presence of distant metastases whatever the size of the primary tumor and the degree of nodal involvement. For patients with stage I disease, there is at least a 90% probability of cure (or rather of disease-free survival to 5 years, after which the survival curve is no different from the curve for the rest of the population). For stage II patients, the probability drops to the 75% range, and for stage III patients to around 35%. The estimated average survival after operation is 3 years, but in general the 5-year survival is lower for patients with cancer of the rectosigmoid or the rectum than for patients with cancer elsewhere in the colon.

A major limitation of surgery in the rectum is that the presence of the bony pelvis and of other vital pelvic organs makes it impossible for the surgeon to obtain radial margins that are as wide as would be desirable. The characteristic pattern of failure after potentially curative surgery is probably associated with this problem, as colon cancers have a higher incidence of recurrence in the abdominal cavity than rectal cancers, in which half of the failures are located in the pelvis. As the rationale for the use of adjuvant therapy in colorectal cancer is based on the patterns of failure after surgery, it is necessary to distinguish between cancers in the colon and in the rectum.

Colon Cancer

For stage I and II disease, the standard surgical procedure is the same, while the role of adjuvant therapy is still disputed despite a large number of trials performed since the 1950s, comprising both irradiation and chemotherapy modalities and many varying regimens. For instance, based on the high incidence of abdominal failure, whole-abdominal irradiation has been tried, although its use is limited by the fact that the tolerance of the whole abdomen is much lower than the dose required for potentially curative treatment of the volume at risk for metastatic disease. As liver metastasis is the most common, and often the only recurrence, much interest has also been invested in regional adjuvant therapy, directed at reducing liver metastases, using either portal vein infusion of cytotoxics or radiation of the liver. Early trials with these modalities showed some promising results, but later confirmatory trials have failed to document a significant reduction of liver recurrences from adjuvant therapy.

A number of large prospective randomized trials have consistently demonstrated benefit for systemic chemotherapy with 5-fluorouracil (5-FU) plus either levamisole or leucovorin. All together, about 4000 patients have participated in these prospective randomized trials, which have demonstrated a reduction in mortality from adjuvant chemotherapy compared to surgery alone of between 22% and 33%. The benefit is clear in stage III patients, while it is less certain for stage II patients. The optimal cytotoxic regimen is not yet clear, however, and many ongoing clinical trials are comparing various postoperative chemotherapeutic or immunotherapy regimens, alone or in combination.

The optimal follow-up monitoring program after potentially curative therapy is an issue of controversy. To date, no large-scale prospective randomized trials have documented the efficacy of a standard postoperative monitoring program, but some general guidelines have been formulated. Standard recommendations comprise history taking plus physical examination supplemented by fecal occult blood testing and sigmoidoscopy every 3–4 months for 3 years, carcinoembryonic antigen (CEA) assays every 2–4 months (despite admitting the absence of evidence of a clear benefit), and yearly X-rays. The same examinations and procedures should be carried out in years 4 and 5, but with a reduced frequency.

For patients with stage IV, or distant metastatic disease, the treatment possibilities are limited. There is some evidence that resection of limited liver metastases may enhance survival in some patients if the resection results in no clinically apparent tumor. Regional chemotherapy against liver metastases has produced higher response rates and increased local toxicity, but no consistent improvement in survival. For these patients, chemotherapy is primarily given with a palliative intent.[1] Most attempts to improve systemic therapy have consisted in empirically adding drugs to the 5-FUs, to which these cancers *do* respond. Overall, there is no demonstrable benefit for all patients treated, but the few patients with an objective response may have a median survival of 16–24 months, compared to a median survival of all the patients concerned of 10–12 months. The dose-limiting effects of bolus 5-FU are mucositis, diarrhea, and leukopenia. The interest is now switching to infusional 5-FU, which has a diverging mode of action and a different pattern of toxicity. From a chemical point of view, the two forms of 5-FU should in essence be considered different.

When modulated by other agents, such as methotrexate or leucovorin, bolus 5-FU has been shown to be more cytotoxic, with a higher response rate, but with variable effects on median survival. Only bolus 5-FU+leucovorin has been shown to be superior to 5-FU alone in prospective randomized trials. A number of clinical trials are currently being carried out with the aim of determining the optimal schedule of 5-FU as a biochemical modulation strategy. For patients not responding to 5-FU, the options are very limited, but some other new chemotherapeutic agents, e.g., irinotecan (CPT-11) and raltitrexed, have been shown to produce some modest responses and stabilization.

For patients with recurrent colon cancer, the picture is very much the same as for stage IV patients. No standard therapy exists, and there is no evidence that standard chemotherapy has improved the survival for these patients, but chemotherapy with single agents, combinations, or new drugs have been used for palliation. Locally recurrent cancer may be resectable, especially if the prior operation was inadequate, as may liver metastases and limited pulmonary metastases, with enhanced survival if resection results in no remaining measurable tumor.

---

[1] For reasons not known, adenocarcinoma of the colon is much less responsive to the various available chemotherapeutic agents (e.g., alkylating or anthracycline agents) than the histopathologically identical adenocarcinomas of other organs, such as breast and stomach.

Rectal Cancer

Treatment of resectable rectal cancers, the extent of surgery (e.g., inclusion of lymph nodes or not), and the options available are very much dependent on the site of the tumor, but there is no uniform definition of resectability, which may for instance also depend upon whether the assessment is made clinically or at the time of surgery. The rectum is usually considered to have three distinct sections of approximately the same length, and overall cure rates for cancers in the lower third are less than for cancers in the upper two thirds. Fewer than one third of the patients require permanent colostomy, and for most patients the primary treatment modality is radical surgical resection. Surgery alone results in cure in about 45% of all patients, mainly because the cure rate is about 75% for patients with no nodal involvement. Few patients with node-positive disease are cured, but approximately one third of these achieve 5-year disease-free survival.

Despite radical surgery, locoregional failure occurs in 20%–50% of patients with transmural or node-positive cancer, and the incidence of treatment failure in the pelvis is directly related to the degree of transmural penetration. A large series of autopsies showed isolated pelvic recurrences in 25% of the patients, but 75% of the tumor-related deaths were associated with tumor in the pelvis. Accordingly, it is assumed that improving local control by using several treatment modalities to manage the primary cancer may reduce cancer-related morbidity and improve survival.

Compared to colon cancer, there is a higher tendency in rectal cancer for first failures to occur *only* in locoregional sites, so the impact of perioperative irradiation is greater in rectal than in colon cancer. Both pre- and postoperative radiation decrease local failure, but a significant improvement in overall survival has not been demonstrated. A decrease in local failures might, however, be considered an important end point in its own right, considering their debilitating effects.

For patients whose cancers have penetrated through the bowel wall or have metastasized to regional lymph nodes (stage II and III), an increase in the disease-free interval and in overall survival has been demonstrated in randomized clinical trials combining radiotherapy and chemotherapy. Following a National Institutes of Health (NIH) consensus conference in 1990, there seems to be general agreement that an appropriately intensive combination of radiation therapy and chemotherapy may offer the greatest survival advantage, even though there is some concern about the toxicity of the combined-modality treatment.[2] There are still a number of unresolved issues, however, such as the exact choice of chemotherapeutic agent or agents that can maximize the benefits while minimizing the adverse effects, the duration of chemotherapy, the scheduling and dosage of radiotherapy, and the optimal

[2] In one of the pivotal trials, severe or life-threatening acute toxic effects occurred in 18% of the patients in the radiochemotherapy arm, and three late deaths were observed.

sequencing of the various modalities. A number of current, large randomized clinical trials are addressing these therapeutic issues.

There is no standard treatment for locally advanced and unresectable[3] disease, but various regimens and modality combinations (e.g., preoperative radiotherapy to convert unresectable to resectable tumor, postoperative radiochemotherapy compared to radiotherapy alone) are being examined in randomized trials or by reporting of case series. Locally recurrent rectal cancer may be curable by radical surgery, possibly combined with radiotherapy. After radical surgery, recurrence in the pelvis may be treated with systemic chemotherapy. A promising experimental approach is regional chemotherapy by internal iliac artery infusion, even though there is so far no evidence that intra-arterial standard chemotherapy with or without resection of liver metastases has improved the survival of patients with recurrent rectal cancer.

The treatment of stage IV, metastatic disease does not diverge from the treatment of metastatic colon cancer. Useful palliation by chemotherapy may be seen in certain patients, whereas radiotherapy is normally the most useful palliative for pelvic recurrences unless prior radiotherapy has been given. A total of 80%–90% of patients treated this way obtain pain relief, although long-term symptom-free survival is rare. If irradiation fails to secure pain control, analgesics should be used for this purpose rather than other cancer treatments.

Economic Evaluations

The published studies on the economics of colorectal cancer cover a wide spectrum, from analyses of screening programs to an analysis of the cost-effectiveness of giving palliative chemotherapy in advanced disease. Most analyses use the terms "colorectal" or "colon," and no explicit distinction between cancers of the colon and of the rectum has been encountered in the retrieved studies.

The study by Taplin et al. (1995), analyzing the associations between the direct costs of cancer treatment and stage at diagnosis, age, and level of comorbidities, has already been described in some detail in the chapter on breast cancer (see p. 54), so here only the results with respect to colorectal cancer will be summarized. The analysis is based on data for 290 incident cases and 1046 prevalent cases for the observational window of 1990 and 1991. The overall result is that the total costs of initial care (the first 6 months after diagnosis) increased with the stage at diagnosis and did not vary with the patient's age, sex, or level of comorbidity, while the terminal costs (the last 6 months of life) did not covary with any of these four vari-

[3] There are prognostic differences between primary and recurrent tumors, but most case series do not report the results separately. Together with the heterogeneous definitions of the disease categories, this may be part of the explanation of the variations in results seen among case series.

ables. The costs of continuing care (the period in between the initial and the terminal phase) increased with stage at diagnosis and level of comorbidity, but were not associated with age or sex. The costs attributable to cancer are found by comparing the case subjects with control subjects without cancer, but the only difference compared to the above analysis of total costs is that, for patients in the continuing care phase, the costs attributable to cancer decreased with age and across levels of comorbidity, partly, of course, because of increasing costs for the control subjects.

Whynes et al. (1993) carried out a similar calculation of the costs of treating colorectal cancer according to the stage of the disease. The study was performed in the context of a large randomized clinical trial of screening for colorectal cancer with a study population of 155,000 individuals, half of which were offered a self-administered fecal occult blood screening test every 2 years, while the other half served as a control group. The trial was initiated in 1981, and patients cancer detected by screening and those presenting with symptomatic cancer in both the study and the control group have been followed up fully. To assess the economic impact of the disease, treatment costs for each patient were calculated over a 3-year period from diagnosis (or until death, if occurring within this period), as it is expected that the large majority of complications and cancer recurrences are likely to occur within 1–2 years of the initial treatment. Up to July 1991, 360 patients, all treated at the University Hospital in Nottingham, UK, fulfilled this criterion, and the cost assessment is based on the case notes for these, all of whom were treated by surgery only.

There were 152 cases in the control group and 208 in the study group, divided into the following: (a) detected by screening, (b) no-response patients (those who did not respond to or refused the offer of screening), and (c) interval patients, i.e., positive responders to screening presenting with symptoms between screening rounds. The costing study is based on the hospital notes for the patients, providing information on the types of diagnostic investigations performed, lengths of inpatient stay (including intensive care), duration and types of operation, radiology, pathology, and electrocardiography (ECG) requests. For the majority of these types of resources or services, unit costs are derived from the University Hospital's financial returns, while the costs of various forms of diagnostic techniques are taken from an earlier study by the same authors. The cost of intensive care is calculated by using a proportional markup over the costs of a normal inpatient day, the markup being based on other empirical studies of intensive care. The authors claim that all the estimated costs are marginal costs, but this claim is not substantiated in the article. The results are expressed in 1990–1991 prices.

The total costs are subdivided into five categories: (1) initial investigation and diagnosis, (2) preoperation, after admission, (3) main treatment, (4) readmission, and (5) other, from readmission to end of follow-up or death. A statistical comparison of the means between the control group and the three study subgroups showed no statistically significant differences (*t* test at 5%) with the following exceptions: (i) the diagnostic costs were higher for the patients detected by screening than for the control group, (ii) the main treatment costs were higher for the no-response group than for the patients detected by screening, and (iii) the total costs were higher for the no-response patients than for those detected by screening. A further inquiry into all the low-cost patients ("low" being defined as costs less than or equal to one standard deviation below the mean of the cost distribution concerned) showed that the majority of these patients in the control group and in the no-response group died before admission or within 6 months after diagnosis, while ten out of 11 low-cost patients in the group detected by screening survived the 3-year follow-up period.

The distribution of costs according to the severity of the disease at diagnosis, assessed according to the conventional Dukes' staging system, is also reported. Between the control and the study groups, the only statistically significant difference is in treating stage C disease. For the combined sample, the mean total costs according to stage are as follows: stage A, £ 2432;[4] B, £ 3242; C, £ 3771; and D, £ 2793. Both A and D are significantly different from B and C. If A and B are combined and C and D likewise, as early and late stage, respectively, the difference between the combined means is not significant. It should accordingly not be expected that screening will lead to large savings in treatment costs, even though the proportion of early-stage patients is much higher in the screening than in the control group. However, if the outcome of the intervention is not taken into account, the conclusion of the analysis may become very misleading. The above-mentioned examination of the low-cost patients may be taken as an indication that the main explanation for low treatment costs in the control group and the no-response group is the early death of the patients. In contrast to this, almost all the low-cost patients detected by screening survived the 3-year follow-up period.

Two other contributions from the group following the screening trial in Nottingham are concerned with costing diagnostic procedures and nursing care, respectively. In Walker et al. (1991), the costs of three different methods of diagnosing colorectal cancers are identified, and the possibilities of minimizing the costs per cancer detected are analyzed. The three diagnostic procedures are colonoscopy (CS), barium enema X-ray (DBCE), and flexible sigmoidscopy (FS), of which only CS is an inpatient procedure, but only in a limited number of cases (about 20%). The costs are assessed from the hospital's point of view. The investigation comprises in each case labor costs (staff time), materials consumed, pathological investigations, inpatient stay (where relevant), and general hospital services. Each of the procedures and their requirements in terms of staff time and materials are described and the assumptions ("typical patients," probabilities from published clinical studies) used in the calculations are clearly stated, and unit prices and their sources

---

[4] With the 1990 purchasing power parity (PPP) of US$ 1 = £ 0.419, the figure for group A becomes US$ 5800.

are given. However, the methods for deriving these unit prices are not explained, so their relevance and validity cannot be assessed.

Expressed in 1989 prices, the average nominal costs of the procedures are determined to be £ 106 for CS (£ 71 if there is no hospital admission, i.e., in 80% of the cases), £ 50 for DCBE, and £ 29 for FS. The expected cost of each procedure may then be determined as the average cost divided by the sensitivity of the test, corrected for the costs of treating the patients with a false-negative test result who will later present with symptoms and for the probability that it will be necessary in some cases to use both endoscopy and radiology. The final cost identification model contains these corrections of the nominal costs, while other modifications which should ideally be taken into account (e.g., the consequences of colonoscopy-induced morbidities and even mortality) are not included, because precise data for these are judged to be too hard to come by. However, even the data for the relative sensitivities of the three procedures are not quite satisfactory, because the clinical evidence is not always consistent, not even with respect to the direction of results. The economic evaluation remains inconclusive because of the wide variations observed in the clinical data.

Walker and Whynes (1990) compare two methods for calculating the costs of nursing care for a sample of 65 colorectal patients in two surgical wards at the Queen's Medical Centre and at the University Hospital in Nottingham. One method is based on average patient costs, where the staffing structure of the wards was costed using hospital data for total employment costs in the National Health Service (NHS; including national insurance and pension contributions). The total nursing costs of the wards, amounting to £ 122,161 per year (1989–1990 prices), were then divided by the number of bed-days per year to determine the average nursing cost per bed-day. The number of bed-days is determined by multiplying the number of possible yearly bed-days by an estimated occupancy rate of 91.7%. By interviewing senior nursing staff, the division of the nursing time between shared care and care for individual patients, was estimated to be 41% and 59%, respectively.

The patient-specific method is based on patient dependency data, which are routinely collected by one of the hospitals according to a four-point scale relating to the patient's ability for self-care. Senior nursing staff were interviewed to estimate the input of nursing effort required for each category of dependency, and these data were translated into nominal workload units, one unit being the care received by the least dependent patient category. By using data for the average dependency mix of the wards and the above-mentioned scaling, the average yearly number of workload units is determined. When divided into the total nursing costs for care for individual patients, this results in an estimate for the nursing cost per workload unit. On this basis, the costs of nursing care for each patient in the sample can be calculated as the sum of the costs of shared care per day multiplied by the length of stay and the sum of the daily nursing workload units received by each patient during the hospital stay.

Given that the two methods of calculating the costs of nursing care described above are based on the same total costs, the mean cost of care for the entire sample estimated by the dependency method and by the average cost per patient are identical at £ 196 (this is about $ 468 in 1990 PPPs) for a mean length of stay of 15 days. The two methods produce highly correlated estimates of nursing cost per patient because of a strong association between length of stay and patient-specific workload units (Spearman rank correlation coefficient, $r=.82$, $p<.01$), but analysis in more detail reveals individual deviations. The modal patient, for instance, requires less care in the earlier and later stages of the episode than implied by the average method, but this is to some extent balanced by higher-than-average requirements in the period immediately following the operation. A wider analysis shows that in more than one third of the cases the estimates deviate by more than 7.5% and that these deviations are equally distributed in both directions. They are not significantly associated with patient length of stay or with the dependency-based cost, while they are associated with the number of patient-specific workload units.

In a somewhat similar methodological vein, Whynes and Walker (1995) examined the extent to which it is possible to take shortcuts in determining the costs of medical procedures, as detailed costing may be a very time-consuming and expensive part of an economic evaluation. Based on their above-mentioned detailed costing study of 360 colorectal cancer patients treated by surgery,[5] they start by showing that, out of the 14 different cost categories considered in the original study, the three (or four) largest account for 89.2% (or 91.6%) of the total costs. However, a more detailed analysis of the individual cases shows that using only the four largest cost categories out of the 14 produces costs estimates in excess of 95% of the true cost in only 45% of the cases. If only the three largest cost categories are used, the corresponding percentage is 22%, and if only two are used the percentage is 6%. It is also shown that the importance of the cost categories differ widely on a patient-by-patient basis. For instance, ±1 standard deviation for ward costs produces a range of approximately 42%–80% of the total, while for operation theater costs the corresponding range is from 8% to 30%. The cost distributions are particularly skewed for investigations and intensive care, while the distributions for ward, operation theater, and other treatment-related costs are closer to normal.

An alternative to using a reduced number of cost items is to approximate treatment costs by means of statistical estimation. One obvious method is to multiply the average cost per patient-day in the general surgery specialty with the length of stay for each patient. The latter variable is available from the patient records, and the cost figure can be obtained from the hospital's accountancy system. An ordinary least squares regression with these two explanatory variables and the original, detailed cost estimates as the dependent variable produces an R^2 of .89, with both variables being statistically significant. If the cost of routine ward care is removed from both the true and the

[5] They estimate that the detailed costing in itself required 1 year of research time.

crude cost figures, resulting in a net cost figure, replicating the regression analysis results in a coefficient of determination of only .31, so that 69% of the variation remains unexplained. The deviation between true net cost and crude net cost seems to be systematic, the implication being that patients with a shorter length of stay tend to generate higher non-ward costs than the average and vice versa for patients with longer stays. The clinical explanation is that, as for other acute interventions, the intensity of care is higher in the early stages of stay and the patients also undergo one or more diagnostic investigations on admission, the costs of which are usually much higher than for an average surgical patient.

One way of improving upon the equation above to obtain a better estimate of the true costs will be to include other cost-event variables (not related to routine ward care) in the equation. By stepwise regression, the equation of best fit is found to give an R^2 of .98 with three significant variables: the product of duration of the operation and the cost per minute of the operation theater, the product of the number of pathology requests and the cost per request, and the product of the average ward cost per day and length of stay. The important thing to note about this equation, however, is that it is only after the detailed costing study has been performed that the analysts were able to estimate the appropriate function. Considering the possible candidates (cost-events), it would have been extremely difficult to predict in advance which of the variables would prove to be the significant determinants of total costs. Even if the variables could have been predicted, the magnitude of the regression coefficients would never have been able to have been.

Yet another possibility is to examine whether the considerable patient-to-patient variability in costs may be explained (in statistical terms) by analyzing the specific clinical and demographic characteristics of each patient. From the list of available variables for the patients and with the total "true" costs (determined by detailed costing) as the dependent variable, the best-fit equation is found by stepwise regression. It contains five significant variables - colostomy performed or not, sex, complications arising during operation or not, age, and early or late stage tumor - but the R^2 is only .19. Factors which common sense suggested would be important, e.g., tumor size, tumor site within the bowel, whether or not a wound becomes infected or bursts, and whether the operation was essentially curative or palliative, appear not to be significant cost determinants. Cost estimates based only on the available clinical and demographic factors would therefore be very misleading, while using only data about the length of stay for each patient and the average cost per patient-day in the surgery specialty leads to a much more precise estimate.

As with many other cancers, the intensity of monitoring and follow-up of colorectal cancer patients after they have been given curative primary treatment is rather controversial. The costs of outpatient and preoperative diagnostics may be considerable and are accompanied by psychological and medical burdens such as the distress caused by false-positive test results and the fears associated with early detection of incurable recurrence as well as the morbidity and mortality related to operations performed on account of positive test results, whether they are true or false. Kievit and van de Velde (1990) have tried to take a number of these factors into account in a decision analysis of the use of CEA monitoring in colon cancer patients after curative resection. CEA appears to be by far the most effective procedure for early detection in colon cancer follow-up monitoring, but the question is whether it increases the patients' quality-adjusted life expectancy and whether the possible increase is worth the costs of CEA monitoring.

The authors use a Markov analysis model, which simulates a follow-up period of 2 years (80% of all colon recurrences occur within 2 years) divided into 24 cycles of 1-month duration. The value of CEA monitoring is estimated by comparing the expected quality-adjusted life-years (QALYs) of a hypothetical cohort of patients monitored by CEA with the expected QALYs of a cohort monitored by symptoms alone. The possible states of the model for both arms are as follows: no evidence of disease; mortality from other causes; suspicion of recurrence, which must be confirmed by operation; if suspicion is false, the result may be no evidence of disease or perioperative mortality; if recurrence is confirmed, operation will again be performed, with risk of perioperative mortality, chance of finding resectable metastases, and risk of finding the recurrence incurable; if no suspicion of recurrence arises (either from symptoms or by CEA), the "no evidence of disease" state continues. The probabilities used in the model and their sources are given explicitly in an appendix, but the references are sometimes quite unspecific (references may be given as "literature," for instance), and the choice of references and actual values are not discussed at all. The expected costs of the strategies are calculated based on costs of diagnosis and treatment in the Netherlands in 1988, where the unit costs have been obtained from the Financial Directorate and from a single hospital. Expected lifetime for the patients is corrected by a quality-of-life factor to obtain expected QALYs, but the derivation of this factor is not explained, except that it is mentioned that it is expressed in time trade-off terms.

The result of the analysis is that, overall, CEA leads to an increase in life expectancy of 7 days (0.3% of life expectancy with monitoring of symptoms only) with an incremental cost of $ 1538.[6] The resulting incremental cost-utility ratio is $ 86,227 per QALY. Sensitivity analyses show that the most favorable effect of CEA monitoring was seen for patients with more advanced tumor stage, for younger patients (under 60), and for lower perioperative mortality rates (under 2%). The maximum expected gain of CEA was 13 days, and the cost-utility ratio varies from around $ 23,000 to $ 5 million, but in some cases CEA may even have a negative influence on the quality of life, because some patients are confronted with their incurable disease at an earlier date.

---

[6] The conversion to US$ is made by the authors themselves, and as it is not mentioned explicitly, it should not be supposed that PPPs have been used; most likely the ordinary exchange rate has been used.

In 1989, the Natinonal Cancer Institute (NCI) in the United States issued a clinical announcement that advised physicians of the benefits of using combination chemotherapy (levamisole+5-FU) as an adjuvant therapy for stage III colon cancer patients after surgery. The announcement was based on two randomized clinical trials that demonstrated a survival benefit and a lower rate of recurrence for patients receiving adjuvant chemotherapy. The relative benefit is on the order of 20%, e.g., increasing the survival rate after more than 4 years from about 50% to 64%. Brown et al. (1994) of the NCI published a study designed to investigate some of the economic consequences of an increased adoption of adjuvant chemotherapy for stage III colon patients. For instance, they calculate a sort of cost-utility ratio after correcting the gain in life expectancy by a quality-of-life factor and also try to estimate a rate of return for the investment NCI has made in the development of the specific combination chemotherapy regimen recommended. However, the technical terms "cost-effectiveness analysis" and "cost-benefit analysis" are used rather misleadingly in the paper, as it is not made explicit, for instance, which alternative the adjuvant chemotherapy regimen of 5-FU and levamisole is actually compared to.

A simulation model was used to examine the costs and benefits of a hypothetical scenario of treatment adoption, where it was assumed that the treatment was available from 1990 to 2000, while the costs and benefits of the scenario are accounted for until 2020. The intention of choosing these periods is to highlight the downstream costs and benefits associated with the assumed treatment adoption. The model is based on various Markov states associated with survival and costs and can generate projections of costs or benefits of a treatment intervention over time when it is applied to a specified hypothetical population, defined by cancer site and stage, age range, and percentage of the target population receiving the treatment. The initial costs of diagnosis and first course of treatment are assigned to the individuals at the time of diagnosis, while terminal care costs are assigned at the time of death and continuous care costs are assigned to each year since diagnosis. The benefits of increased survival expectancy and reduced recurrence of adjuvant chemotherapy are adjusted for quality-of-life considerations by weighing these clinical benefits against the clinical costs due to the toxicity of the adjuvant chemotherapy. To achieve this, time after surgery is divided into three phases: (1) time during which toxic effects are experienced, (2) time without toxic effects or symptoms, and (3) time during systemic relapse.[7]

In the baseline analysis, it is assumed that 25% of the patients receive adjuvant chemotherapy in 1990 and that this adoption rate has increased to 80% in 1993, at which level it remains throughout 2000. The clinical results on survival benefit and recurrence reduction from the National Intergroup Trial are incorporated, and estimates of costs of initial and terminal care costs are taken from another study and inflated to 1990 prices. Estimates for

[7] The approach used for quality adjustment is very much like the Q-TWiST method introduced by Gelber and colleagues (see, e.g., Gelber et al. 1991; Goldhirsch et al. 1989).

other cost factors are obtained in a highly nonrigorous way from diverse sources. There is no explicit identification of a viewpoint for the analysis, but the cost of adjuvant therapy is reported to include an estimate of lost earnings (or the value of time) due to 26.5 treatment-related lost workdays (4 h per treatment). The total cost of adjuvant chemotherapy thus calculated is corrected (on the basis of the experience from the clinical trials) by a factor of 0.75 to correct for patients not undergoing the full adjuvant therapy due to toxicity or early death. The duration of the phases "time with toxic effects" and "time with systemic relapse" is found by extrapolating the survival and recurrence curves from the trial to the simulation study, and time without either is found by subtraction of these estimates from total survival. The three phases are assigned quality weights by arbitrary assumptions, which are rationalized by the findings of a few other studies, based on informal surveys of expert opinions and not on preferences stated by (potential) patients.

The baseline analysis results in a gain in expected years of 1.9 per patient treated, which amounts to 11.6 life-years per death averted, because the life-years saved by using adjuvant therapy are not evenly distributed among the treated patients. Using the assumed utility weights (0.8 for time with toxicity and an average of 0.5 during the period of systemic relapse), the gain in expected quality-adjusted lifetime is approximately 1.8 years. If both future costs and future gains in life are discounted by 6%, the cost per life-year saved is calculated to be $ 2094 (expressed in 1990 dollars). After quality adjustment, using the variable values given above, the cost-utility ratio becomes $ 2260/QALY.[8]

Finally, the authors attempt a calculation of the economic return on the investment in research on adjuvant chemotherapy in colon cancer that the NIH has made. They do this by considering the return on this investment to consist of "the economic value of the colon cancer deaths averted" due to the adjuvant therapy minus the net costs associated with the therapy, measured in the same way as for the cost-effectiveness computations above. They call this a cost-benefit analysis, measuring the value of averted deaths by the conventional Human Capital approach of measuring the discounted value of lost earnings. However, this whole approach to technology assessment is so contentious and the data are so weak that this part of the analysis is probably better left ignored.

Glimelius et al. (1995) examined the cost-effectiveness of primary chemotherapy versus BSC in nonoperable patients with advanced gastrointestinal cancer, of whom the majority had colorectal cancer. The economic evaluation was carried out within a clinical trial with prospective collection of cost and effectiveness data. Primary chemotherapy was etoposide+leucovorin+5-FU for patients under 60 and 5-FU+leucovorine for patients aged 60

[8] Oddly enough, this result is not stated in the text and must be calculated by the reader, while the changes in the ratio produced by varying some of the assumptions in sensitivity analyses are given.

and over. BSC, given in both randomization groups, consisted of attempts at relieving any symptoms by radiotherapy, pain killers etc., and psychosocial support, while chemotherapy was allowed in the BSC group if requested or if palliation was not obtained otherwise. This strategy is allowed, because it is believed to mirror clinical practice, where chemotherapy would presumably only be given to selected patients and not routinely.

Survival was measured from the time of randomization with a maximum follow-up of 3.5 years. The patients' quality of life was measured by structured interviews according to a questionnaire which is claimed to have been shown to be reliable and valid in several tests. In order to have a favorable quality-of-life outcome, the patient should either have improved or have an unchanged high quality of life for at least up to the second evaluation, i.e., for a minimum of 4 months. The collection of cost data excluded prescribed outpatient drugs for concomitant disorders and used the following categories: cytostatics (including antiemetics), administration of cytostatics (including costs for cytostatic-induced toxicities), radiotherapy, surgery, outpatient visits, and inpatient hospital stay. The costs incurred for home care given by the local social authorities are not included, because they could not be accurately assessed for all. For a sample of patients, the costs of home care were equal in the two groups (at about SKr 3500). Unit prices for the various types of resources are given in 1992 SKr, but the sources of these cost data are not explicitly stated and the claimed distinction between average and incremental[9] costs is not substantiated. Moreover, the perspective of the analysis is not explicitly stated, while it is claimed that the costs of all medical care given by the medical community were calculated and used in the analysis.

A total of 33 patients were randomized to chemotherapy and 28 to BSC, but of these 17 patients ultimately received chemotherapy. Median survival was 9 months in the chemotherapy group and 4 months in the BSC group, which was not significantly different, as the study was underpowered. Radiotherapy was given in the same proportions in each group (to nearly all patients, with a mean of 30 Gy per patient), and the overall toxicity of the treatments was equally low, except for alopecia. The overall incremental survival with chemotherapy was 102 days, and after quality adjustment the gain for the chemotherapy group was estimated as 108 days (58% of the chemotherapy group had favorable quality-of-life outcomes compared with 29% of the BSC group). The total cost for the BSC group was SKr 96,000, while it was SKr 143,000 for the chemotherapy group,[10] leading to incremental costs of a quality-adjusted year of survival of SKr 157,000.

---

[9] This is one of many examples of confusion between the terms "marginal" and "incremental" costs. "Marginal costs" refer to the costs of providing yet another patient with a given treatment, while the term "incremental" should preferably be reserved for the costs incurred by changing from one treatment to another. Usually, one is interested in the increment in marginal costs when changing between the treatments compared.

Concluding Remarks

Table 1 summarizes the main characteristics of the economic assessments of treatments against colorectal cancer described and briefly discussed in this chapter.

Among the studies retrieved for this survey, there are very few actual economic evaluations in colorectal cancer in the proper sense of assessing both the costs and outcomes of interventions with identical objectives, and none of these are very convincing, because the study designs or/and the data used are rather poor. In recent years, a number of new cytotoxic drugs have been marketed as alternatives to the conventional 5-FU regimens. In relation to these, most of the new drugs have a comparatively high price associated with claims of equal efficacy but less side effects or, conversely, a gain in efficacy but at the expense of more frequent and serious adverse events. The appearance on the market of these alternatives will no doubt be accompanied by economic evaluations.

Comparing the studies concerned with assessment of the costs of patient management according to the stage of disease at diagnosis underlines the importance of taking variations in outcome into account if the results are intended to inform decisions about screening or other early detection policies. Focusing on costs alone may lead to erroneous conclusions, as shown by Whynes et al. (1993). This can serve as a reminder that the consequences or outcomes of choices are just as important as costs in economic assessments.

Another interesting paper by the same group of researchers demonstrates that using shortcuts in cost calculations may lead to very imprecise and unsatisfactory results compared to detailed microcosting attempting to determine the real marginal costs of the resources consumed. Obviously, the cost calculation methods used in most of the economic evaluations of the management of cancer patients (and of health care in general) are seriously lacking, but it is also clear that using a microcosting procedure will be very time-consuming and beyond the scope of most of the analyses initiated. As usual in economics, a trade-off has to made between an extra effort (costs) and the expected gain in terms of more precise and/or relevant results. In principle, this trade-off is itself amenable to economic analysis assessing the value of the gain in information compared to the costs of obtaining it.

[10] Using 1990 PPPs, these amounts become approximately $ 12,800 and $ 19,000, respectively.

Table 1. Main characteristics of economic assessments dealing with colorectal cancer

Reference	Disease category	Treatments examined	Main characteristics of the study
Taplin et al. (1995)	All stages	All treatments given (i.e., those covered by Medicare)	Do treatment costs vary with stage at diagnosis? Third-party payer perspective (Medicare) Retrospective data for patients enrolled in HMO to find costs attributable to cancer; pooled time series and cross-section analysis to simulate longitudinal (incidence) cost data Costs rise with stage at diagnosis for the initial and the continuing care phase (until 6 months prior to death), no relation in terminal care
Whynes et al. (1993)	All stages	Surgery and all tests, examinations, and hospital stays related to this	Do treatment costs vary with stage at diagnosis? Hospital perspective Retrospective analyses of hospital notes for 360 patients treated with surgery, comprising all care and services provided over a 3-year period from diagnosis (or until death, if occurring earlier) No statistically significant differences between costs for patients diagnosed at an early or late stage of disease; however, low cost found in patients diagnosed at a late stage often due to early death, while many screening-detected low-cost patients survive at least 3 years
Walker et al. (1991)	All patients	Three different diagnostic methods: colonoscopy, barium enema X-ray, flexible sigmoidscopy	Expected cost of each diagnostic procedure (i.e., nominal cost corrected for sensitivity and the cost of later treatment of patients with a false-negative test result) Hospital perspective Calculations comprise labor cost and materials consumed for "typical" patient, sensitivity figures from the literature, treatment of patient with false-negative test result Only nominal cost figures given, results on expected costs too inconclusive because of wide variations observed in clinical data
Walker and Whynes (1990)	All patients undergoing surgery	Nursing care given to patients in surgery wards	Compares two methods of calculating the costs of nursing care for such patients: an average-patient method and a patient-specific method Hospital perspective Average-patient method based on bed occupancy rates, while patient-specific method based on individual dependency data for a patient sample; total costs are the same for the two methods Resulting cost measures highly correlated, due to strong association between length of stay and patient-specific workload units; more detailed analysis reveals significant deviations

Table 1 (continued)

Reference	Disease category	Treatments examined	Main characteristics of the study
Whynes and Walker (1995)	All patients	Surgery and all tests, examinations, and hospital stays related to this	Feasibility of shortcuts in costing procedures to avoid time-consuming detailed costing Estimates based on the detailed costing study mentioned above (Whynes et al. 1993) Shortcuts examined are restriction to a few main cost categories, statistical estimation, and patient clinical and demographic characteristics None of the shortcuts really satisfactory, some highly dependent on preceding detailed costing Reliance on available clinical and demographic data may be very misleading; much more precise estimates obtained by using average cost per day in surgery ward multiplied by individual data on length of stay
Kievit and van de Velde (1990)	All resectable patients	CEA monitoring as follow-up of primary treatment	Cost-utility analysis of monitoring of CEA compared to symptoms only Hospital perspective, not explicit Markov model decision analysis, with probabilities from the literature and costs from public authorities and a single hospital; survival adjusted by a quality-of-life factor, not explained CEA leads to a very low increase in life expectancy (7 days) and a high cost-utility ratio of around $ 86,000/QALY; results highly variable depending on assumptions
Brown et al. (1994)	Stage III colon cancer	5-FU+levamisole as adjuvant therapy	Examines various economic consequences of a regimen of adjuvant chemotherapy Social perspective (by including productive time lost to treatment) Simulations by a Markov decision-making model; clinical data from large clinical trial, cost data from a previous study, inflated; utility values assumed Gain in expected quality-adjusted survival is estimated as 1.8 years, and the calculated cost-utility ratio is very low
Glimelius et al. (1995)	Advanced disease, nonoperable	Primary chemotherapy versus BSC	Cost-utility analysis of primary chemotherapy vs. BSC Third-party payer perspective (not stated explicitly) Clinical data and resource utilization data from 61 patients in clinical trial, sources on unit costs not clear, patient utilities from trial using a particular questionnaire Chemotherapy compared to BSC results in gain in quality-adjusted survival (insignificant because the study was underpowered), and the result is a relatively modest cost-utility ratio

CEA, carcinoembryonic antigen; 5-FU, 5-fluorouracil; BSC, best supportive care; QALY, quality-adjusted life-year.

Prostate Cancer

Prostate cancer is second only to lung cancer as a cause of cancer deaths, and it is the most common cancer among men in the United States and many other westernized societies. About 30% of men older than 50 have latent prostate cancer (i.e., autopsies show that they harbor foci of cancer within the prostate), and this high prevalence makes it the most common malignancy in humans. One out of six men will develop prostate cancer during their lifetime, and the risk increases with age, being 42% for a man at the age of 50 years, whose risk of dying of the disease is below 3%. The median age at diagnosis is 72 years, and many patients, especially those with localized tumors, will die from other causes without having suffered significant or any disability from their tumor. The incidence of latent carcinoma of the prostate increases considerably with age, with estimates of 70% of men over 70 years of age having histologic evidence of cancer, while there is little geographic or racial variation. On the other hand, the clinical incidence shows a tenfold difference according to race or geography. In the chapter on the "Epidemiology of Cancer," the average incidence for the EU countries was cited as being 28 per 100,000, while it is around 17 in the United States and less than 3 in Hong Kong.

The incidence and mortality from prostate cancer has been rising steadily since 1970. This increase seems to be partly caused by the increased use by general practitioners of more efficient screening tools, such as measurement of levels of prostate-specific antigen (PSA), a serum tumor marker; in addition, the increased use of transurethral resection for benign prostatic hyperplasia may have led to an increased frequency of chance discovery of localized prostate cancer. Even taking these factors into consideration, there appears to have been an increased incidence of prostate cancer. As the incidence increases more rapidly with age than for any other cancer and as the average age of men is rising in many countries, the number of men with clinically evident cancer is expected to rise steadily over the coming decades.

The latent cancers found in autopsies appear to be cytologically and histologically similar to the cancers detected clinically, while there are important differences between the two types in the volume, grade, and invasiveness of the tumor. Most of the cancers found at autopsy are small and well differentiated and show no tendency to invade normal structures. These observations are in accordance with a hypothesis about the pathogenesis of prostate cancer being a multistep process, in which the latent cancers have only progressed through some of the steps necessary for a fully malignant expression. A major challenge in the management of prostate cancer is to find objective criteria to differentiate between the latent and the clinically overt forms of the disease, because the treatment may lead to significant morbidity, which it would be desirable to avoid for men who have cancers that will not affect them during their lifetime. However, there are current controversies with regard to the most appropriate staging system and the optimal treatment for each stage of the disease.

The value of screening and early diagnosis is also controversial, as results are not yet available from ongoing randomized trials aiming to determine whether or not early diagnosis has a positive impact on overall survival or disease-specific survival. State-of-the-art treatment provides prolonged disease-free survival for many patients with localized disease, while it is usually not curative for locally advanced disease. Metastatic disease is not curable. From analyses of the pathologic features of tumors found at autopsy, it is estimated that 80% of these are truly latent, i.e., clinically unimportant. Of the clinically important cancers, nearly half are advanced at detection, while about 40% are early stage (curable) and about 10% are focal, well-differentiated stage 0 tumors that are perhaps clinically unimportant. For early-stage, local disease, some treatment groups prefer a strategy of deferred treatment because of the high rate of intercurrent death from causes other than prostate cancer and the significant morbidity associated with current treatment options. For patients with established metastatic disease, cure is not possible, but by various means of androgen ablation[1] a regression of the tumor and reduction of cancer-related symptoms may be achieved.

Considering the morbidity induced by treatment and the associated psychological burden for the patient and the costs for society, the ability to differentiate accurately at the level of the individual patient between clinically important and unimportant tumors is of the utmost importance. This depends largely on the accuracy of the diagnostic instruments used (i.e., their specificity, sensitivity, and predictive value).[2] Currently, there is a high incidence of clinical understaging, and a large proportion of patients will develop disseminated disease after undergoing local therapy. The main prognostic factors for the outcome of primary therapy are baseline PSA level and tumor grade (e.g., according to the Gleason grading system), both of which are inversely related to outcome. Other prognostic factors are the size of the tumor, clinically and pathologically determined (cT, pT), and the involvement or not of pelvic lymph nodes.

---

[1] The term "ablation" refers to the removal of a body part (traditionally by cutting) or, more recently, the negating of a bodily function by chemical means (often hormonal treatments).

[2] *Sensitivity* (true-positive rate) is the proportion of patients with the disease who have a positive test result. *Specificity* (true-negative rate) refers to the proportion of patients without the target disease who have a negative test result. The *predictive values*, positive and negative, respectively, refer to the proportion of patients with a positive (or negative) test result who actually have (or do not have) the disease.

Treatment Options

The most commonly used staging system is the TNM system, which takes into account the fact that many cancers are diagnosed as the result of an abnormal PSA value (T1c). PSA is often considered to fulfill many of the ideal requirements for an optimal tumor marker for prostate cancer, including effectiveness in early detection of clinically important disease, staging, and monitoring of the patients after treatment. The use of PSA for diagnostic testing was allowed by the American regulatory authorities (Food and Drug Administration, FDA) in 1994. There are certain concerns about overdetection because of a dramatic increase in incidence of prostate cancer accompanied by a shift to earlier stage disease, but there are also data showing that PSA screening detects clinically important and potentially life-threatening disease in some patients. A number of approaches to improve the predictive accuracy[3] of PSA testing are under investigation, including a determination of age-specific cut-off values, because there is an expected increase in PSA value by age, independent of disease.[4]

One of the critical issues in staging is whether or not the tumor is confined to the prostate gland. Prostate cancer that is no longer confined to the organ is generally not curable, while localized disease may be cured, and patients successfully treated may expect a survival rate equal to a cohort of age-matched men without prostate cancer. This is the basis for the interest in early detection, as all prostate cancers are confined to the organ at the inception.

For tumors confined to the prostate, i.e., stages T1a–T2b,N0, the three primary treatment strategies are as follows:
1. Radical prostatectomy
2. Definitive radiation therapy
3. Watchful waiting or deferred therapy

Despite a very large number of studies, there is no clear-cut evidence in the literature of the superiority of any of these treatment options. To a considerable extent, however, this is due to poor study designs, the inherent biases in case series of selected patients, lack of randomized studies of comparably staged patients, diverging definitions of failure, and differences in the intensity and periodicity of monitoring outcomes.

Several population-based studies with more than 10 years of follow-up show excellent survival without any treatment in patients with well- or moderately well differentiated tumors clinically confined to the prostate gland, irrespective of the patient's age. However, the authors of a recent structured

---

[3] Typical rates observed in patient series are as follows: sensitivity, 55%–79%; specificity, 59%–68%; and positive predictive value, 40%–49%; thus there is plenty of room for improvement.

[4] PSA is prostate specific and not prostate cancer specific, and PSA values may be elevated by any prostate disease, e.g., benign prostatic hyperplasia (BPH).

review of more than 12,000 papers[5] attempting to compare the treatment strategies conclude that poor reporting and factors indicating selection bias in all series make a valid comparison of the strategies impossible, and proponents of any one of the strategies cannot point to the literature for any convincing support. Many series show the best results in 10-year disease-specific survival from radical prostatectomy (over 90%), the next best from careful observation (85%–90%), and the worst from radiation (75%–80%). However, results such as these should probably rather be seen as an indication of selection bias in the series, as it is medically highly unlikely that radiation should worsen the disease-specific survival.

Provided that the treatment option and not observation is chosen and that the patient is fit for either modality, there is a choice between radical prostatectomy and irradiation. For similarly staged patients, there are no differences in 10-year end points. Outcomes vary inversely with pretreatment PSA level and tumor grade (Gleason score). Reported complication rates for each of the modalities vary significantly, e.g., from 25% to 89% for impotence and from 2% to 47% for incontinence. In addition to causes such as differences in the experience of the treatment teams and case selection, a factor such as variations in definitions of complications and events should probably be invoked in order to explain such immense diversity in complication rates. Frequently made statements to the effect that younger patients should preferably be treated by surgery because they will live longer or that radiation shows late failure cannot be corroborated with empirical data of a good quality.

The management of patients with detectable PSA after radical surgery or with rising PSA levels after radiation therapy is controversial and the subject of ongoing trials, inter alia in the European Organization for Research and Treatment of Cancer (EORTC). After successful radical prostatectomy, no PSA should be detectable, so detectable PSA in such patients is an indication that they probably have subclinical micrometastases. For radiation therapy, the goal is to achieve (and sustain) a post-therapy decline in PSA to below 1 ng/ml, and failure to achieve this may be the result of either resistant cells within the primary tumor or micrometastases. It is often unclear whether detectable PSA after surgery or rising PSA after radiation is caused by local recurrence or distant metastases, but the choice of treatment modality depends critically on this. However, early elevations of PSA (less than 1 year after treatment) tend to be associated with distant metastases, while late elevations more likely are associated with local recurrence.

For locally advanced clinical disease (stages T2c, T3, T4), the outcomes with radical prostatectomy alone are generally poor, and many patients are likely to develop adverse features preventing them from undergoing radical prostatectomy. Such patients can often be identified in advance, e.g., as patients with poorly differentiated tumors and bilobar tumors, who have a more than 70% likelihood of having positive nodes or positive seminal vesicles. Under such

[5] Only slightly more than 1% of these provided what was considered acceptable information about the case series or trial concerned.

circumstances, surgery is not advisable, and external beam radiation is the standard of treatment with which any new method must be compared. One promising new approach is conformal radiotherapy, which provides an opportunity to increase the dose to the prostate. Another possibility is to combine external beam radiation with hormonal treatment to achieve androgen ablation, and recent data from randomized trials tend to favor this option. There are no randomized trials showing an advantage of hormonal treatment alone.

Since the beginning of the 1940s, where it was observed that androgen ablation caused regression of prostate carcinoma, the standard treatment of advanced, metastatic prostate cancer has been castration. A total of 90%–95% of the androgens originate in the testicles, while the remainder are synthesized in the adrenal gland. Castration may be achieved by surgical removal of the testes or by using various chemical agents, in which case the castration is usually reversible (in contrast to surgical castration). There are controversies with respect to the optimal timing (early versus late) and to the optimal type of castration (combined androgen blockade versus monotherapy).

Current clinical practice is guided by the results of several large-scale randomized trials that have shown equivalent antitumor effects of many different chemical agents that block the production of androgens. The duration of response generally varies from 12 to 18 months, but roughly 20% of the patients show no evidence of disease after 5 years of follow-up. What differs between the various agents is the profile of side effects, which include loss of libido, impotence, gynecomastia, fatigue, loss of muscle tone, hot flashes, and changes in personality. Surgical orchiectomy is considered the gold standard, but, given the choice, most patients prefer to select a medical approach first.

The controversy regarding the optimal timing of hormonal therapy is determined by the fact that hormonal therapies are not curative and that three different types of cells exist in a prostate tumor mass. Androgen-dependent cancer cells require a continuous critical level of androgen stimulation in order not to die. Androgen-sensitive cells do not die in the absence of androgen, but their growth rates are decreased. Androgen-independent cells are completely autonomous of the level of androgens, and they neither die nor slow their growth following androgen ablation, no matter how complete. Prostate cancers progress from androgen-dependent to androgen-independent states and, in doing so, they begin to synthesize and secrete PSA in the absence of androgen. Rising PSA values will usually precede symptomatic relapse or progression by several months, and by this lead time in the natural history of the disease one can distinguish between two distinct groups of patients with diverging prognoses and tolerances of the toxicities associated with hormonal therapy.

The prognosis of patients is assessed by various schemes, e.g., by monitoring the PSA values after initiation of hormone therapy, while pretreatment PSA does not appear to be correlated with outcome. Patients whose PSA values do not normalize within 6 months after therapy being initiating are considered to be high-risk patients and will normally be evaluated early for treatments directed at the hormone-independent cell population. Conversely, patients with a good prognosis may be offered treatment options with the aim of minimizing toxicity as an overriding concern.

Until quite recently, chemical castration was usually accomplished by exogenous estrogens, but because of their severe cardiovascular complications these agents are no longer used frequently as monotherapy, while there are numerous ongoing studies on their effect in combination with other agents such as the taxoids or as radiosensitizers. Luteinizing hormone-releasing hormone (LHRH) analogues, adrenal enzyme synthesis inhibitors, and antiandrogens are newer agents of interest. The antiandrogens comprise two classes, steroidal, e.g., cyproterone acetate and megestrol acetate, and nonsteroidal, e.g., flutamide and bicalutamide (Casodex), which are mainly of clinical interest because they potentially preserve potency, while their antitumor effect must currently be considered inferior to conventional castration. The results of additional studies and longer follow-up are awaited, however.

Despite its apparent rationality, combined androgen blockade or maximum androgen blockade, in which both sites of production of androgen (testicles and the adrenal gland) are targeted is a controversial concept which has still not been definitively settled. The combinations considered include combining a nonsteroidal antiandrogen (e.g., flutamide) with orchiectomy or with an LHRH analogue. When compared to monotherapy in large international trials, there have been both positive and negative results and meta-analyses showing no significant benefit. The results of the largest trial ever evaluating this concept are currently awaited. A meta-analysis of more than 1000 patients treated in randomized trials comparing orchiectomy alone with orchiectomy plus an antiandrogen (nilutamide) showed a statistically superior response rate in the combination group, but no statistical improvement in survival. Another meta-analysis of more than 5000 patients in 22 randomized trials comparing conventional surgical or medical castration with maximum androgen blockade (castration plus the prolonged use of an antiandrogen) showed no significant improvement in overall survival associated with the combination therapy.

Apparently, however, the results should be differentiated according to the patients' prognosis as determined, for instance, by their performance status and the degree of metastatic spread. For patients with a poor prognosis, no matter how this is defined (e.g., widespread metastases and a poor performance status), responses are typically short, and combined androgen blockade has in no study been shown to give a significant advantage in comparison with the LHRH analogues or orchiectomy alone. In contrast, in patients with minimal disease (i.e., good performance status and limited metastases), a significant survival advantage for the combined androgen blockade is seen.[6] These results are interpreted by some to support the idea of early ver-

[6] In the NCI Intergroup I study, which has been very influential on the practice pattern in the United States, the survival advantage of combined androgen blockade for the group with minimal disease (15% of the enrolled patients) was 10 months or more than a 50% gain compared to the control group.

sus late androgen ablation in patients with no symptoms but rising PSA values, but this is still controversial, and some physicians continue to defer treatment until symptoms are documented.

Intermittent therapy in patients with low-volume tumors has given intriguing results. The idea of intermittent hormonal therapy is that stem cells that survive the removal of androgen will remain sensitive to subsequent deprivation of androgen if they are allowed a period of proliferation in an androgen-containing environment. Patients are thus treated for 2–3 months beyond the time point of maximal response, and subsequently all hormonal therapy is stopped. As the toxicities of androgen ablation diminish after discontinuation of hormonal therapy, the PSA level will increase steadily. At a predetermined level of PSA (rise), hormonal therapy is restarted and the cycle is repeated. Several such cycles have been observed in clinical trials, and patient tolerance has been documented to improve, but it is still uncertain whether cycling increases the overall time that the tumor remains responsive to androgen ablation or even decreases it. A large randomized trial has recently been started to investigate these ideas.

For hormone-refractory tumors (i.e., hormone-insensitive and androgen-independent tumors), nonhormonal approaches are required. The traditional view has been that chemotherapy has no role to play in androgen-independent prostate cancer, because no randomized trials have shown a survival advantage of any single agent or combination of cytotoxics. This assessment of the potential of chemotherapy is derived mainly from the pre-PSA era, but with PSA monitoring more patients are identified earlier in the course of disease and are referred to treatment prior to the development of symptoms, and this may increase the chances of responding to chemotherapy. As a result, a number of cytotoxics are being reevaluated in ongoing studies, with promising preliminary results being observed with high-dose chemotherapy using drugs such as cyclophosphamide and doxorubicin, supported with hematological growth factors (the colony-stimulating factors, CSFs; see the chapter on "Supportive Care II: Hematological Support," this volume). Chemotherapy also seems to have a useful role in palliative treatment, in which external beam radiation and bone-seeking radioisotopes are important modalities.

Among the approaches to management of prostate cancer under intensive current investigation are several that are not primarily directed at killing cancer cells. These include immunologic approaches, angiogenesis inhibition, and differentiation of tumor cells. Therapies that modulate the patients' immune function by means of cytogenic genes such as interleukins and interferons are being tested on patients with a high probability of relapse after definitive local therapy or with rising PSA but no other clinical signs of disease. Angiogenesis refers to the fact that growth of a tumor mass beyond a certain size requires the formation of new blood vessels. By inhibiting angiogenesis, already metastasized tumors may thus be prevented from continuing to grow, in addition to reducing the rate of metastatic progression. Several agents with the potential to inhibit angiogenesis are under investigation, as are agents which may promote the differentiation of tumor cells (e.g., retinoids). This may be used to slow the rate of progression of disease, allowing patients to remain asymptomatic despite the persistence of tumor.

Economic Evaluations

According to Vahrenhorst et al. (1994), few areas in medicine generate more controversy than prostate cancer, the confusion being largely due to the variable natural history of the disease and its occurrence in a population usually of advanced age and with many competing causes of death. Economic assessments have until now only been performed in connection with studies comparing various forms of hormonal treatment in advanced disease, while economic factors have not yet been included in studies published on treatments aimed at curing localized prostate cancer. Apart from a number of screening studies, which are not included in this review, there is also a study calculating the costs of treatment, and this will be the first one described.

The direct hospital costs of prostate cancer treatment were calculated by Carlsson et al. (1989), inter alia to provide background information for the appraisal of new treatment or screening programs. All cases of prostate cancer treated at a specific hospital since 1973 were identified, and all patients dying in 1984 and 1985 (a total of 101) were selected for the assessment, which was based on a classification of the patients according to stage and treatment and an extraction of all medical data from the patients' medical records. All hospital visits and stays and all investigative or therapeutic procedures performed were recorded and dated, even for hospital stays at other departments necessitated by the prostate cancer. Unit prices used for the costing were based on the hospital's accounting system and on the authors' own calculations. However, no details are given about these calculations or about the validity of the accounting costs of the hospital. The effect on survival was calculated for each individual by comparing the time from diagnosis to death with average life expectancy of men of the same age. For all cases, the average loss of life was 4.3 years, varying from 10.7 years for patients under 70 years at the start of treatment and 1.5 years for patients aged 80 years or over. In 44 of the cases, prostate cancer was the primary cause of death, while 39 died of cardiovascular disease and 18 of other causes.

The average total costs were SKr 78,800, with a median of SKr 50,100, indicating a very skewed distribution.[7] The average total costs were SKr 120,000 for those dying of prostate cancer and only a third of this, i.e., SKr 45,500, for those dying of other causes. The treatment costs are low for patients living less than 1 year after diagnosis, i.e., about SKr 20,000, and high for patients living 6 years or longer, i.e., around SKr 100,000. The costs of hospitalization (including "hotel costs") account for 72% of the average total, while tests account for 2%, radiology for 5%, surgery for 4%, and chemotherapy and other drugs

[7] All costs are given in 1985 SKr; converted by the PPP of 1985, the mean and median are approximately $ 17,800 and $ 11,300, respectively.

(e.g., analgetics or antibiotics) for 17%. The costs per patient are fairly concentrated around the period just before death, which is partly a reflection of the dominant management strategy, which until 1985 was rather conservative, so that only symptomatic patients were given active treatment.

The study by Taplin et al. (1995) on the associations between cancer treatment costs and stage at diagnosis, age, and comorbidities, which has already been mentioned in the chapters on breast and colorectal cancer, also examines these associations in prostate cancer, with results given in 1992 US$. By using a "time window" of 2 years, pooled cross-section and time-series data are used to estimate the total Medicare-reimbursed treatment costs for a cohort of cancer patients, while the net costs of cancer are found by subtracting the Medicare costs found for an age- and gender-matched cohort of control subjects from the total costs for the cancer patients. In prostate cancer, the average total costs are about $ 26,000, with about 60% falling in the terminal phase (the 6 months before death) and almost 40% in the initial phase (the 6 months after diagnosis) and the last few per cent spent in the 3-month period of continuing care in between. The total costs of initial care did not vary with stage or comorbidity, but they did decrease with age. Total continuing care costs did not vary with stage or age, but they were significantly higher for patients with a high level of comorbidities. The costs of terminal care did not vary with any of these variables.

The net costs of cancer care are determined for the initial and continuing care phases, but not for the terminal phase, as this would require knowledge of the costs of terminal care for patients dying of causes other than cancer from other sources. The average net costs of initial care are about $ 6900, and they vary with the stage at diagnosis, being highest for regionally advanced cancers and lowest for distant metastases and tumors of unknown stage. The average costs of continuing care were $ 200 and were similar across stages. The net initial care costs decreased significantly with age, but were not related to the patients' level of comorbidity, while increasing comorbidity decreased the net costs of continuing care significantly.

Licht and Klein (1994) published a study with the aim of assessing the impact on costs and postoperative morbidity of a policy of early discharge from hospital after radical retropubic prostatectomy. The data used for the study concern a case series of bilateral pelvic lymphadenectomy and radical retropubic prostatectomy performed by a single surgeon with a standardized technique on patients with clinical stage I and II disease. The case series consists of 272 consecutive patients, operated on between July 1989 and April 1994. From February 1993, a policy of early discharge was promoted by the hospital, and 101 of the patients were operated during this period. Before the policy shift, patients were admitted the day before operation for preparation and postoperative pain was managed with either intravenous or epidural patient-controlled analgesia, diet was slowly initiated and advanced, patient mobilization was slow, and the patients were not discharged from the hospital before a certain threshold level of lymphatic drainage was reached. After the policy shift, the patients were admitted on the day of surgery, having been prepared at home, all patients were started earlier on a diet which was more rapidly advanced, the patients were actively ambulated several times a day, and the lymphatic drains were removed earlier. Management of pain was identical, however.

Length of stay and complications were considered for the two groups, while the costs were examined by studying the development over the years in the two diagnosis-related groups (DRG) relevant for the patient group, i.e., radical retropubic prostatectomy with (DRG group 334) or without (DRG group 335) comorbidity or complicating conditions. The patients treated before the policy shift are represented by the DRG groups up to 1992, and the patients treated after the shift by the DRG groups for 1993 and 1994. An index for the development in the mean cost per day and the mean cost per patient was constructed by assigning the hospital-associated charges (excluding the physician's professional fees) the value 1.0 for 1989.

The median length of stay was 8 days (range, 5–20 days) before the policy change and 5 days after the change (3–11 days), while the overall complication rate was equal for both groups, as was the proportion who experienced major complications such as deep venous thrombosis, pulmonary embolism, or sepsis. A fall in the mean length of stay for the two DRG groups was also observed. The mean cost per day increased slightly each year, but there was no significant difference in the costs per day for the two DRG groups. In parallel with the reduction in the length of stay, there was a reduction of about 30% in the average hospital costs for the patients in both DRG groups from before to after the policy change.

A number of studies concerned with the costs and effects of various forms of hormonal treatments in advanced disease have been published. It seems that there is a considerable variation in the clinical course of the disease, no matter which hormonal treatment is chosen, and this may of course result in great variations in the costs of treatment, because with most hormonal treatments (except surgical castration, of course) the principle is to continue the treatment as long as the patient responds. This leads to some confusion among certain analysts regarding what is cost-effective and what is not and even about the meaning of the term "cost-effectiveness."

The following studies are all very rudimentary, based on the most easily available data and often rather crude assumptions which are hardly ever discussed or justified. In no case has the economic assessment been based on prospectively collected data from clinical trials comprising both effectiveness and cost variables. All of these studies should rather be considered as preliminary exercises based on the data readily at hand, which may be useful in order to gain an idea about the quantitative relations and about the most important data to collect in a prospective trial, but which should in no way be considered definitive.

Henriksson and Edhag (1987) aimed at comparing the direct costs of treating advanced prostatic cancer with oral estrogens or orchidectomy (surgical castration). They assumed equal effectiveness of the two alternatives and based their cost calculations on the case records of 122 consecutive patients recruited at a single institution between 1980 and 1984 and randomly assigned to one of the two treatments. Orchidectomy was a little more costly during the first year, about SKr 32,000 versus 28,000 for estrogen therapy.[8] The dominating cost item in orchidectomy is the operation itself, which is a one-time event, while the costs for the drug in estrogen treatment continue for the rest of the patient's life, or at least as long as he responds to treatment. Depending on the patients' survival, the costs of the two strategies will of course eventually become equal, the exact breakeven point depending on the assumptions chosen with respect to the incidence of side effects of estrogen therapy.

The main adverse effect of oral estrogen therapy is cardiovascular morbidity, probably because estrogen has an effect on the coagulation factors. Because of a high first-pass metabolism, one must increase the dosage of estrogen roughly tenfold when it is administered orally compared to parenteral treatment, so oral estrogen therapy is no longer considered ethical. Henriksson and Stege (1991) performed a cost comparison between parenteral estrogen therapy and conventional hormonal therapy (oral estrogen or orchidectomy) on the basis of a case series of 44 patients receiving parenteral estrogen compared with a historical control group receiving oral estrogen or orchidectomy. The costs for inpatient care, outpatient care, and for drugs, seen from the hospital's perspective, are included.

No differences in the tumor response rates among the three groups are seen, but during the first year of treatment the incidence of cardiovascular complications was 25% in the oral estrogen group and 0% in the other two groups. The interesting difference is therefore between parenteral estrogen and orchidectomy, the total average costs of which are calculated as being around $ 2900 and $ 8200, respectively. Oral estrogen is in between the two, at $ 6800.[9] The main factor explaining the difference is inpatient care, where orchidectomy is nine times costlier than parenteral estrogen. The combined yearly costs of the drug and of district nurse visits to perform the injections are about $ 550 for continuous parenteral estrogen therapy, so the breakeven point between the costs of the two alternatives is about 9 years. However, patients with advanced prostate cancer usually do not survive this long, so surgery will almost certainly be more expensive.

Rutqvist and Wilking (1992) compared orchidectomy to treatment with LHRH analogues in advanced prostate cancer. The total costs of orchidectomy were calculated based on the average length of stay for patients undergoing orchidectomy in a single institution in Stockholm, Sweden, during the years 1981–1986. This average length of hospital stay (about 8 days, criticized by other analysts for being much too long) was multiplied by an average daily cost for hospital stays provided by the hospital authority (differentiated according to department, general surgery or urology). To this are added the average costs for two outpatient visits, one before and one after surgery. Average costs for outpatient visits are also provided by the hospital authority.

---

[8] With the PPPs of 1985, these amounts correspond to about US$ 6000 and 7000, respectively.
[9] 1989 prices; the authors' own conversion to US$, probably using 1989 exchange rates.

The total cost of LHRH treatment is found by multiplying the monthly drug costs (in 1990 Swedish retail prices) plus the cost of an assumed monthly visit by a district nurse to inject the depot LHRH by the mean treatment time observed in a British randomized clinical trial comparing orchidectomy with a depot LHRH analogue. The mean treatment time observed was between 19 months (patients dying or discontinuing treatment before end of follow-up) and 23 months (for patients still in treatment at the end of follow-up). The cost of orchidectomy was found to be £ 2580,[10] while the costs of LHRH analogue treatment vary between £ 2760 and £ 3380, i.e., between 7% and 31% more than the cost of orchidectomy.

The costs of a policy with an initial period of treatment with an LHRH analogue followed by surgery after 3–36 months were also calculated. For instance, an initial LHRH analogue treatment period of about 2 years followed by orchidectomy would result in average costs of £ 1900, i.e., 26% lower than the cost if all patients were operated on immediately. Moreover, surgery would be avoided for about 85% of the patients. This policy of initial LHRH analogue treatment combined with deferred surgery is declared by the authors to be the most cost-effective policy for castration.

Nicol et al. (1993) compared the average costs of orchidectomy, an LHRH analogue, and an LHRH analogue plus flutamide by assuming that the mean survival of the patients is 2 years regardless of the treatment. In this case, surgical castration was found to be by far the cheapest alternative, i.e., about four times cheaper than the LHRH analogue and five times cheaper than the combination of LHRH and flutamide. These authors suggest that endocrine therapy should be restricted to patients unsuited for surgery or with an expected survival of less than 6 months.

Vahrenhorst et al. (1994) provided estimates of the expected costs of treatment for six alternative hormonal therapies in prostate cancer based on the regimens recommended by a Swedish regional health authority. Unit prices are given, but their derivation is not described or explained, except that average wholesale prices are used for drugs and that, for the orchidectomy, an inpatient hospital stay of 4 days is expected. A time span of 36 months is used, and for all treatments except orchidectomy the total costs increase with the expected survival (or treatment period). The breakeven point between orchidectomy and all the other treatments occurred at around 12 months, meaning that when expected survival is more than 1 year, orchidectomy is clearly the least costly alternative, while with a shorter survival time treatment with high-dose parenteral estrogen is the least costly alternative.

Hillner et al. (1995) estimated the cost-effectiveness of total androgen blockade with flutamide in metastatic prostate cancer (M1 disease). As described above, 20%–25% of prostate cancer patients present with metastatic disease at first diagnosis, in which case the cornerstone therapy is either surgical castration (orchidectomy) or medical castration using LHRH analogues.

[10] With the 1990 PPP, this corresponds to around US$ 6200.

These therapies are equally effective, with about 70% of the patients responding, and it is controversial whether adrenal androgens can add anything to this. Some recent trials seem to indicate, however, that an improvement of up to 20% in median survival can be obtained by adding an antiandrogen such as flutamide to either orchidectomy or LHRH therapy. The survival and economic impacts of these alternatives are examined in a decision theoretic model with transitions occurring at 3-month intervals. After the initial cycle, the patients move to either one of the following four possible states: (1) response to therapy (complete or partial remission), (2) no progression (stable disease), (3) progression, or (4) death. After each subsequent cycle, the patient may continue to respond to therapy, have disease progression, or die. Patients beginning a cycle with progressive disease are assumed to have a constant risk of dying, and non-cancer-related death risks are based on standard age-adjusted mortality tables.

Two hypothetical cohorts of patients are considered, one with severe disease and the other with minimal metastatic disease (i.e., no involvement of long bone, rib, or skull). The primary data source for transition probabilities used in the model is the estimated survival curve from a large Intergroup trial in the United States. The benefit of flutamide is assumed to be to reduce the rate of progression from either response or stable disease to progressive disease. After progression, flutamide is assumed to be stopped, as survival after progression seems to be the same independent of flutamide. The relative efficacy of flutamide in reducing deaths was estimated from the trial to be 25%, while orchidectomy and LHRH are assumed to be equally effective and differ only with respect to cost. The costs are considered from a third-party payer perspective, specifically all the direct costs paid by Medicare and other such insurers. There was no attempt at estimating true costs or individual patient charges. The costs of orchidectomy were based on Medicare reimbursement, assuming an outpatient procedure, and drug costs were based on average wholesale prices, including a visit to the physician's office for LHRH analogues. For each health state, the costs of ongoing care were based on Medicare payments. A time span of 7 and 10 years for severe and minimal disease, respectively, was assumed, and costs and benefits appearing in the future were discounted by 5%. No serious attempt was made to assess the quality of life of the various health states, although the impact of some arbitrary quality-of-life adjustments were explored.

For patients with severe disease, the average survival benefit was estimated to be 4 months, implying an incremental cost of $ 20,000 per year. For patients with minimal disease, 13.5% of the patients in the Intergroup trial, the estimated benefit was 5.2 months and an incremental cost per life-year gained of $ 25,300 if orchiectomy was the alternative and around $ 30,000 if it was an LHRH analogue. For any given efficacy assumption for flutamide, the incremental costs were always higher using LHRH than using orchiectomy, due to the delayed progression in the flutamide cohort, leading more patients to require ongoing LHRH therapy. Sensitivity analyses with variations in the efficacy (from 10% to 50% relative reduction in the rate of disease progression) show that the results of the analysis are very sensitive to changes in the costs and duration of flutamide use.

Another study of metastatic disease in prostate cancer was carried out by McEwan et al. (1994), who aimed to assess the impact of a new radiopharmaceutical, Metastron, on the costs of managing prostate cancer patients with bone metastases. The cost assessment was based on a partial, retrospective analysis of the 29 patients that were recruited by a single center in a multicenter clinical trial of Metastron versus placebo. Metastron was administered on an outpatient basis, and no special radiation precautions were required. Meaningful pain palliation occurred in about 75% of the patients about 10 days after administration and lasting for around 3–6 months. If effective in the individual patient, it was administered on multiple occasions. The toxicity was limited to occasional mild thrombocytopenia.

The analysis was based on a retrospective assessment of the management needs of the two groups of patients (14 randomized to Metastron, 15 to placebo), from the time of entry into the trial and for their remaining lifetime. Data were collected from the review of trial records for each of the patients and from charts from the referring hospital, the cancer clinic, and any other hospitals to which the patients may have subsequently been referred. Cost items assessed were classified as direct (analgesics, steroids, anti-inflammatory drugs, radiotherapy, hormone therapy, outpatient visits, and blood transfusions) and indirect (e.g., X-rays, bone scans, hematology, biochemistry, days in hospital). Hospital admissions for "obviously nononcological care" and for social problems were excluded, as were general practitioner or specialist office visits and visits by district nurses, as these data were not retrievable by retrospective analysis. The costs of Metastron and the initial radiotherapy were *not* included in the analysis. Unit cost data were derived from a number of sources, such as wholesale prices for the pharmacy for drugs, charges taken from the provincial health insurance plan's fee schedules, more or less offical rates for outpatient and day-patient visits, and updated costs from earlier studies.

There was no significant difference in median or total survival (the differences going in opposite directions), and no differences in the cost items grouped under the rubric "indirect costs" or in total inpatient costs. However, the costs related to direct therapy and tertiary inpatient stay showed marked differences, the total of these cost items for the Metastron group being about 40% lower than the total for the placebo group. There were wide variations among the individual patients on each arm, but the mean costs for radiotherapy and drugs were significantly smaller for the Metastron group, indicating a significant fall in the requirements for additional radiotherapy and analgesics. The total costs of care per patient were CAN$ 16,570 for the Metastron group and CAN$ 23,700 for the placebo group (with the PPP of 1990, these amounts correspond to US$ 14,400 and 20,600, respectively). The cost per week of survival was around $ 350 in the Metastron group and $ 560 in the placebo group. If the cost of Metastron was also considered in the analysis, the difference in costs between the groups seems to disappear, as the 1991 cost of a standard dose of Metastron was deemed to be approximately equivalent to the saving in the direct management cost in this group.

Oesterling (1993, 1995) discussed the clinical usefulness of the tumor marker serum PSA in relation to other diagnostic and staging tools such as biopsies, pelvic lymphadenectomy, and radionuclide bone scans. For each of these tools, the sensitivity and specificity compared with PSA is discussed on the basis of various case series, most of them provided by the author and coworkers. While it is conceded that reliance on PSA alone and eliminating most of the tests using these other diagnostic and staging tools may lead to a certain number of cases not being detected, it is argued that, in general, the proportion of cases missed will be very low and that the large majority of cases missed will be of favorable pathology and of no clinical significance for the patients.

By eliminating the majority of tests using staging tools such as prostate biopsies, staging bilateral pelvic lymphadenectomy, and radionuclide bone scans, it will obviously be possible to save resources and obtain financial savings, at least in the very short run. Oesterling reports some very crude and preliminary calculations of the financial savings that would be made possible by more or less complete elimination of these supplementary tests. Multiplying the average cost or charge per test avoided by the expected annual number of tests performed in a country such as the United States (based on data for the incidence of prostate cancer) inevitably results in impressive figures amounting to hundreds of millions of dollars.

The optimal use of diagnostic tools and staging procedures is obviously an important question amenable to economic analysis, since it is a matter of balancing the benefits in terms of information obtained and the value of this information (in terms of probabilities for action which would not be available without this information) on the one hand with the costs of obtaining this information on the other hand. However, the approach used by Oesterling is too crude and approximative to warrant further discussion. Nevertheless, this kind of "back-of-an-envelope" calculations may serve the purpose of arousing the interest in a given subject and may pave the way for more rigorous analyses based on better data.

Concluding Remarks

Table 1 contains a summary of the main characteristics of the economic assessments of treatments for colorectal cancer that have been discussed in this chapter.

Economic aspects have not yet been integrated in studies published on treatments aimed at curing localized disease. The main treatment alternatives are radical prostatectomy and radiation, which seem to be equally effective. The actual costs of these alternatives are not known, and new trials are also currently considering the relative merits of radiotherapy and radical prostat-

Table 1. Main characteristics of economic assessments dealing with colorectal cancer treatments

Reference	Disease category	Treatments examined	Main characteristics of the study
Carlsson et al. (1989)	All patients	All treatments given	Determination of costs of standard treatment Hospital perspective, not explicitly stated Retrospective examination of medical records for all patients treated at a particular institution and deceased in 1984–1985; all hospital stays and procedures counted, including those performed in other departments but related to the cancer; unit prices from hospital's accounting system and authors' own calculations; effect on survival estimated by comparison with average life expectancies; around 40% died of the disease Very skewed cost distribution; average total costs highest for those dying of prostate cancer, three times higher than for those dying of other diseases; costs are higher the longer the patient survives, fairly concentrated around the period just before death; hospitalization accounts for 72%, chemotherapy and other drugs 17%
Taplin et al. (1995)	A cohort of patients with all stages of disease	All treatments given, i.e., those covered by Medicare	Do treatment costs vary with stage at diagnosis? Third-party perspective (Medicare) Retrospective data collection for patients enrolled in HMO to find costs attributable to cancer; pooled time series and cross-section data analysis to simulate longitudinal (incidence) cost data Of the average total cost, almost 60% falls in the terminal phase (6 months before death), almost 40% in initial phase (6 months after diagnosis), and the rest in between; average costs attributable to cancer in the initial phase vary with stage at diagnosis and with age; net costs of continuing care do not depend on stage or age, and net costs of terminal care are not assessed
Licht and Klein (1994)	Patients undergoing radical prostatectomy	Early discharge from hospital vs. normal stay	Impact on costs and morbidity of policy change, earlier hospital discharge after operation Third-party payer perspective Retrospective series of 272 consecutive patients operated on by the same surgeon before and after the policy change; length of stay and complications in the two groups considered; costs examined by analyzing the development in the relevant DRGs over the years Median length of stay reduced from 8 to 5 days, while the overall complication rate is unchanged; average hospital costs fell by 30%
Henriksson and Edhag (1987)	Patients with advanced disease	Orchidectomy vs. oral estrogens	Cost-minimization analysis Hospital perspective, not explicitly stated

Table 1 (continued)

Reference	Disease category	Treatments examined	Main characteristics of the study
			Cost calculation based on examination of case records for 122 consecutive patients in single institution, randomly allocated between the two treatments; these are assumed to have the same efficacy The costs are a little higher for orchidectomy during the first year, about 15%; with a longer time perspective, drug therapy will eventually become the most costly, as this is usually continued as long as the patient responds or until death; the exact breakeven point depends on the assumptions regarding incidence of side effects of estrogen therapy
Henriksson and Stege (1991)	Patients with advanced disease	Parenteral estrogen vs. oral estrogen or orchidectomy	Cost-minimization analysis Hospital perspective Case series of 44 patients receiving parenteral estrogen compared with historical control group (limited to orchidectomy because of high incidence of cardiovascular complications), no difference in tumor response rates Orchidectomy is almost three times more costly than parenteral estrogen, mainly because of in-hospital care; breakeven point between the two is 9 ears, but few patients survive that long
Rutqvist and Wilking (1992)	Patients with advanced disease	LHRH analogues vs. orchidectomy	Cost-minimization analysis Hospital perspective Average length of stay after orchidectomy in one institution multiplied by average daily hospital costs plus two outpatient visits; mean treatment time with LHRH analogue from randomized trial, retail price for drug plus assumed monthly visit by district nurse to perform injection The costs of LHRH 7%–31% higher than the costs of orchidectomy, depending on assumptions; a policy of 2 years of LHRH followed by orchidectomy is calculated to cost 26% less than operating all immediately, in addition to sparing surgery in about 85% of the patients
Nicol et al. (1993)	Patients with advanced disease	Orchidectomy vs. LHRH analogue vs. LHRH analogue+flutamide	Cost-minimization analysis Perspective not stated Model calculations with mean survival assumed to be 2 years regardless of treatment; costs of antihormonal drugs based on drug prices and recommended dosages; costs of orchidectomy from secondary sources Orchidectomy found to be four to five times less costly than the two alternatives

Table 1 (continued)

Reference	Disease category	Treatments examined	Main characteristics of the study
Vahrenhorst et al. (1994)	Patients with advanced disease	Six alternative hormonal treatments	Cost-minimization analysis Hospital perspective, not explicitly stated Model calculation with time span of 3 years; for orchidectomy an inpatient hospital stay of 4 days is expected; unit prices used are given, but their derivation not explained, except that wholesale prices are used for drugs With the antihormonal drugs, increased survival implies increased costs, while the costs of orchidectomy is not influenced by survival; the break-even point is 12 months, i.e., if the patients survives 1 year or more, orchidectomy is the least costly; with shorter survival, parenteral estrogen therapy is the least costly alternative
Hillner et al. (1995)	Patients with metastatic disease	Total androgen blockade vs. orchidectomy or LHRH analogue alone	Cost-effectiveness analysis Third-party payer perspective (Medicare) Markov state transition model with four states (complete or partial response, no progression, progression or death), each state assumed to last 3 months; two hypothetical cohorts of patients, one with severe, the other with minimal metastatic disease; transition probabilities from large intergroup randomized trial; costs calculated are only the Medicare reimbursements; fixed time span Survival benefit of 5.2 months in minimal disease and 4.0 months in severe disease; incremental costs depend on whether the alternative is LHRH or orchidectomy alone; always highest if LHRH is the alternative regardless of the efficacy assumed for flutamide; results are very sensitive to changes in costs and duration of flutamide use
McEwan et al. (1994)	Patients with metastatic disease	Radiopharmaceutical vs. placebo	Cost-minimization analysis Perspective not explicitly stated Retrospective assessment of management needs of 29 patients randomized to either radiopharmaceutical or placebo; data from trial records and hospital charts for all cancer-related admissions; unit cost data from several sources, e.g., wholesale prices for drugs, fee schedules from public heath insurance plan, updates of other studies; costs of radiopharmaceutical not included Total costs of care lower for the radiopharmaceutical group, especially due to lower direct costs (e.g., analgesics, anti-inflammatories, steroids, radiotherapy), indicating reduced need for pain management; difference disappears when including approximate cost of radiopharmaceuticals

LHRH, luteinizing hormone-releasing hormone; HMO, health maintenance organization.

ectomy compared with a wait-and-see policy. Another current problem is the development of conformal radiotherapy, which allows a safe increase in the radiation dose and possibly therefore an improved local control and improved survival. In all these cases, the costs of the various treatments should be determined and should be given the same amount of consideration as the relative effectiveness in the decision about treatment strategies.

As stated above, none of the studies concerned with the costs and effects of various forms of hormonal treatments in advanced disease should be considered as much more than preliminary exercises in cost calculations, based on the crudest data. The clinical evidence is that roughly the same clinical results concerning time to disease progression and survival can be expected for the large majority of patients no matter what hormonal treatment is chosen. The duration of treatment will also be roughly the same, no matter whether it is started early or late in primarily asymptomatic patients. In most cases, systemic treatment is given for 1–3 years.

It is clear that, when no differences in effectiveness have been shown, cost considerations take on major importance, and the studies above have documented that the expected costs may vary considerably according to the treatment chosen. However, it should also be made clear that patient preferences and quality-of-life issues should be explored and emphasized in the choice of treatment, especially when the alternatives include surgical (irreversible) versus medical (reversible) castration.

Genitourinary and Gynecological Cancer

A limited number of publications concerning cancers of the genitourinary system and gynecological cancers have been identified and retrieved. The studies comprise economic assessments of bladder, testis, and ovarian cancer treatments. As the number of studies is quite small, they have been collected in this single chapter.

Bladder Cancer

Urinary bladder cancer is a fairly common disease, the fourth most common in men and the ninth most common in women. The incidence is increasing slightly, while the mortality rate of patients with the disease is decreasing. The presenting symptom is typically blood in the urine, and the stage at diagnosis is superficial in 75% of the cases, invasive disease in 20%–25%, and metastatic disease in up to 5%. Median age at diagnosis is 65 years, and one fifth of the patients die within 1 year after being diagnosed. Most often staging is performed using the TNM classification, and the most important distinction is whether the disease is confined to the organ or not. If there is nodal disease, outcomes without systemic therapy are poor, with 5-year survival rates from 4% to 35%. For patients with metastatic disease, median survival is 6–9 months, and practically no one survives to 5 years.

For superficial disease, the standard treatment is complete endoscopic resection or transurethral resection (TUR). Virtually all patients will develop new tumors, and 30% of these will progress to higher stages, so patients are followed at 3-monthly intervals after the first TUR. Intravesical chemotherapy with cytotoxic or immunologic agents (e.g., bacille Calmette-Guérin, BCG, an antituberculosis vaccine used as a kind of immunotherapy) or cytokines is sometimes used for these patients, especially for patients in which disease has shown a particularly marked tendency to recur with new tumors. For patients with carcinoma in situ, the standard treatment is surgical removal and BCG, usually for 6 weeks. The possible role of maintenance BCG is controversial, as uncertain benefits must be balanced against the frequent toxicities of this treatment. The recurrence risk is associated with tumor type and grade, the length of follow-up, and treatment given.

Economic Evaluations

Only two fairly early articles containing economic assessment of treatments for bladder cancer have been identified and retrieved for this survey. One is a study aiming at calculating the costs of intravesical chemotherapy, a sort of "local chemotherapy" (as opposed to the usual systemic type), where the cytotoxic drug is instilled directly into the bladder for 1 h (or a few hours). This direct instillation, which should reduce the adverse side effects of the cytotoxics, is then repeated any number of times with a typical periodicity of 6–8 weeks. The other study is concerned with the effectiveness and costs of various types of investigations that may be used for the diagnosis and staging of invasive bladder cancer.

Smith (1985) aimed to calculate the costs of intravesical chemotherapy from the hospital's and from the patient's perspective. However, there is no actual attempt at valuing the patients' costs, which might comprise inter alia the costs of travel, subsistence, and sometimes loss of earnings. The costs from the hospital's perspective are calculated on the basis of a number of assumptions, without any attempt at relating these to actual patient data or to data gathered from the literature. The unit prices used for costing of the various procedures involved in the management of a "typical" treatment course are given (in very round numbers), but there is no explanation of the origin of these figures.

The procedures performed in the initial clinical evaluation of the patient are taken from what was prescribed in EORTC clinical trials at the time of the study; the same is true for the examinations performed before each cycle of chemotherapy. The number of instillations and the periods between these may vary widely, and depending on the regimen chosen for the calculations the calculated total costs vary between £ 433 and £ 1508. Converted with the purchasing power parities (PPPs) of 1985, these amounts translate into $ 1000 and $ 3600, respectively.

Hunt and Woodhouse (1987) attempted to determine what they call the cost-effectiveness of different types of clinical tests and procedures that are more or less routinely used to diagnose and stage invasive bladder cancers. The different procedures are costed using figures published by the Department of Health and Social Services (from 1982) as unit prices. The effectiveness of the procedures is determined by examining a case series of one hundred consecutive patients from a single institution. Histologically determined staging and grading data are used to determine the effectiveness (actually measured as the sensitivity, i.e., the proportion of patients with the target disorder who show a positive test result) of each procedure.

The sensitivities found for the diagnostic procedures are 41% for culture of midstream urine (MSU), 59% for urine cytology, and 71% for intravenous urogram (IVU), making the cost of a positive result vary from very low for MSU (actually reported as negative!) to £ 10 for urine cytology and £ 30 for IVU. The sensitivities reported for the staging procedures are even lower, from 13% for a lymphangiogram to 5% for bone scans and 1% each for liver scan and chest X-rays. The authors dismiss bone and liver scans, but recommend lymphangiograms, with a cost of £ 550 per positive result, because they consider them of value in identifying patients who are incurable and who may therefore be spared radical local treatment and be given palliative radiotherapy instead.

Concluding Remarks

Table 1 summarizes the main characteristics of the studies described in the former paragraph.

These two studies do not contribute significantly to the common knowledge concerning the economic consequences of the various treatment possibilities in bladder cancer. This is not so much because of their somewhat obsolete data, but primarily because of poor study designs and data of dubious quality. Almost any new study in bladder cancer including economic vari-

Table 1. Main characteristics of economic assessments dealing with bladder cancer treatments

Reference	Disease category	Treatments examined	Main characteristics of the study
Hunt and Woodhouse (1987)	All patients	Various procedures for diagnosing and staging	Cost-minimization analysis approach Perspective is not explicitly stated Effectiveness of procedures assessed as their sensitivity found by comparing test results with histological stage and grade data for case series of 100 consecutive patients from one institution; unit price figures based on update of data from government publication; the cost of a positive result found by dividing the unit price of a procedure with the sensitivity rate Lowest cost for a positive result for a diagnostic procedure is found for culture of midstream urine followed by urine cytology; reported sensitivity rates for staging procedures extremely low, all under 15%; only lymphangiograms recommended, due to their value in identifying incurable patients that may be spared radical treatment
Smith (1985)	Patients with invasive disease	Intravesical chemotherapy	Determination of costs of treatment Hospital perspective Analysis based on assumptions not related to actual patient data; procedures for initial clinical evaluation and the examinations before each cycle of chemotherapy taken from prevailing standard protocols; sources of cost data not supplied, data approximative Wide variations in the number of instillations and the periods between these; depending on the regimen chosen for the calculations, the costs vary by a factor of three

ables would seem to be a step forward and, considering that bladder cancer is actually one of the most common malignancies, it is surprising that so little has been published.

After a large number of clinical trials with intravesical chemotherapy and intravesical BCG, it is beyond doubt that these treatments, with varying combinations of cytostatics and many different regimens, reduce the risk of superficial recurrence greatly, often by about 50%, from a natural risk of recurrence of superficial bladder cancer of around 40%. Despite all these trials, however, it is still unclear whether intravesical chemotherapy or BCG contributes to prolonged survival, because the trials have been focused on short-term tumor control, optimal regimens and dosages etc. and because the trials tend to select patients with a good prognosis.

It would therefore be very interesting to have performed a large simple trial (as suggested by Hall 1994), including as many "ordinary" patients as possible and also including variables on costs and quality of life. By this kind of trial, it would be possible to obtain an idea of the costs of a possible survival benefit in terms of resources consumed and in terms of possible reductions in patients' quality of life because of the inconvenience and toxicity of repeated treatments and the consequent admonition of being ill.

Testis Cancer

Testicular cancer is the most common malignancy in men aged 15–35 years, and its incidence seems to be growing in several countries. In the United States in the mid-1980s, the average age-adjusted incidence rate was 4.7 per 100,000, more than double the rate of 2 per 100,000 seen in the 1930s. A similar trend with a doubling (or more) of the incidence has been noted in several European countries. In the 1990s, testicular cancer has become one of the most curable solid neoplasms, with a very high survival rate as opposed to a survival rate of 10% in the 1970s. This large improvement is generally considered to be due to a combination of more effective diagnostic techniques, improvement in serum tumor markers, effective regimens of combination chemotherapy, and modifications of surgical techniques. The overall survival rate for all stages of testicular cancer is expected to rise to well over 80% in the 1990s and approaching 100% for patients with low-stage disease.

Testicular cancer is broadly divided, according to a histologic classification, into seminoma and nonseminoma types, where seminoma is the most common single germ cell tumor, accounting for about 40% of all tumors. This classification is used for treatment planning, as seminomas are more sensitive to radiation.

A variety of clinical staging systems have been advocated, the principal differences among staging systems for seminomas and nonseminomas relating to the roles of surgical lymph node sampling and serum tumor markers. The mainstay of the various systems is the following classification system:

- *Stage I:* Tumor limited to the testis with no spread through the capsule or the spermatic cord
- *Stage II:* Clinical or radiologic evidence of tumor extension beyond the testicle, but contained within the regional lymph nodes
- *Stage III:* Disseminated disease with metastases above the diaphragm or visceral disease

Clinical staging is rather inaccurate, as for instance about a quarter of patients with clinical stage I disease are understaged by all available modalities of nonsurgical staging. About the same fraction of clinical stage II patients are downstaged by histologic staging. Treatment decisions are determined by the staging, but the reverse may also be true, as the extent of staging may be dependent on the therapy possibilities considered, as for instance a greater effort will be made to exclude patients with any evidence of regional lymph node involvement if a strategy of careful surveillance is considered. Retroperitoneal lymph node dissection remains the only modality that can accurately distinguish between pathological stage I and stage II patients. However, even with the large proportion of clinically understaged patients, it is considered a problem that more than 70% of the patients undergoing retroperitoneal lymph node dissection are found to have pathologic stage I disease and therefore receive no therapeutic benefit from the operation.

Seminomas

The overall cure rate for patients with seminomas in all stages is now over 90% in most treatment centers. For patients with stage I disease, the standard treatment is surgical removal of the testicle followed by radiation in modest doses to the regional lymph nodes. Prophylactic radiation of the lymph nodes is used even for patients with a negative lymphangiogram or CT scan because of the risk of occult nodal spread (seen in approximately 15% of the patients). As an alternative to prophylactic irradiation of all patients, a strategy of surveillance (with frequent determination of serum markers, chest X-rays, and CT scans) and possible salvage therapy by radiation or chemotherapy is under clinical evaluation. However, it has not as yet been possible to identify a subset of clinical stage I patients who are at low risk for occult para-aortic metastases.

Stage II seminomas are usually divided into bulky (tumors >5 cm) and nonbulky disease for treatment planning and prognosis purposes. For the nonbulky tumors, the current standard treatment is the same as for stage I disease, as it is no longer considered necessary to use prophylactic radiation of the mediastinum and neck. For patients with a bulky tumor, radical orchiectomy is followed by cisplatin-based combination chemotherapy or by radiation to the abdominal and pelvic lymph nodes. Stage III seminomas are usually curable, with the standard treatment being radical orchiectomy followed by combination chemotherapy. Various combinations of cytotoxics are possible, but they all contain cisplatin. However, single-agent carboplatin has also been tried in these patients with results considered to be excellent.

There is not much debate about the proper strategy for patients presenting with stage III seminoma, while the proper management of patients with bulky, but localized seminoma (stage IIB) is debated. The cure rate with the common cisplatin-based combination chemotherapy regimens is at least 90%, but it is equally logical to treat these patients with initial radiation therapy alone, with a probable cure rate of 70%–90%. Most failures of this modality can be salvaged by subsequent chemotherapy. Another controversial issue is the proper management of patients with bulky tumors who have a residual mass after chemotherapy, which may require additional therapy, e.g., in the form of postchemotherapy regional lymph node dissection. It has been reported that the size of the residual mass does not correlate well with active residual disease and that most of these residual masses do not grow. Some centers therefore consider that a viable alternative to active treatment would be careful surveillance with frequent tumor marker and CT evaluations, even when the residual mass is 3 cm or larger. A current cooperative study between some of the antagonists in this controversy may contribute to its resolution.

Nonseminomas

Tumors which have a mixture of seminoma and nonseminoma components should be managed as nonseminoma. For nonseminomatous tumors, removal of the testis by an inguinal approach is the definitive procedure for local treatment and pathologic diagnosis. The inaccuracy of clinical staging by lymphography and/or CT or magnetic resonance imaging (MRI) scanning, where patients with a negative result on either test have a 25%–30% risk of having microscopic involvement of the lymph nodes, is a problem, and surgical staging by dissection of the retroperitoneal lymph nodes is often required. A nerve-sparing lymphadenectomy with modified retroperitoneal lymph node dissection, which preserves fertility in more than 90% of patients, is a possibility, and it appears to be as effective as the classical non-nerve-sparing procedures in preventing retroperitoneal relapse.

The cure rate for patients with pathologically confirmed stage I disease is about 96% with surgery alone. Careful follow-up examinations are necessary for the first 2 years after definitive local treatment, generally with monthly chest X-rays and tumor markers for the first year and bimonthly for the second year. However, there is concern about the fact that approximately 70% of the patients (those who are found to be pathologic stage I) will have no therapeutic benefit to offset the costs and risks of dissection of the regional lymph nodes. In addition, 5%–10% of patients relapse outside the field of retroperitoneal lymph node dissection. Careful surveillance is therefore considered an attractive alternative, and several large surveillance programs have been undertaken throughout the world. Surveillance for these patients should be considered an active form of treatment, with careful follow-up studies being mandatory. In several of these series, a relapse rate of about 30% is seen, and a death rate of 7% is observed for those relapsing. The problem then becomes one of identifying patients at low risk for metastases, and several series have evaluated prognostic factors associated with relapse. The most important factors seem to be the presence of vascular or lymphatic invasion and the local T stage.

Stage II nonseminoma is considered highly curable, with a cure rate of 95% or more. Standard treatments comprise radical orchiectomy with regional lymph node dissection plus adjuvant cisplatin-based chemotherapy or careful surveillance. A large randomized study comparing these options concluded that, although adjuvant chemotherapy will almost always (>95% of cases) prevent relapse, careful observation for relapse (seen in 49% of the patients followed, almost all of whom could be effectively treated, however) will lead to an equivalent cure rate. Another option, especially for patients with large, unresectable residual masses, is radical orchiectomy followed by chemotherapy and delayed surgery for removal of residual masses and close observation. Various cisplatin-based chemotherapy regimens are in common use, and some, including high-dose chemotherapy with autologous bone marrow transplantation (BMT), are under clinical evaluation.

Stage III nonseminomas are usually (70%) curable with standard chemotherapy regimens, but clinical trials aiming at identifying equally effective, but less toxic combinations are in progress. Patients who are not cured with standard chemotherapy usually have large, bulky metastases. In selected cases, surgery should be used after chemotherapy to remove residual masses, to determine whether viable tumor cells remain, and to prevent regrowth of teratomas present in some of these masses. Some recommend surgical resection of all residual masses in patients who have normal tumor markers after responding to chemotherapy, because neither the size of the initial tumor nor the degree of response to chemotherapy appears to identify patients with residual teratoma or carcinoma. However, this approach is controversial and there is no evidence of improved survival.

In addition to identifying equally effective, but less toxic chemotherapy regimens, clinical trials are also in progress evaluating the use of high-dose chemotherapy with autologous BMT. This strategy has also been used with some success in patients with cisplatin-refractory disease, where durable complete remission may be achievable for 10%–20% of the patients and with even greater success in patients who relapse after an initial response. In general, the decision on further treatment for patients with recurrent testicular cancer depends on factors such as the specific cancer, prior treatment, site of recurrence, and individual patient considerations. The standard initial salvage regimen is cisplatin-based combination chemotherapy, which can induce long-term complete response in 20%–45% of these patients. In some selected patients with chemotherapy-refractory disease confined to a single site, surgical resection may result in long-term disease-free survival.

Economic Evaluations

The majority of the cost analyses and economic evaluations in testis cancer identified and retrieved for this survey are concerned with determining optimal follow-up policies. Ciatto et al. (1986) calculated the costs of performing routine X-rays as a follow-up test for stage I/II testicular seminoma patients and the costs per asymptomatic lung or mediastinal relapse (or intrathoraic metastases, ITMs) detected by this means. The data come from a retrospective review of a series of 253 patients treated for stage I/II seminoma and systematically followed up by chest X-rays. The data are from 1958 to 1982.

Primary treatment after orchiectomy was radiotherapy alone, after which a follow-up program was initiated, consisting of clinical examination and chest X-ray every 3 months in the first year, every 6 months in the second year, and yearly after that. The minimum follow-up for the patients in the study was 3 years, and the frequency of asymptomatic ITM detected by chest X-ray was evaluated according to the stage of the disease at first diagnosis and the disease-free interval. Without any sources of cost data provided, the cost of a chest X-ray is estimated to be $ 50, which is supposed to cover both the costs in the outpatient facility, the patient's travel expenses, and the social costs due to the loss of work activity in order to attend the hospital for the test.

In these patients, 18 ITMs (13 asymptomatic) were detected by chest X-rays, 14 of which in the first year of follow-up, with the detection rate clearly related to stage at first presentation (1.4% in stage I, 12.5% in stage IIB). The costs of each asymptomatic ITM detected were much lower in the first year of follow-up, i.e., $ 4200, than in the successive follow-up, i.e., $ 130,000, and tenfold lower for stage IIB patients than for stage I patients, i.e., $ 1600 versus $ 14,000. The authors conclude that routine chest X-rays should not be carried out for stage I patients and that detection of asymptomatic ITMs is so infrequent and the cost per detected case so high that this policy should not be continued after the second year of follow-up.

Munro and Warde (1991) used a Markov model to simulate and assess a large number of follow-up policies for surveillance of patients with stage I nonseminomatous tumors of the testis. The surveillance programs analyzed (instead of prophylactic treatment of the retroperitoneal lymph nodes) are taken from the literature and contain two distinct elements: (1) a hospital visit with history taking, physical examination, chest X-ray, and serum tumor markers and (2) CT scanning. The nine different policies differ with respect to the periodicity and to whether CT scanning is performed and how often. In addition to the policies taken from the literature, a hypothetical maximum policy (visit plus CT scan every month for 2 years), a minimum policy (visit only every 3 months), and a "no follow-up" policy are also considered. No information is given about the sources of the probabilities used for this part of the analysis.

A Markov model with a cycle length of 1 month and 24 cycles was set up (i.e., 2 years of follow-up, as late relapses are very rare in testis cancer). The model contains three states, well, false negative, and false positive, between which the patients cycle, and two absorbing states, alive and dead. A number of assumptions are specified, inter alia about the rates of false-positive and false-negative results. The probability of relapse is governed by a monthly probability of relapse, based on data for the true relapse rates of patients on the different surveillance policies. For the probabilities used, the authors refer to four different publications without giving any actual data. Relapsing patients (and also those with false-positive results) are assumed to be treated with a standard chemotherapy regimen of bleomycin+cisplatin+etoposide, with outcome probabilities taken from a single study of this regimen. The probability of 2-year survival is assumed equal to the probability of cure.

The cost calculations are carried out from the perspective of the government, and to a certain extent they are based on time and motion studies, calculations of the costs of capital for CT equipment, etc. However, no detailed information is provided on the sources of data or the methods used for calculations of unit costs, and the ranges of cost data and probabilities used in the sensitivity analyses are very wide indeed, which indicates quite a low quality of the data.

The surveillance policies clinically used are assumed to be equally effective, but they result in costs varying from almost $ 3000 to $ 5300 per patient. The hypothetical "no follow-up" policy is least effective, but surprisingly costly, due to the costliness of the salvage chemotherapy. By assuming a life expectancy for cured patients of 40 years, the incremental costs per year of life saved for cured patients is calculated to vary from about $ 1500 to $ 23,800, i.e., by a factor of 15. Comprehensive one-way and multiway sensitivity analyses show that the rank ordering of the policies is not influenced by varying the effectiveness data assumed, while overall costs (but not the rank ordering) are quite sensitive to changes in assumptions. It is concluded that, based on 2-year survival data, a policy with no CT scans but monthly visits in the first year and bimonthly in the second is just as effective as policies using scanning, but far less costly.

Berdel et al. (1987) reported on the local experiences in a Munich university hospital with a particular 5-year follow-up program for patients with stage IIB/IV nonseminatomous testis tumor. The patients were followed up closely, inter alia with chest X-rays, abdominal CT scans, and tumor markers, with varying periodicity over the 5-year period. The report was based on a retrospective analysis of 7 years of follow-up of patients who had received adjuvant cisplatin-based chemotherapy after primary surgery. All patients achieving a complete response after adjuvant chemotherapy entered the follow-up program, and the retrospective analysis comprised 185 of the 197 patients entering the follow-up program from 1979 to 1985 (three patients lost to follow-up, nine still in treatment at the time of analysis).

Cost data are given without any explanation of the sources or their calculation, except that they are based on information from the German insurance funds. The perspective of the assessment is not clear either, but it seems to be the hospital's perspective. The cost per patient for the follow-up program varies from $ 850 per year for the first 2 years to $ 260 per year for years 4 and 5. The data cover a period of follow-up of 326 patient-years, costing a total of $ 215,000, of which about 50% are due to the CT scans performed.

Out of a total of 20 relapses, 14 were found by one or the other of the examinations included in the follow-up programs in asymptomatic patients in complete response. A success rate of approximately 10% is postulated (14 relapses detected by the follow-up program in 138 patients in complete response), and the cost per relapse detected is given as $ 18,000. All the relapsing patients detected through the examinations in the follow-up program were able to obtain a second complete remission, while this was possible for only one of the six patients presenting with symptoms of a relapse. The authors conclude by recommending a close follow-up of these patients.

Sharda et al. (1996) analyzed the choice of optimal management strategy for early-stage testicular seminoma after inguinal orchiectomy using a cost-minimization approach. Standard treatment is adjuvant irradiation, but this policy has been questioned in recent years because of concerns about the potential toxicity of radiotherapy and surgical evidence that only a small proportion of the patients harbor occult lymph node metastases. An alternative strategy of observation might be considered, as this has been shown not to lead to any decrease in overall survival, in particular because early relapses can generally be salvaged successfully by either chemotherapy or radiotherapy.

A model is set up, with frequencies of events derived from a number of international case series. Costs are calculated under the assumption that all the patients in each alternative – adjuvant radiotherapy or observation – are managed in exactly the same way. For the observation arm, a constant recurrence rate of 1.5% every 6 months for 5 years is assumed. Recurrences in the pelvic and para-aortic nodal regions (80% of all) are assumed to be treated with a standard radiotherapy regimen, while the remaining 20% of recurrences in sites such as the inguinal nodes, the mediastinum, or the lungs are assumed to be treated with a standard cisplatin-based chemotherapy regimen. All patients in the observation group are followed with a regimen commonly reported in the literature.

For patients receiving adjuvant radiotherapy, a constant recurrence rate of 0.5% every 6 months for the first 5 years is assumed, based on several case series. Early recurrences are most frequent outside the irradiated area and are assumed to be effectively managed by three cycles of a standard chemotherapy regimen with bleomycin+cisplatin+etoposide. The follow-up schedule assumed for this group is also one commonly reported in the literature, somewhat less intensive than the one for the observation group, especially because the latter was examined regularly with CT scans of the abdomen/pelvis. The only complication of radiotherapy noted was mild nausea, managed by oral antiemetics. A major issue of concern, the possible development of secondary tumors in the irradiated area, was left out of consideration because of a lack of unambiguous data.

The calculations of the costs of treatment were based on an examination of inpatient hospital and physician charges for a small number of patients (n=5) treated either with chemotherapy for recurrrence or with postorchidectomy radiotherapy in the authors' university hospital. All charges not associated with or resulting from the diagnosis of seminoma and its treatment were excluded. An incidence of febrile neutropenia of 40% in the chemotherapy-treated patients was assumed and an average charge for hospitalization for this was included in the calculation. For inpatient hospital stays, a cost-to-charge ratio for the institution was assumed, while the costs of physicians are calculated at 80% of the charges, because the average reimbursement amounts to this. The perspective chosen was stated to be that of the payer (e.g., the health insurer), and follow-up costs were calculated for a period of 5 years. The future costs were not discounted.

The baseline result, stated in the original charge figures, was an average cost in the observation group of $ 27,000, while it was about $ 19,500 in the group receiving adjuvant radiotherapy. Two thirds of the costs in this group occurred up front due to the radiotherapy, while follow-up costs accounted for 26% and salvage chemotherapy for 7%. For the observation group, follow-up accounted for 91% of the average total costs and CT scanning alone for 70%. The decision not to discount the cost figures[1] may therefore have an important impact on the cost comparison. The results are not very sensitive to variations in the recurrence rates assumed for the two groups, and no other sensitivity analyses are reported.

Baniel et al. (1995) compared the costs of two different management strategies for clinical stage II nonseminatomous testis cancer patients considered to be clinically equivalent in terms of survival, but not with respect to side effects. The strategies were nerve-sparing peritoneal lymph node dissection (RPLND) with adjuvant or delayed chemotherapy (in the case of relapse) versus primary chemotherapy with postchemotherapy surgery for residual disease. The calculations were based on a model with follow-up for 5 years. The model included the common observation of clinical overstaging, i.e., that more than 20% of patients with clinical stage II disease will turn out to be stage I patients after surgery and pathological examination.

Data on effectiveness and adverse effects of the treatments were taken from case series from the authors' university hospital and others. The selection of the actual data used is neither described nor discussed. The costs of RPLND surgery, chemotherapy, and follow-up were estimated on the basis of local costs and management protocols of the hospital, but when these were considered inadequate, other sources for cost data were evaluated and used for the calculations. Again, the actual choice of data and its motivation is not always entirely clear, and the perspective of the analysis is not made explicit.

The estimated costs of treatment were $ 47,400 for the chemotherapy group and $ 29,300–34,800 for the RPLND group, a statistically significant

[1] A flawed argument is used to justify this decision, referring to an expectation that the inflation in medical charges will correspond to the general inflation rate in the economy. The economic argument for discounting, however, is based on a postulate of *time preference*, i.e., that the economic agents attach a higher weight to events in the near future than to events in the more distant future. In economic evaluations (and economic analyses in general), it is always implied that the expected inflation is deducted from the nominal amounts before any data analysis, so that these are always conducted in real terms.

difference ($p<.05$), mainly due to the high price of chemotherapy, which is given as \$ 31,500, while the cost of primary RPLND is \$ 16,000. In addition, the follow-up of patients managed with chemotherapy alone is more costly because of the need for repetitive CT scans of patients who have obtained a complete response in order to monitor the retroperitoneum. This is not necessary for the RPLND patients. Another factor is the indirect cost, where the expected average per patient is about twice as high with primary chemotherapy as with RPLND, as the data show that the average time lost from work is about 13 and 7 weeks, respectively.

A comparison of the expected side effects of the two modalities show that RPLND is favored on all counts, with lower morbidity and mortality, lower risk of late relapse, and a higher quality of life (based on estimates of anxiety/depression and sexual dysfunction). A deficiency of both modalities is the need for double therapy, as about 35% of the operated patients will need chemotherapy later, while 20%–33% of the patients treated with primary chemotherapy will undergo surgery later.

Shibley et al. (1990) reported what they (unjustifiably) call a cost-benefit analysis of the benefits of using a cisplatin-based chemotherapy regimen PVB (cisplatin+vinblastine+bleomycine) for the treatment of advanced-stage testicular cancer. The idea is to determine the benefits of the treatment in terms of the expected future earnings of those patients that survive because of this treatment and compare this value with the costs of treatment plus the costs of developing the regimen. The reduction in indirect costs, which is the measure of the benefits of treatment chosen for the analysis, is calculated by using the traditional Human Capital approach commonly used in cost-of-illness (COI) analyses (see the chapter on "The Economic Burden of Cancer" for a description of this method and a critique of the use of this capital value as a proxy measure for the benefits of treatment to be used in a cost-benefit analysis).

The number of new testis cancer cases in the United States in 1987 was estimated by multiplying the proper incidence rates (for stages II and III of both seminomas and nonseminatomous tumors) by the male population of the United States in 1987. The number of treatments were then determined by multiplying the number of new cases with the percentage of patients with each cancer type who received chemotherapy, according to a national survey of patterns of care for testicular cancer. For each of the four cancer types, the increase in survival with PVB chemotherapy compared to the expected survival before the use of this regimen was estimated based on the survival rates from several clinical trials. An estimated total of 331 lives were saved in the whole country in 1987 because of the use of PVB chemotherapy.

This survival gain is then subdivided into age-groups for the purpose of calculating the expected future earnings of the survivors. The values used for the calculation reflect the life expectancy of each age-group and the pattern of average earnings and labor market participation over their remaining lifetime. Total pretax income figures are used, and a discount rate of 6% is used to calculate the net present value of the expected future stream of earnings.

This calculation results in a net present value for 1987 of $ 166 million, which represents the benefits of the PVB regimen.

The costs are calculated as the increase in charges for chemotherapy compared to the chemotherapy regimens used before the advent of PVB plus an estimate of the costs of the investment in research and development of the PVB regimen made by the American NCI over the period 1971–1987, the entire lifetime of the project. Cost estimates for the earlier chemotherapy regimens were obtained from historical data, and for the PVB regimens they were based on information from different oncology centers. The difference between these two is multiplied by the incidence in 1987 advanced-stage testicular cancer in order to determine the total cost increase due to PVB. A total of $ 16 million results from this calculation.

The costs of the research and development of the PVB regimen incurred by the NCI were found by identifying the funding given for applied research of this regimen for each year from 1971 to 1987. The historical cost figures were then converted to constant 1987 dollars by means of a sector-specific price index. The calculated net present value of the investment in research and development was calculated as $ 56 million. Based on the figures reported, the authors conclude that it is clear that the yearly benefits of the PVB combination exceed the incremental costs and that the investment in this regimen has obviously been worthwhile.

Concluding Remarks

Table 2 summarizes the main characteristics of the economic assessments of testis cancer treatments discussed in this chapter.

As for so many other cancers, the economic assessments that have appeared in the field of testis cancer are quite disparate, focusing on distinct groups of patients and divergent issues of patient management, and this makes an overall assessment difficult, except for the obvious possibility of pointing out questions which need to be investigated. Among others could be mentioned a serious economic evaluation of the costs and benefits of cisplatin-based chemotherapy in patients with locally advanced disease compared with a realistic alternative such as initial radiotherapy alone, i.e., one of the controversial clinical issues. The one economic study focusing on cisplatin, in an "historical" comparison with traditional chemotherapy, is a curious example of the result of linking various forms of available secondary data into a chain of reasoning with a certain air of "economic analysis" about it. The outcome of this exercise, in terms of a return-on-investment figure, may have pleased many, but the analytical approach is flawed.

Of the actual treatment choices analyzed, the most clear-cut result is seen for lymph node dissection (RPLND) versus primary chemotherapy in patients with stage II nonseminatomous disease. The two strategies are assumed to be equally effective, but RPLND is found to be much less expensive and more favorable with respect to adverse events and therefore assumed to

Table 2. Main characteristics of economic assessments dealing with testis cancer treatments

Reference	Disease category	Treatments examined	Main characteristics of the study
Ciatto et al. (1986)	Stage I and II patients	Follow-up with routine X-rays	Determines the costs of this strategy and the costs of each case of metastases detected Perspective not explicitly stated Retrospective evaluation of a case series of 253 stage I and II patients followed by routine X-rays after surgery and radiotherapy; assesses number of asymptomatic intrathoraic metastases found in this way, according to stage at diagnosis; an approximate cost figure, supposed to cover costs in the outpatient facility as well as travel costs and production loss, is used, no sources provided Number of (asymptomatic) metastases found in the case series was small; the cost per find was much lower in the first year of follow-up compared to later years of follow-up, and a tenfold lower for stage IIB patients compared to stage I was found
Munro and Warde (1991)	Stage I non-seminomatous patients	A variety of follow-up policies, varying with respect to CT scan or not and to the periodicity	Cost-effectiveness analysis Third-party payer perspective (government) Markov state transition model, 2-year perspective (cure assumed after 2 years); effectiveness data (sensitivities, specificities) taken from diverse publications supplemented with assumptions (hypothetical policies of maximal and minimal surveillance); unit cost data partly based on time and motion studies and calculations of costs of capital, but insufficient information on sources; large variance in cost data for sensitivity analysis; 40 years life expectancy after cure assumed Hypothetical minimal follow-up policy least effective, but costly, due to costs of salvage chemotherapy; incremental costs per year of life saved vary by a factor of 15 and are lowest with a policy of no CT scans but monthly visits the first year and bimonthly the second; results are very sensitive, but not the rank ordering of policies
Berdel et al. (1987)	Patients with stage IIB–IV disease	Comprehensive follow-up program (chest X-rays, abdominal CT scans, tumor markers)	Determines the costs of a follow-up program and of identifying asymptomatic metastases Hospital perspective, not explicitly stated Retrospective analysis of all patients included in the surveillance program of a particular institution over a 7-year period; unit costs based on data from insurance funds, no details on calculation methods

Table 2 (continued)

Reference	Disease category	Treatments examined	Main characteristics of the study
			70% of all relapses in asymptomatic patients in complete response were found by one of the procedures in the follow-up program; over 10% of asymptomatic patients in complete response were found to have metastatic disease, and these could all obtain a second complete remission, which is rarely possible in patients with symptomatic relapse
Sharda et al. (1996)	Patients with early-stage disease	Adjuvant irradiation vs. observation	Cost-minimization analysis Third-party payer perspective Model-based analysis with frequencies derived from several international case series; for each group, a constant rate of recurrence per time period is postulated, three times higher for the observation group; treatment of recurrences and follow-up regimens based on reports in the literature; costs of treatments calculated based on hospital and physician charges for five actual patients treated in the authors' hospital; a cost-to-charge ratio is assumed; future costs are not discounted Average costs of observation 35% higher than for adjuvant irradiation; the time profile of costs differs greatly, two thirds of the costs in the radiotherapy group occurring up front, 90% of the costs in observation group due to follow-up; comparison may be influenced by decision not to discount
Baniel et al. (1995)	Patients with stage II nonseminatomous disease	Lymph node dissection (RPLND) vs. primary chemotherapy	Cost-minimization analysis Perspective not made explicit Treatments are equally effective, but adverse effects differ; data on effectiveness and adverse effects from case series; cost calculations based on local costs and management protocols of the authors' hospital Estimated treatment costs are 50% higher for the chemotherapy than for the RPLND group; follow-up is also more costly for the chemotherapy group (due to repetitive CT scans) and the loss of production is twice as high; with respect to expected side effects, RPLND is again favored on all counts and is also assumed to lead to a higher quality of life

Table 2 (continued)

Reference	Disease category	Treatments examined	Main characteristics of the study
Shibley et al. (1990)	Patients with advanced disease	Cisplatin-based vs. traditional chemotherapy	Cost-of-illness analysis Societal perspective Differences in survival from several randomized trials; estimated incidence of new cases in US multiplied by estimated proportion receiving chemotherapy multiplied by survival gain from cisplatin to estimated number of lives saved; net present value of expected future incomes calculated after subdivision of survivors in age-groups and using average life expectancy; costs equal ized to increase in charges for chemotherapy plus estimate of the costs of the investment in developing cisplatin-based chemotherapy; the costs of investment are found by summing the yearly funding for applied research updated to 1987 prices by a special price index The calculations result in the postulate that the net present value in 1987 figures of the benefits of the cisplatin-based regimen is three times higher than the net present value of the extra costs of using this regimen plus the investment in developing and investigating it

CT, computed tomography; RPLND, nerve-sparing peritoneal lymph node dissection.

be preferable in quality-of-life terms as well. However, the practical relevance of the treatment choice posed for this analysis must be doubted, as the standard treatment regimens are considered to be radical orchiectomy with regional lymph node dissection *plus* cisplatin-based adjuvant chemotherapy *or* careful observation. The other study concerned with a treatment choice (adjuvant irradiation in early-disease patients versus observation) gives equivocal results because of the problematic decision not to discount future costs in an analysis, where the patterns of costs over time vary considerably between the two choices.

Determining an appropriate research design for analyzing the difficult question about optimal follow-up strategies after treatment of patients in various disease stages is a complex task. The popular approach of examining a case series of patients and trying to determine the costs of finding one recurrent case is certainly too simplistic, as it does not take into account many costs, e.g., of false-positive and false-negative findings. Modeling will surely be needed, and an interesting study is found for stage I nonseminomatous patients, which focuses instead on the costs per year of life saved, which is a more relevant outcome for economic evaluations. However, the results are very sensitive to variations in the assumptions, and better data are necessary to resolve these uncertainties.

Ovarian Cancer

Three major types of ovarian cancer are distinguished by their clinical and pathological features: (1) epithelial carcinomas, which alone account for 90% of the ovarian cancers, (2) stromal carcinomas, (3) and germ cell tumors. The vast majority of newly diagnosed patients are postmenopausal women with a median age of 63 years. Most of the patients are diagnosed at an advanced stage of disease, and 70% of the patients with epithelial carcinoma have stage III or IV disease at diagnosis. In contrast, 70% of the women with germ cell tumor have stage I disease at diagnosis. During the last 20 years or so, the incidence has increased slightly, while the survival rate has increased by over 20% (about 8 percentage points), mainly due to the development of curative cisplatin-based chemotherapy regimens. The lifetime risk for women of developing ovarian cancer is about 1.5%, while 1% of all women will die of the disease.

Patients with early-stage disease and well-differentiated tumors are usually treated by a comprehensive staging laparotomy without any adjuvant therapy, and the 5-year survival rate for these patients is over 90%. For patients with an unfavorable prognosis, the question about optimal management is much more controversial, and a number of ongoing randomized trials are under way in an attempt to clarify and possibly settle this issue. Current interest centers on brachytherapy with intraperitoneal radioisotopes, cisplatin-based chemotherapy regimens, and deferred treatment. Randomized trials of radioisotopes versus cisplatin-based chemotherapy have shown no clear difference in survival, but less adverse effects of chemotherapy. The most important problem with radioisotopes is gastrointestinal toxicity. Preliminary results from an ongoing randomized trial of deferred treatment versus adjuvant cisplatin has shown no difference in overall survival, but a clear advantage for cisplatin with respect to disease-free survival.

For patients with advanced disease, the standard management is debulking or cytoreductive surgery and adjuvant chemotherapy. There are no prospective randomized trials assessing the value of cytoreductive surgery in these patients, but several case series indicate a significant impact, even though some recent meta-analyses of such series give somewhat conflicting results. There are some speculations that the variations in the apparent effect of maximal cytoreduction may be due to variations in the biology of the tumors. The hypothesis is that less invasive tumors, which will allow debulking surgery to result in the smallest size of residual disease (e.g., <2 cm), may also be more sensitive to chemotherapy.

A current concern is the potential value of neoadjuvant chemotherapy, i.e., giving cytotoxics before cytoreductive surgery. The anticipated advantage of this is that the cytoreduction achieved by chemotherapy will make the following surgery smaller and easier, therefore requiring a shorter period of hospitalization of the patient. This will presumably make this treatment less costly and will allow a faster recovery of the patient's quality of life. There are as yet no randomized clinical trials assessing these potentials, but the initial experience with cisplatin-based regimens indicates that neoadjuvant chemotherapy is just as efficacious as the normal adjuvant therapy.

With respect to chemotherapy, the new agent paclitaxel in combination with cisplatin or carboplatin has come to be considered the optimal therapy as of the mid-1990s, but a number of issues concerning the role of paclitaxel still remain to be determined. These include the importance of the dose and schedule (duration of the infusion) and the potential of adding other agents to the combination of paclitaxel and cisplatin/carboplatin (e.g., cyclophosphamide and ifosfamide). Most of the previously untreated patients achieve complete remission after induction chemotherapy, but most of those in complete clinical remission and up to half of those with surgically confirmed remission will ultimately relapse. The patients with the highest risk of relapse are those with large-volume disease before chemotherapy and those with poorly differentiated disease. Recurrence before 6 months indicates a bad prognosis, while patients recurring later have a rather good prognosis.

For patients with recurrent disease with a good prognosis, a secondary cytoreductive surgery gives an important survival gain of about 6 months compared to no cytoreduction. The optimal chemotherapy is paclitaxel if the prior treatment did not contain this, possibly even as single-agent therapy for patients relapsing after paclitaxel+cisplatin (PC). With previous standard chemotherapy regimens, it has been established through randomized trials that intraperitoneal chemotherapy is better than intravenous administration, with longer survival, less toxicity, and higher rates of complete remission. Equivalent trials with the current standard paclitaxel-based regimens are under way. Experimental treatment approaches comprise high-dose chemotherapy with hematological support, previously with autologous BMT, but increasingly with peripheral blood stem cell transplantation (PBSCT). Other approaches are testing other new cytotoxic agents (e.g., gemticabine) or aim at reversing the development of drug resistance.

Economic Evaluations

Etzioni et al. (1996) calculated the direct COI of ovarian cancer by means of the incidence approach, in which the stream of costs arising over the course of disease is assessed as a capital value at one point in time, i.e., when the disease is incident (at the time of diagnosis). The source of cost data is the database linking Medicare claims with epidemiological data from the SEER cancer registry database mentioned in the chapter on "The Economic Burden of Cancer," so the data concern women above the age of 65, diagnosed with ovarian cancer between 1973 and 1989 (inclusive). Only cases with epithelial ovarian cancer were chosen, as the study is a preliminary to a cost-effectiveness analysis of a screening method which is specific to this type of ovarian cancer. Different patients in the database have cost data covering different periods in the disease process, so there is a pooling of cross-section and time-series data, which the authors term a "synthetic cohort." The Medicare data comprise both charges and the amounts actually paid by Medicare, which are roughly two thirds of the charges. The calculations are based on the payments, which are considered as costs.

The average 15-year postdiagnosis costs are estimated by a so-called Kaplan-Meier sample average estimator, which is intended to take account of the problem of censoring, i.e., that the proportion of patients surviving from the start of one time interval (here, months are used) to the start of the next is generally not known, as follow-up may be terminated for some reason or another while the patient is still alive. The costs attributable to ovarian cancer are estimated by calculating the corresponding costs for a group of matched control subjects without the disease. In 1990 dollars, the attributable costs by stage of the disease at diagnosis range from about $ 21,000 for local cancer to about $ 32,000 for both regional and distant cancers. For an early-stage patient with 3 years' survival after the diagnosis, a very distinct U-shaped curve is observed, with very high costs immediately after diagnosis and in the months just before death and rather small costs in the intermediate period.

Two papers concerned with the cost-effectiveness of PC chemotherapy compared to standard regimens have been identified and retrieved, both based on the Gynecologic Oncology Group study 111 (GOG-111; McGuire et al. 1996). The results of this trial indicate that PC increases median survival of advanced ovarian cancer patients from 24 months to 37 months (54%) compared to the standard regimen of cisplatin+cyclophosphamide (CC).

Covens et al. (1996) used a highly simplified modeling approach to calculate the costs of applying the PC regimen based on a calculation of the costs of using the standard CC regimen. To determine cost-effectiveness ratios, it was assumed that PC increases average survival time by 50% compared to the standard.

The determination of the costs of the CC regimen was based on a retrospective examination of the patient charts for 18 patients with advanced ovarian cancer undergoing first-line CC chemotherapy at a particular regional cancer center after debulking surgery. The cost of the cytoreduction was not included, as it does not depend on the chemotherapy regimen. One of the criteria for inclusion of patients in the review was a minimum follow-up period of of 3 years after initial diagnosis. Data collection was limited to hospital- and cancer clinic-based care at the cancer center and days of hospitalization in any other hospital. The number and type of all medical consultations, medical procedures, laboratory tests, and drugs were recorded. A Ministry of Health perspective was used for the costing of the resource utilization data, based on official rates for physician fees for consultations and procedures and the costing system of the cancer center.

A basic assumption of the modeling approach to determining the costs of the PC regimen was that the entire 50% increase in survival time achieved by the PC patients occurs during the first follow-up phase after initial chemotherapy. In addition, it was assumed that the frequency of use per day of the various resources was constant for each day of the follow-up period, so that the observed resource utilization can be linearly extrapolated to the increase in the first follow-up phase, which is attributed to the survival gain of 50%. The treatment costs in all the following phases (e.g., relapse, new course of chemotherapy, relapse, terminal stage) were assumed to be identical for the two regimens, so the difference in total costs between them were essentially determined by two factors: (1) the difference in the costs of the cytotoxics used for chemotherapy and (2) the increase in resource utilization caused by the prolongation of the first follow-up phase assumed for the PC patients. The model-determined cost of the PC regimen is justified by comparison with the costs calculated on the basis of chart reviews of four patients treated with the PC regimen at the center.

The average overall survival gain for the PC group was 7.8 months compared to the CC group. The difference in average total cost per patient was an increase for the PC group of about CAN$ 13,000, which translates into an incremental cost-effectiveness ratio of around CAN$ 20,000.[2] More than three quarters of the cost difference between the regimens were caused by the higher acquisition price of paclitaxel ("overheads" for the costs of administering the drugs were determined as a fixed percentage of their acquisition price). The stability of the results was assessed by several sensitivity analyses, based on variations in the survival gain, in unit costs of drugs and hospital days etc. The results are quite sensitive, varying by a factor of 4–5, although the direction is not changed.

Messori et al. (1996) used the data from the GOG-111 trial in a so-called lifetime approach to economic evaluation, in which both costs and outcomes of treatment are extrapolated in the long run to cover the whole life span of the patients. Specifically, it was assumed that long-term follow-up costs are identical for the two arms, so that the cost determination was limited to the first-line treatment. The long-term outcomes in terms of survival were determined by analysis and extrapolation of the survival curves published in the paper reporting the GOG-111 trial. Both costs and outcomes were normalized to a population of 100 patients.

The GOG-111 publication comprised data from 4 years of follow-up. At this time point, the residual survival rate was 31% for the PC group and 25% for the CC group. By careful measurement of the height of the published survival curves every 3 months from month 3 to month 48, the numerical values necessary for describing the time course of a survival curve were estimated using Gompertz' law. By iterating a nonlinear weighted least square regression analysis, the best fitting curves for the PC and CC groups, respectively, were then determined by the criterion of minimizing the root mean squared error. The fitted survival curves were then extrapolated until all the patients had died, and the area under the curves was determined by standard numer-

[2] Costs are reported in 1993 Canadian dollars; after conversion with the PPP of that year, the cost-effectiveness ratio amounts to around US$ 16,000.

ical integration.[3] By this method, a survival gain of 46 years per 100 patients was estimated for the PC group.

The cost calculations comprised only the direct costs related to the administration of the first-line chemotherapy, i.e., administration of drugs (including their acquisition costs), hospitalization or day-hospital for the intravenous infusion, and the costs of treating episodes of febrile neutropenia (the incidence of FNE in the GOG-111 trial was 15% in the PC group and 8% in the CC group). It is claimed (without any substantiation, however) that costing was done from the social perspective. The unit cost figures were taken from a variety of sources without any explanation or justification. Thus drug acquisition prices are taken from the Red Book for the United States market, while the cost of 1 day of hospitalization (for administration of PC) and for day-hospital (for infusion of CC) were taken from two previously published studies from different countries. The cost of treating an FNE was taken from one of these studies.

By this method, an incremental cost of US$ 902,000 per 100 patients was calculated, and combining this with the estimated survival gain, an incremental cost-effectiveness ratio of US$ 19,600 results. Several sensitivity analyses were performed, but the estimated result appears to be rather stable, with the biggest change occurring if the extrapolated parts of the survival curves are excluded from the analysis (by this procedure, the cost-effectiveness ratio is reduced by around 20%).

Concluding Remarks

The main characteristics of the economic assessments of ovarian cancer treatments discussed in this chapter are summarized in Table 3.

One of the few instances of directly comparable economic evaluations is found in ovarian cancer, where two studies use the same clinical trial as their source of clinical efficacy data. The overall conclusion of the two studies is the same, namely that the gain in survival for patients with advanced disease from PC compared to CC is obtained at the expense of considerably higher direct treatment costs. Even the cost-effectiveness ratios estimated are similar, but this must be considered a mere coincidence, because the costing principles and unit cost data applied differ fundamentally.

Several other economic evaluations of the substitution of paclitaxel for cyclophosphamide in cisplatin-based chemotherapy regimens for this patient group are under way. Thus this is a rare chance of seeing whether the initial results are corroborated by (approximate) study replications in different settings and of carrying out comparative analyses of the economic evaluations

---

[3] For both curves, the extrapolated right tails contribute relatively little to the estimated area under the curve: 9% for the PC group and 15% for the CC group (this has a very long tail and actually cuts the PC curve at 60 months and a residual survival rate of about 15%, becoming the most favorable thereafter).

Table 3. Main characteristics of economic assessments dealing with ovarian cancer treatments

Reference	Disease category	Treatments examined	Main characteristics of the study
Etzioni et al. (1996)	All patients with epithelial ovarian cancer	All treatments	Cost-of-illness analysis, incidence approach Third-party payer perspective (Medicare) Source of cost data is the database linking SEER data with Medicare claims; pooling of cross-section and time series data; problem of censored cost data solved by so-called Kaplan-Meier sample estimator; costs attributable to ovarian cancer found by comparing with a group of matched controls without the disease According to stage at diagnosis, costs for regional and distant spread are about 50% higher than for local disease; for patient diagnosed with local disease, costs follow a distinct U-pattern over the survival period
Covens et al. (1996)	Patients with advanced epithelial ovarian cancer	Cisplatin-based chemotherapy with PC vs. CC	Cost-effectiveness analysis Ministry of Health perspective Efficacy data from randomized trial, showing a 50% improval of median survival from PC compared to CC; costs of CC regimen based on examination of charts for 18 patients; costs of PC derived from costs of CC by simple model based on assumption that all the gain in survival is to be found in a delay of first relapse; unit prices are official fee rates and charges The overall result is an increase in survival from PC associated with higher costs, more than three quarters of the cost difference being due to the high acquisition price of paclitaxel; the results are very sensitive to changed assumptions, but the direction does not change
Messori et al. (1996)	Patients with advanced epithelial ovarian cancer	Cisplatin-based chemotherapy with PC vs. CC	Cost-effectiveness analysis Societal perspective Long-term outcome found by extrapolating the survival curves from randomized trial; long-term follow-up costs assumed to be identical, so cost determination limited to direct costs of first-line treatment, i.e., administration of drugs, hospitalization, day-hospital, and costs of febrile neutropenic episodes; unit figures are derived from various sources, e.g., catalogue prices and published studies By the extrapolation method, a survival gain of 46 years per 100 patients is found for PC, associated with higher costs; the baseline results appear rather stable in sensitivity analyses, with biggest change if using only the censored data

PC, paclitaxel+cisplatin; CC, cyclophosphamide+cisplatin.

performed. As these new economic evaluations have not yet been finalized and published, however, it is still too early to contemplate such analyses, which will therefore be left as an exercise for the future.

Hematological Malignancies

There is a large variety of hematological malignant diseases, of which only the main forms will be included in this description. The *leukemias* are characterized by the proliferation of a single type of malignantly transformed cell in the patient's hematopoietic (blood-forming) system, while the *lymphomas* are malignant tumors of the lymph system. The incidence of the individual hematological malignancies is rather low, but their combined incidence is only exceeded by the incidence of the five to six most common solid tumors. Further, their significance for the understanding of the disease mechanisms in oncology in general and for the development of new treatment regimens has been disproportionate to their relatively modest incidence.

Leukemias

Leukemia entails a greatly increased production of useless white blood cells, usually immature cells which are not able to perform their normal functions. Some rare forms of leukemia can also attack the progenitors of red blood cells and of platelets. In the leukemias, the growth of white blood cells is so great that it takes place at the expense of other types of blood cells, so anemia and bleedings are common and early symptoms of leukemia.

The white blood cells are of various types, and an important distinction is made among the leukemias depending upon which type of white blood cells are afflicted. *Lymphocytes* are a part of the specific immune defense. These cells can recognize, fight, and destroy foreign entities that enter the human body, especially viruses, but also other antigens such as transplanted organs. This process happens either through the creation of antibodies (B lymphocytes) or through the binding of the white blood cells to the intruding body (T lymphocytes). If lymphocytes are involved, the leukemia is called *lymphocytic*. The *granulocytes* are white blood cells in the nonspecific immune defense, which can attack many different types of intruding bodies, but mainly bacteria. In the *myeloid* leukemias, the disease begins in immature *myeloid (myeloblast) cells*, which would normally develop into granulocytes.

Another distinction is made between *acute* leukemias, which are rapidly progressing diseases where the growth concerns mainly very immature white blood cells, the so-called blasts, and *chronic* leukemias, which are slowly progressing diseases dominated by blood cells that bear a greater resemblance to mature, differentiated cells. According to these two dimensions, the four main forms of leukemias may then be distinguished: acute (AML) and chronic (CML) myeloid leukemias, and acute (ALL) and chronic (CLL) lymphocytic (or nonmyeloid) leukemias.

In 1993, the incidence of all leukemias together was about 10 per 100,000 individuals in the United States. Leukemia accounts for nearly one third of all cancers in children, but less than 10% of the newly diagnosed cases per year occur in children, so the disease affects far more adults. ALL is the most common form in children, accounting for three quarters of all new cases, while it is the least common form in adults (6%). AML is the most common form in adults (54%), and accounts for one fifth of all new cases in children; thus 95% of childhood leukemia cases are acute. For children and adults combined, AML is five times more common than ALL. The variability in incidence among countries or even regions within countries is very much smaller for this than for most other cancers. For adults, nearly half of the new cases are chronic, with CLL accounting for a fourth of all cases and CML accounting for 15% of all cases. The 5-year survival rates for some types of leukemias have improved quite considerably during the last 30 years or so. The most impressive improvement in survival rates is seen for young children aged 2–10 years with ALL, for whom the 5-year survival rate has increased from about 50% in the mid-1970s to more than 70% in the late 1980s.

Acute Leukemias

Acute leukemias seem to arise when the normal process of cell maturation (differentiation) is interrupted at a very early (blast) stage of the cell's life. The result is an accumulation in the bone marrow and also in the blood of blast cells, i.e., immature, nonfunctional blood cells which are not able to carry out the various specialized functions of normal, differentiated blood cells. Ultimately, the leukemia cells replace most of the normal hematopoietic cells, producing the symptoms of the disease, of which the most prominent is bone marrow failure and the consequent infections, bleedings, and anemia.

The acute leukemias are the most carefully studied and characterized of all tumors, despite a relatively modest incidence of 5 per 100,000. This intensive research effort may partly be due to the very high fatality rate of untreated disease (a 90% mortality rate within 1 year of diagnosis), which requires immediate institution of treatment upon diagnosis. Partly, it may be because the disease itself has many resemblances with the major complicating factors in the treatment modalities of other tumors, especially chemotherapy but also radiotherapy. The intensive study of the disease, in combination with recent discoveries with regard to the functioning of the hematopoietic system (the role of growth factors, stem cells, and progenitor cells), the existence of oncogenes, and other factors have given many valuable biologic and therapeutic insights.

The cornerstone of treatment for both diseases is chemotherapy, which is used for induction of remission of the tumor and for postremission therapy. The overall goal is to eradicate the tumor cells and restore normal hematopoiesis. Induction therapy aims at attaining complete remission by causing severe bone marrow hypoplasia with very high doses of chemotherapy. This will allow the residual normal stem cells the opportunity to regrow faster than the leukemia cells and to restore normal neutrophil and platelet counts and hemoglobin level in the patient's blood. The attainment of complete remission is a necessary step in a curative strategy, and the ability to attain this has been directly correlated with survival.

Supportive care is absolutely essential in the induction therapy phase of acute leukemias, because both the disease and the treatment interfere with the patient's ability to produce red and white blood cells and platelets, which leaves the patient at great risk of life-threatening infections and fatal bleeding. The primary causes of death in leukemia patients are infections and serious bleedings, and advances in supportive care measures are important factors in the improvements of the care of leukemia patients seen in recent years. Supportive care may include transfusions of red blood cells and platelets and aggressive empirical antimicrobial therapy from the very first signs of infection. The need for empirical antimicrobial therapy of patients with infections is not disputed, but there is considerable controversy about the value of many newer measures in supportive care, such as infection prophylaxis, the use of protected or isolated environments, and the use of the hematopoietic growth factors (the colony-stimulating factors, CSFs) to accelerate the recovery of neutrophils.

Postremission therapy aims at preventing relapse and achieving actual cure. Normally, the clinical response to induction therapy is of a temporary nature, because it fails to achieve adequate cell death, and leukemia cells survive the initial treatment. Several approaches to postremission therapy exist and have been examined in a number of studies. *Consolidation therapy* is the term used to refer to postremission regimens given immediately after induction therapy and with doses similar to those used in induction. *Intensification therapy* aims at eradicating minimal residual disease with high doses of cytotoxics, while *maintenance therapy* refers to the administration of weaker doses of cytotoxics over prolonged periods of time, e.g., 2 years or more.

Currently, standard induction therapy for AML is based on a combination of cytarabine (Ara-C) and an anthracycline (e.g., idarubicine) with complete remission rates of 50%–75%. Cytarabine is the most important drug in the treatment of AML, and a large part of the clinical research in this field in the last 20 years has been concerned with improving the efficacy of this drug by combining it with various other cytotoxics, changing its dose and schedule etc. Dose intensification of cytarabine is the central idea of many recent trials, but this invariably results in greater toxicity, which to a certain extent may limit the use of this strategy (especially for elderly patients). The use of hematopoietic growth factors (CSFs) may support the intensification of the chemotherapy by allowing a faster recovery of the patient's neutrophil count, but this option is still the subject of clinical trials.

The benefits of postremission therapy have been demonstrated by several randomized trials, but the optimal form of this therapy is somewhat controversial. A clear benefit has been shown for brief courses of intensive consolidation compared to long-term maintenance therapy with lower doses, so currently interest centers on intensification of postremission therapy, while maintenance therapy is considered as of no interest in AML. One possibility for obtaining a dose intensification is the use of bone marrow transplantation (BMT)[1] in order to rescue the patient from the consequences of bone marrow failure after being given myeloablative doses of chemotherapy (possibly in combination with whole-body irradiation) in order to maximize cell death. Several recent comparisons between high-dose cytarabine regimens and BMT have consistently shown no difference in overall survival, while the BMT group has a lower relapse rate but higher morbidity and mortality.

Eventually, most AML patients relapse and die from the disease, with a median survival of only a few months after a second remission has been achieved. For patients in first relapse or second remission, BMT has been shown to prolong the period of disease-free survival. The optimal timing of BMT is controversial, but in any case, most patients are not candidates for either of the two types of BMT, and for these patients the goal is to obtain a second remission. The worst prognosis is for patients relapsing before 12 months after first remission, and the very early relapsers are not likely to respond to any known chemotherapy. A second remission is achieved for 30%–50% of the patients, while the prognosis for patients failing this is very bad and response to salvage regimens is rare.

The treatment of ALL normally consists of four main elements: induction, consolidation, and maintenance therapy plus prophylaxis of relapses in the central nervous system (CNS).[2] Standard induction regimens include four or five agents, based on additions to a combination of vincristine and prednisone, without any evidence of superiority of any particular of these. Complete remission rates of 65%–85% are reached, but only about a quarter of the patients prove to be cured of the disease by the induction.

Consolidation therapy is given with many different drugs in varying sequences, most often with cytarabine included in the combination. The evidence from randomized trials of the value of consolidation is very limited, although most authors believe it to be beneficial. In pediatric ALL, prolonged maintenance therapy for 2–3 years has been clearly documented to be necessary, while its value for adults has been less clearly demonstrated, although the evidence is suggestive. Such protracted maintenance chemotherapy is a

[1] See the chapter on "Supportive Care II: Hematological Support" for a more complete description of the use of allogeneic or autologous BMT as supportive care.

[2] The CNS is one of the so-called sanctuary sites, into which systemically administered cytotoxics do not penetrate easily, because of the brain-blood barrier. This leads to an elevated risk of local relapse.

unique feature of ALL among all the cancers treatable by this modality, where the treatment courses normally stretch over 3–6 months. Without CNS prophylaxis, the cumulative risk of CNS involvement is about 35% over the course of disease. Prophylaxis with intrathecal chemotherapy (possibly combined with whole-brain irradiation) reduces this incidence to 10%, without any demonstrated impact on the risk of systemic relapse or on overall survival.

In the treatment of relapsed patients (60%–70% of those obtaining complete remission) and of patients refractory to the current standard induction regimens (10%–25% of all patients), numerous regimens have been used, the most successful of which seems to be a combination of high-dose cytarabine and an anthracycline, with complete remission rates of about 70%. However, most patients relapse again, and each successive response tends to be briefer than the preceding one. The potential of allogeneic BMT seems more limited in ALL than in AML, because there is a high relapse rate among patients surviving the transplantation, while this is an uncommon event in AML. Two large randomized comparisons of allogeneic BMT and standard chemotherapy for ALL patients in first remission showed no differences in overall survival. Autologous BMT in these patients is considered experimental but not very promising, as both randomized and nonrandomized evidence so far has shown no survival benefit compared to standard chemotherapy.

Many investigators are examining the potential role in the management of acute leukemias of several modern noncytotoxic agents designed to alter the biology or growth of the leukemia cells or to kill them by immunologic means. Generally, there are promising clinical results with nonspecific immunostimulators such as interferon and interleukin (IL)-2 and genetically engineered humanized antibodies, but so far the evidence of efficacy has not been corroborated by results from randomized clinical trials.

Chronic Leukemias

In the chronic leukemias, too many mature white blood cells are produced and accumulated in the body. Early in the disease, the cells retain some ability to differentiate and perform essential functions, but over longer periods of time these abilities seem to be lost, the cells becoming more abnormal and less functional. These diseases develop slowly and often with no symptoms. CLL is the most common leukemia, with an annual incidence of about 3 per 100,000 in the United States, and together they account for over 40% of all leukemias. The incidence of CLL is clearly age related, with an average age at diagnosis of 60 years compared with 45 years for CML. Twice as many men as women are affected by CLL, while there are no sex differences in the incidence of CML.

In CLL, the lymphocytes multiply very slowly but in a poorly regulated manner, and they live much longer than normal and are unable to perform their proper functions. The lymphocytes accumulate in blood, bone marrow, lymph nodes, and spleen, resulting in an enlargement of the organs and decreased bone marrow function. The natural course of CLL varies greatly, with rapid progression in some patients and very slow and asymptomatic progression in others. The ability to identify the two types of patients has improved in recent years. The median survival of untreated patients is believed to be approximately 6 years. The observation that many patients can live for long periods without requiring therapeutic intervention, coupled with the assumption that older patients cannot tolerate aggressive chemotherapy and the fact that CLL cannot be cured with current chemotherapy, has led to a generally conservative attitude to treatment, which is usually palliative in character.

The standard treatment of CLL is chlorambucil, with or without prednisone. Several trials comparing this combination or chlorambucil alone with several other regimens and in various doses and schedules of administration have been performed, with median survival up to around 6 years. Until the end of the 1980s, no cytotoxics other than the alkylating agents (particularly chlorambucil) and corticosteroids had been shown to have any activity in CLL, so no effective salvage regimen was available for patients not responding to or becoming refractory to the traditional treatments. Recently, however, the purine analogues, particularly fludarabine, have been shown to have considerable activity in both refractory and previously untreated CLL patients. In comparative trials with conventional treatments, fludarabine has been shown to achieve a much higher response rate and a significant gain in event-free survival but without any difference in overall survival. A number of studies of various combinations of purine analogues are under way, and strategies to increase their activity by reducing their major toxicities (myelosuppression and immunosuppression leading to opportunistic infections) are being examined.

CML is a form of chronic leukemia that eventually progresses to an acute phase. The disease has three distinct phases: an initial chronic phase, a transient accelerated phase, and a blast phase. In the initial chronic phase, abnormal granulocytes multiply but usually retain their ability to differentiate and perform specialized essential functions. Some patients go through a transient accelerated phase in which the cells gradually lose this ability and blast cells accumulate; in the blast phase, more than 30% of the cells in the blood or bone marrow are blast cells. If the blast phase occurs abruptly, it is referred to as a "blast crisis," which is very similar to aggressive acute leukemia, although more difficult to treat. Most patients are diagnosed in the chronic phase of the disease, and the median survival from diagnosis is about 4 years. CML is invariably a fatal disease with conventional therapy, but some patients may have a prolonged course.

Patients in the chronic phase with nearly normal blood counts may receive no further treatment other than careful monitoring until progression occurs. Chronic-phase patients respond well to standard chemotherapy, usually with one of the two agents busulfan or hydroxyurea. Recent studies indicate that hydroxyurea is superior and should be preferred. These patients may lead normal lives, although some treatment of symptoms may be required (e.g., resection of a severely enlarged spleen). It has recently been shown that interferon may control blood counts and enlarged spleen and may result in prolonged remission. Some recent randomized trials comparing interferon and conventional chemotherapy have shown a significant survival gain in the interferon group, but this difference is not seen invariably in all studies.

The only existing potentially curative treatment of chronic-phase disease is high-dose chemotherapy with whole-body irradiation and allogeneic BMT. Over 4,000 patients with CML have received allogeneic BMT. For patients undergoing BMT in the chronic phase of disease, the disease-free 5-year survival rate is 50%–60%, and fewer than 20% of patients have relapses. The best results are seen for young patients and those undergoing BMT within 1 year of diagnosis, but the optimal timing of BMT in these patients is controversial, as it involves weighing the risks and potential benefits of early BMT against the risk of delaying the BMT (i.e., the risk of the disease moving into a progressive phase, mainly blast crisis). For clinically stable patients, there is a relatively constant risk of transformation into the acute phase of 25% per year. Some prognostic factors have been identified, and early allogeneic BMT is recommended for patients with average or poor prognosis. Following the preliminary data indicating the possible benefits of interferon, some centers delay BMT for about 1 year in order to see whether the patient responds to interferon. If this fails, the patient can subsequently be referred for allogeneic BMT.

However, more than half the patients are not eligible for allogeneic BMT or are not responsive to interferon. In these patients, intensive chemotherapy supported by autologous BMT has been studied for the last 10 years. When the preparations used for reinfusion are purged (removal of the leukemic cells from the autologous cell transplants), complete remission is achieved in 20% of these patients, but it is usually of short duration (median, 12 months). Patients in the accelerated phase or in blast crisis have a poor prognosis with conventional treatment, i.e., intensification of the chemotherapy regimen which they received in the chronic phase. Median survival is less than 3 months, and few survive past 1 year. Allogeneic BMT is generally not very successful in these patients, with a relapse rate of approximately 60%, but a minority of 10%–20% of these patients may achieve long-term disease-free survival.

Lymphomas

Malignant lymphomas are cancers in which the malignant cells are in the lymph system of the body, i.e., the anatomic basis of the immune apparatus. As there is lymph tissue almost all over the body, lymphomas can start in almost any part and the cancer can spread to almost any organ or tissue, including the liver, bone marrow, and spleen. There are two major subgroups of lymphomas, Hodgkin's disease and non-Hodgkin's lymphomas, the latter of which are also sometimes called lymphocytic lymphomas, because 98% of these lymphomas are of lymphocytic origin. Non-Hodgkin's lymphomas are about five times more frequent than Hodgkin's disease.

In the EU countries, the incidence of the lymphomas is barely high enough to rank it among the ten most common cancers, but in the United States the incidence is much higher, ranking them as the fifth most common cancer in men and one of the cancers with the largest increase in incidence over recent decades, with a 50% increase in incidence from 1973 to 1988. The impact of the disease in terms of loss of expected life-years and also economically (because of the loss of production as determined in cost-of-illness studies, COI; see "A Brief Introduction to Economic Evaluation") is, however, much higher than the ranking according to incidence suggests, because the average age of the lymphoma population is low (42 years). Part of the increase in incidence can probably be ascribed to lymphomas developing in association with acquired immunodeficiency syndrome (AIDS), but in the United States there has been a steady increase of about the same relative size in all age-groups. For Hodgkin's disease, the prognosis has been greatly improved, with a fall in mortality of 50% from the mid-1970s. In contrast, the mortality rates for non-Hodgkin's disease have been slightly increasing, despite apparent improvements in therapy.

Non-Hodgkin's Disease

Non-Hodgkin's lymphomas are a very heterogeneous group of malignancies of the lymph system with widely divergent patterns of behavior and responses to treatment. Before the advent of modern techniques such as genetic analysis and immunophenotyping, it was assumed that non-Hodgkin's lymphoma was a single disease with a wide spectrum of clinical manifestations and histological characteristics. This belief led to multiple classification systems being used around the world, making international comparisons very difficult. At the beginning of the 1980s, an international collaborative group developed a common classification, the Working Formulation, in which each of ten specific subtypes of lymphomas were further subdivided into three prognostic groups, i.e., low, intermediate, and high grade.

However, it has since become clear that each of these subtypes contain several distinct diseases with varying etiology, natural course, response to treatment etc. Recently, the International Lymphoma Study Group reached consensus about a new classification system, the Revised European-American Classification (REAL), containing the diseases which are recognizable with the currently available (imperfect) analysis techniques and understanding of the immune system. This new classification distinguishes three major categories of malignant lymphomas: B-cell neoplasms, T/natural killer (NK)-cell neoplasms, and Hodgkin's disease. This classification includes both lymphomas and lymphocytic leukemias, as these are in many cases merely different manifestations of the same neoplasm. The diseases in the main categories, B- and T/NK-cell neoplasms, are further subdivided according to their natural course, being classified as indolent if survival is measured in years and as aggressive or highly aggressive, respectively, if survival is measured in months or weeks. In adults, 85% of new cases are B-cell lymphomas and 15% T/NK-cell neoplasms, while in children two thirds are T/NK-cell neoplasms.

Another international collaborative effort has been working on the development of a prognostic factor model with data from patients with aggressive disease treated from 1982 to 1987 with a doxorubicin regimen. Increasing age is an important factor augmenting the risk. Low-risk patients over 60 years old have a 5-year survival of 56%, while this rate is 83% for patients 60 years old or younger. The corresponding risks for high-risk patients are 21% and 32%, respectively.

Choice of treatment strategy for the non-Hodgkin's lymphoma patients depends on the specific type of neoplasm, the stage of disease, and the prognostic status of the patient. Given that, according to the REAL classification, the clinical grouping of non-Hodgkin's lymphomas comprises 19 different entities, the current options and results are not easily summarized. Only two of these entities comprise a large number of patients, however, each accounting for about a third of newly diagnosed adult lymphomas, and these two will be summarized below. The residual third of the patients is spread fairly evenly over the remaining 17 disease entities. In general, the options for patients with indolent disease include a "wait and see" policy with careful follow-up, radiotherapy alone, chemotherapy in various forms (single agent or combination, mild or aggressive), or antibiotics. Patients with aggressive disease are treated with combination chemotherapy, possibly supplemented with radiotherapy. Patients with highly aggressive disease are treated with regimens also used in ALL, including prophylaxis of CNS relapse.

A total of 35% of adult patients have indolent disease in the form of follicular B-cell lymphoma. For patients with early stage (I and II) localized disease, the treatment of choice is radiotherapy, while several randomized trials have failed to show an improvement in overall survival from the addition of combination chemotherapy. Relapse-free survival rates at 10 and 20 years of around 40% are seen. The treatment choice for patients with advanced disease is controversial. They respond to single-agent and combination chemotherapy, radiotherapy, and combined modalities, but the duration of complete remission is short, with a median of 2 years. Nonetheless, many series have reported median survival periods of more than 9 years. The approach to treatment diverges between a conservative with no immediate treatment followed by palliative chemotherapy or radiotherapy at disease progression and an aggressive approach with combination chemotherapy, radiotherapy, or both. In terms of overall survival, there is no evidence supporting one or the other of these approaches.

More than a fourth of the follicular lymphomas undergo a transformation to a more aggressive subtype of disease with a more diffuse (less differentiated) pattern and more large cells. Reported median survival periods after such transformation vary from 2 to 12 months, with most longer-term survivors having been treated with doxorubicin-containing chemotherapy.

Several new agents are under investigation in the treatment of indolent follicular lymphomas. The purine analogues, including fludarabine, alone or in combination, have resulted in high response rates. A number of studies suggest a significant benefit of interferon-α in these patients, e.g., used as a maintenance therapy after standard combination chemotherapy. High-dose chemotherapy with stem cell transplantation in the form of autologous BMT has been used both for recurrent follicular lymphomas and as primary treatment for newly diagnosed patients with advanced disease. The preliminary results are considered promising, but the potential value of this treatment has not yet been determined precisely.

A total of 30% of the patients have large B-cell lymphoma, which is an aggressive disease. The optimal treatment for patients with early stage (I and II) disease is controversial, but the efficacy of combination chemotherapy has been well established. There is also some support for a combined modality with adjuvant radiotherapy, which may allow a reduction in the number of cycles of chemotherapy. For patients with advanced disease, combination chemotherapy is the treatment of choice. Recent randomized trials have shown no gain from so-called second- and third-generation chemotherapy regimens compared to the first-generation regimen developed in the 1970s, which is still the standard induction therapy. However, the 5-year survival rates are no higher than 35%–40%, and there is a great need for experimental treatments.

Careful selection of the patients for experimental treatment is necessary and possible due to the aforementioned risk factor analyses. Thus low-risk patients have a 5-year survival rate with standard therapy of 73% and thus have far less to gain from participating in experimental treatments than high-risk patients with a 5-year survival rate of 26%. In particular, younger high-risk patients are considered candidates for experimental treatments, as they are expected to tolerate intensive treatment better. The experimental approaches so far have focused on increasing the doses of chemotherapy with or without additional radiotherapy and hematopoietic stem cell support. The intensified therapy is either given as induction or consolidation therapy. It is still too early to give a final evaluation of either of these approaches.

Hodgkin's Disease

About one sixth of all patients diagnosed with malignant lymphomas have Hodgkin's disease, in which the cancer cells have a very characteristic form. The special multinuclear giant cells seen in the patients were described by Reed and Sternberg around the year 1900, but Thomas Hodgkin is credited with the original recognition in the 1830s that the disease should be considered as a primary disease and not as a secondary response to inflammation. The incidence of this disease has been falling slightly, but this is mainly due to a more accurate diagnosis of the lymphomas. The treatment regimens used and the prognosis for the patients are much better than for patients with the other lymphomas, as more than 75% of all newly diagnosed adult patients are curable with radiation therapy and/or chemotherapy. Improvements in both these treatment modalities during the last decades have brought about a decrease of about 65% in the mortality of Hodgkin's disease patients in the United States, which is more rapid than for any other malignancy. The most important prognostic factors for any given patient seem to be the presence or absence of systemic symptoms, the stage of disease, and the quality and suitability of the treatment administered.

The stage plays a critical role in the selection of treatment and the recommended staging procedures are extensive, comprising biopsy, CT and MRI scanning, and sometimes laparectomy in addition to history taking and physical examination. Some of the possible staging procedures, in particular laparectomy, may cause severe morbidity, and their use should be guided by considerations of the probabilities that a more precise staging will enable a significant reduction of the treatment given.

For patients with the most localized disease (there is per definition involvement of lymph nodes in lymphomas), i.e., stages IA, IB, and IIA, radiotherapy is considered the treatment of choice. Other options are chemotherapy alone or combined with radiotherapy. For stage IIB patients, in whom the risk of occult abdominal disease is considerable, the optimal choice is considered to be combination chemotherapy, possibly supplemented with radiotherapy. For patients with disseminated disease (stage III or IV), combination chemotherapy with one of three equally effective drug combinations and schedules should be the treatment of choice. Some trials indicate, without being definitive, that a combined modality with chemotherapy followed by radiotherapy might be superior, but this depends on the degree of dissemination of the disease. Radiation is especially indicated for areas with initially bulky disease. With the excellent survival rates obtainable with current treatments, ongoing trials are concerned with minimizing treatment-related side effects, while no major improvements in survival are foreseen.

Patients who relapse after initial radiation therapy have a good prognosis, because salvage combination chemotherapy results in 10-year disease-free and overall survival rates of about 57% and 80%, respectively. However, patients relapsing after initial combination chemotherapy have a rather poor prognosis, especially if they relapse within the first 12 months after the initial treatment. Late relapsers (later than 12 months) have long-term survival rates with salvage chemotherapy of 22%–45%, while the long-term survival rate for early relapsers is only 11%. For (the majority of) patients with more than limited nodal recurrence following initial chemotherapy, participation in one of the ongoing clinical trials using high-dose chemotherapy and autologous BMT and/or peripheral blood stem cell transplantation (PBSCT) is recommended. Some earlier trials of these regimens have resulted in a 3- to 4-year disease-free survival rate of 27%–47% Other experimental treatments which have shown promising potential, although the experience with them is not extensive, include radiolabeled immunoglobulin therapy and monoclonal antibodies.

Economic Evaluations

By far the majority of the published studies are concerned with adult AML, which is not unexpected considering the epidemiology of the disease and the orientation of the clinical research being performed. Only few studies dealing with lymphomas have been published (and most are treated in other chapters of this report, especially in the following chapter on supportive care).

Tenvall et al. (1994) calculated the direct and indirect COI in Sweden due to AML using the traditional Human Capital-based approach to COI analyses. The calculations were based on a multistage model of the disease and treatment process, showing the flow of a given cohort of patients through the various possible stages and end points. All patients were assumed to receive induction chemotherapy after diagnosis. Some achieved complete remission, others died as a result of the toxicity of the treatment, and some were refractory (this group is not followed any further). The patients in complete remission received consolidation therapy, and of these some died, while others survived this initial phase of the treatment. Of these, some had an early relapse, while others received maintenance chemotherapy and/or allogeneic or autologous BMT. In each of these groups, a number of patients relapse, and this is the end point of the model.

The probabilities and rates for the transitions between the various phases of the model were taken from a number of different sources, most often by taking a round number more or less midway between the extreme values found in studies in the literature with no further justification or discussion. An overall complete remission rate of 70% was assumed (45% after one course of induction therapy); the refractory rate was 15%, and the mortality rate was 10% under each course of induction and 3% under consolidation therapy, resulting in 15% of the patients diagnosed dying during initial therapy. For patients surviving this, a rate of early relapse and death of 15% was assumed.

The cost estimates are based on information about treatment procedures and their costs from a recent Swedish retrospective study of 18 patients receiving autologous or allogeneic BMT and on records of accounts from Swedish regional hospitals and assumptions. Thus it was assumed that each patient received 1.45 induction courses, with an average treatment time of 42 inpatient days and an average cost of about SKr 380,000, and so on for all the other stages of the model. The calculations were performed for 1989, when 275 patients were diagnosed with AML in Sweden. For the 36% of the patients that were under 65 years, indirect costs were calculated based on the average income per day, including non-wage labor costs. Morbidity costs were calculated based on assumptions about the average length of sick leave for patients in the various stages. Mortality costs due to premature deaths (before the age of 65) were calculated according to the actual deaths of AML at various ages by means of life expectancy tables for the general population and data on the average yearly incomes of the different age categories. All direct costs were assumed to occur within 1 year of diagnosis, while indirect costs were discounted by a rate of 5%.

The average total cost was estimated to be about SKr 1.7 million per diagnosed patient.[3] For all the 275 patients in 1989 combined, the direct costs were estimated to be SKr 225 million, divided into 130 million for initial therapy, 51 million for relapse, and 19 million for maintenance therapy. Total indirect costs are a little higher, i.e., SKr 236 million, most of these, 213 million, or 775,000 for the average patient, being due to premature mortality.

The costs of obtaining a complete remission for AML patients with a conventional induction chemotherapy (daunorubicin+cytosine arabinoside, DNR-AraC) were calculated by Marie et al. (1992a,b), based on a retrospective examination of patient charts and notes for 15 patients treated in one institution between 1987 and 1989. The patients were hospitalized in a single room without laminar air flow, and the costs were evaluated from the first day of hospitalization to achievement of CR, which 11 patients obtained after the first induction and four patients after the second, which was given 28 days after the first. A total of 228 different cost items were identified. Laboratory costs (89 items) were determined based on the total number of tests for each patient using the official national price list for hospitals and clinics for each item. Supportive treatment (135 items) included blood and platelet transfusions, antibiotics, intravenous fluids, antiemetics etc., costed by using the full price charged by the pharmacy and the blood bank. The cytotoxic drugs were costed by using the full price charged by the pharmacy. General costs of hospital accommodation, including a proportion of the administrative costs shared by all patients admitted, were based on figures provided by the hospital administration.

Basic resource utilization data are taken from the EORTC AML8 trial, which showed that for patients obtaining complete remission in one course the average length of hospitalization was 33 (±5) days, with 16 (±8) of these on antibiotics. The number of transfusions given was ten (±4) for blood and 41 (±18) for platelets. Similar data, including the range, are given for patients needing two courses to obtain complete remission. The estimated costs were approximately[4] US$ 16,700 (±4400) for one induction course and US$ 37,000 (±5000) for two. The greater than proportional increase when going from one course of induction chemotherapy to two was primarily due to the need to increase the level of supportive care, e.g., transfusions and antibiotics, while the increase in ordinary hospitalization costs were less than proportional. The data shows that the direct costs per day for an AML patient do not diminish with the length of stay, and the total costs are strictly correlated with the duration of hospitalization. For patients obtaining complete remission in one course, general hospitalization costs represent about 57% of the direct costs, and the total drug costs about 11%. The cytotoxics

[3] About US$ 225,000 if the PPPs of 1990 are used for the conversion.

[4] The cost calculations in FF were converted to US$ by the authors, using the mean exchange rate during the study period.

themselves accounted for about 12% of all the drug costs or 1% of the total direct costs.

A somewhat more comprehensive costing study for AML patients was published by Brodin and Stalfelt (1993), based on a retrospective extraction of information for 54 newly diagnosed AML patients treated in a specific hospital during 1981–1988 (accrual ended in September 1987, but follow-up continued to the end of 1988). The study aims at including all the activities performed in the management of the patients, except the costs for BMT (only one patient). Most of the patients were treated with standard combination chemotherapy regimens, and patients achieving complete remission were given maintenance chemotherapy with various regimens. In both cases, the regimens varied according to the patient's age (over and under 60). Patients who relapsed were given new courses of induction therapy, and all patients were given supportive treatment, comprising prophylactic treatment with acyclovir, nystatin, and allopurinol, intensive antibiotic therapy, and blood products, whenever needed, and often dental hygiene services were required.

Dates of admission and discharge from the oncology center or from relevant local hospitals were registered, and the frequency and amount of each item of care and treatment were registered. Altogether, 304 types of activities were registered and subsequently grouped into one of 14 different cost groups for each day of active treatment; days on which no active treatment was given were registered as being without costs. For the costing, the prices that most laboratories or departments had for internal billing were used, as they are believed to be good approximations of the average costs for the tests and other activities and also to give a better reflection of the marginal costs for the individual patients than if the total overhead costs of the service departments involved in the management of AML patients had been included. Costs that could not reasonably be assigned to an individual patient were included in so-called basic costs, including general administrative and technical services and bed service costs, including food, laundry, cleaning, transport etc. Patient-specific costs, e.g., for laboratory tests, X-rays etc., were allocated to the individual patients and then added to the basic and bed service costs, which were calculated according to the dates of admission and discharge.

A total of 59% of the patients achieved complete remission, and for these patients the median survival was 87 weeks, while it was about 7 weeks for the patients not achieving complete remission. Fourteen patients were still alive when the data collection stopped, and these had survived for at least 14 months. The average cost per patient was about SKr 303,000 (about US$ 40,000 if the PPPs of 1990 are used), with the highest individual costs being SKr 962,000 for a patient surviving nearly 5 years after diagnosis. For the 40 patients that died during the observation period, the median survival was 25 weeks and the average total costs SKr 285,000 (median, 245,000). For those of the patients who achieved complete remission, the median survival was 56 weeks and average total costs were SKr 446,000, while the corresponding figure was 153,000 for the patients not achieving remission. The average cost per patient decreased with increasing age, reflecting a decreased probability of achieving complete remission.

A couple of studies focus on calculating the costs of treatment in childhood leukemias, one of them (Baranko 1994) being limited to a comparison of the costs of the protocol-mandated laboratory and radiographic examinations up till 5 years after diagnosis for two clinical trial protocols in ALL. This calculation, which shows consistent and rather high differences in the charges for all patients, is very partial and therefore of only limited interest, as it excludes charges for medications, hospitalization, professional fees for physician services etc.

Phillips et al. (1991) attempted to estimate the impact in terms of resources consumed and treatment results of the intensification of treatment in childhood AML that has taken place during the 1980s. The estimation was based on a retrospective examination of the case reports for an unselected case series of all patients referred to treatment at the authors' institution. The patients are divided into two groups, comprising children treated between 1972 and 1982 and those treated between 1983 and 1987, respectively, because the management strategy was changed at the beginning of the 1980s. The clinical and hematological features at presentation were compared in the two groups, and the length of time spent in hospital and the number of courses of chemotherapy were calculated for each child; in addition, the possible need for antifungal therapy with amphotericin B was noted.

Patients in the earliest treatment group (n=99) had received a variety of schedules of combination chemotherapy drug regimens. They were largely managed on an outpatient basis after (or even during) the first course of induction chemotherapy, and those who developed neutropenia were given empirical intravenous antibiotic therapy, while there were no strict guidelines concerning commencement of systemic antifungal therapy. Only four patients in this group underwent allogeneic BMT. Patients in the later group (n=53) had for the most part been on a protocol for a clinical trial, receiving more intensive treatment with induction therapy (cytarabine + daunoru-bi-cine + oral thioguanine), consolidation therapy with the same regimen but reduced dose, and later a maintenance regimen plus several other forms of support treatment. All episodes of fever and neutropenia were investigated and treated promptly with broad-spectrum intravenous antibiotics, and children with persistent fever of unknown origin received intravenous amphotericin B. A fifth of these patients received BMT. All patients were followed up until 1990.

The authors considered the two groups to be comparable, despite significantly more children under the age of 2 in the later group. Between the two periods, an improvement in the outcomes of treatment was seen, with an increase in event-free survival from 12% to 45%, a fall in the rate of early deaths from 13% to 7%, and a fall in the rate of cytotoxic failure from 20% to 6%. The relapse rate was more than 50% in the earlier group, while it was about one third in the later group at the end of the (much shorter) follow-up. The improvements in outcome were accompanied by the following increases in resource utilization, which have not been valued in pecuniary terms: The *median* number of days in hospital increased from 35 to 170, of antibiotic courses from two to seven, of antifungal courses from none to three, and of days with total parenteral nutrition from none to 55. Analysis of the children in the later group showed no relationship between the outcome and presenting leukocyte count, sex, or FAB type (the French–American–British classification of leukemias), but younger children had a significantly better prognosis (p=0.04).

Two studies are concerned with determining the relative cost-effectiveness of the two cytotoxic drugs idarubicin and daunorubicin, in combination with cytarabine (cytosine arabinoside) in the treatment of AML. Pashkoet et al. (1991) based their analysis on the data from a single-institution randomized trial of the two combination drug regimens in first induction treatment (and second induction, if one induction was not enough), while postinduction treatments and the treatment offered to nonresponders were not included. Computerized clinical reports for each of the 120 patients in the trial were used to determine the consumption of resources on an individual basis, from the first day of induction therapy to the time when remission status was determined or until death or hospital discharge, whichever occurred first. The calculation only comprised the use of hospital resources, but even these are not complete, as physical, occupational, and respiratory therapy were excluded due to lack of data. The cost calculation was based on estimated average national hospital charges (cost plus markup) for each item. Laboratory charges were taken from a list of national medical laboratories, marked up to reflect hospital charges, and medication prices were derived from the average wholesale price, again marked up to reflect hospital charges. All other prices were derived from a proprietary national survey of hospitals.

With 60 patients that could be evaluated in each group, the overall rate of complete remission was higher in the idarubicin group and their survival was significantly longer, 19.7 vs. 13.5 months in the daunorubicin group. Four patients in each group died during the induction therapy. The mean total charges per patient in the first induction therapy and in the intermediate period before a possible second induction therapy were significantly higher for the idarubicin patients, while the average charges for idarubicin patients in the second induction therapy were significantly lower. Overall, the total charges per treated patient showed almost no difference, but the mean charge per complete remission achieved becomes significantly lower for idarubicin, about \$ 74,600 vs. 102,000 for the daunorubicin group. Based on the median survival of the patients that could be evaluated, the hospital charges per year of life were \$ 36,300 for the idarubicin patients and \$ 52,700 for the daunorubicin patients. The sensitivity of the results was investigated using the nonidentical results of two other randomized trials (both favoring idarubicin), but the overall conclusion of the analysis is not affected by this. Thus idarubicin seems to be a dominant solution, offering an improvement in outcome at no extra cost.

Essentially the same conclusion was reached by Lobo et al. (1991) using a rather unusual analysis design. From a retrospective study of the case notes of ten patients with AML, 160 specific cost items were identified and categorized into one of four groups: general costs, diagnostic costs, chemotherapy costs, and costs of supportive treatment. In order to determine the unit cost of each of these 160 items, a prospective time and motion study was conducted for 1 month on one patient. Using these data and the rather detailed data on patient management from the MRC9 trial comparing the two regimens with idarubicin and daunorubicin, respectively, the total costs of one and two cycles of induction therapy were calculated. The MRC trial, with 268 patients, yielded the mean length of stay in hospital, the mean number of transfusions of blood and platelets, and the mean number of days that antibiotics were given during one and two cycles of induction therapy. The frequency with which each cost item (e.g., routine hematological and biochemical tests, chest X-ray) was given during one cycle (32 days) and two cycles (56 days) was determined, and by multiplying this with the unit prices determined, the total costs of treatment in one or two cycles were calculated.

These total treatment costs were then used to determine the relative cost-effectiveness of idarubicin and daunorubicin based on the efficacy data from four international randomized trials, which all came out in favor of idarubicin, but only in one case with a statistically significant difference (at 5%). The calculations are performed with data for each of the four trials individually and with a weighted average, the weights being determined by the relative number of patients that could be evaluated in the trials. However, all the results go in the same direction, so only the result with the averaged data will be described. The overall treatment costs per patient were almost identical for the two regimens, idarubicin being 5% cheaper. The higher cost of cytotoxic chemotherapy with idarubicin (about £ 600 per patient) was more than offset by lower general, diagnostic, and supportive treatment costs. The average cost per complete remission was about £ 28,000 for idarubicin and £ 35,400 for daunorubicin, equivalent to $ 67,000 and $ 84,000 respectively.[5] No data are given for a more final and less intermediate outcome, such as the gain in survival, with or without quality adjustment, but the analysis gives support to the notion that idarubicin offers a therapeutic gain at no extra cost, sometimes even with a saving in cost.

Welch and Larson (1989) performed a cost-effectiveness analysis of the relative cost-effectiveness of BMT compared to chemotherapy in AML patients, based on a retrospective analysis of a case series of 111 adult patients, who were all enrolled (between 1978 and 1982) at the time of diagnosis of AML (this procedure is claimed to reduce the potential selection bias). A total of 90 of the patients achieved complete remission after induction chemotherapy. If a related donor was available, BMT was offered at this time; if not, two courses of consolidation therapy were given, followed by two courses of intensification chemotherapy and thereafter monthly maintenance chemotherapy. The cost-effectiveness analysis was limited to the 41 patients

[5] No time period is given for the cost and price data; 1990 PPPs are used for the conversion.

who received induction chemotherapy at one single institution, of which 17 underwent transplantation, 19 had chemotherapy, and five were eligible for, but refused, transplantation and were excluded.

Five cost items were counted in the case records and used in the analysis: hospital days with and hospital days without intensive care, number of laboratory tests, number of radiological examinations, and number of procedures in operating room. An econometric equation including these variables, but excluding professional fees, was formulated to express total charges as a linear function of these variables. The model, the parameters of which are not explained in the paper, however, is used to avoid problems with varying cost-to-charge ratios if data are collected from more than one institution (a quarter of the admissions were from hospitals other than the main one), so the charge estimate used should provide a more resource-based measure of costs. Effectiveness was measured as the patients' survival time after induction therapy, and the cost-effectiveness of BMT was expressed both relative to chemotherapy and to a hypothetical "no treatment" alternative (implicitly assuming immediate death of the patient if no treatment is provided). All cost figures were adjusted to 1989 prices using a 5% discount rate.

The 5-year survival rates were 59% and 26% in the BMT and chemotherapy groups, respectively (marginally significant), while after 5 years of follow-up, the average length of survival was 3.3 years (BMT) and 2.2 years (chemotherapy). Over the same period, the chemotherapy group had seven hospitalizations vs. 4.6 for the BMT group and also spent 10% more days in hospital, although the BMT group spent significantly more time in intensive care, as they were routinely treated in intensive care units regardless of their general health. All other cost items were remarkably similar. Average total treatment costs were $ 193,000 for the BMT group and $ 136,000 for the chemotherapy group, while the estimated costs per additional year of life were about $ 60,000, regardless of whether the comparison was chemotherapy vs. nothing, BMT vs. nothing, or BMT vs. chemotherapy. At the time of study, all the survivors had been in complete remission for at least 7 years, so they were assumed to be cured, and cost-effectiveness was estimated based on normal life expectancy. The estimated costs per additional life-years were $ 22,900 for chemotherapy vs. nothing, $ 16,600 for BMT vs. nothing, and $ 10,000 for BMT vs. chemotherapy. If the gain in survival from BMT relative to chemotherapy is 40% or higher, BMT is a dominant solution, giving a survival gain at no higher cost. Otherwise, there is a positive trade-off between the survival gain and higher costs, i.e., a survival benefit can be achieved but only at the expense of an increase in costs.

Finally, a study by Ozer et al. (1989) on the use of interferon-alfa-2b in the treatment of hairy cell leukemia should be mentioned. This disorder, accounting for 2% of all leukemias in the United States, is a chronic lymphoproliferative disease characterized by the presence of leukemic cells with hair-like villous projections in the bone marrow and blood, various degrees of cytopenia and splenomegaly, and multiple defects of cellular immunity. The initial treatment of choice has been splenectomy, resulting in clinical improvement in 80%–90% of patients, about half of which, however, have subsequently developed disease progression and not responded well to chemotherapy, but suffering from the increased risk of opportunistic infections due to chemotherapy-induced immuno- and myelosuppression. Long-term survival of conventionally treated patients is reported to be about 50%, while the remainder of the patients usually die within a few years of diagnosis, the usual cause of death being infections. Interferon has induced an objective response in about 75% of the patients and minor hematological improvement in another 15%. The treatment leads to reduction in the incidence of severe hemorrhages and recurrent severe infections and to improved survival expectancy.

The study population comprised 128 patients with progressive disease treated with interferon in seven medical centers between 1982 and 1985 and was compared with a group of historical controls (believed to be eligible to receive the interferon protocol, had it been available, and therefore highly comparable to the interferon patients) who received standard treatment at two other hospitals during the 10-year period before 1982. The study patients received long-term, low-dose, self-injected interferon three times a week for at least 6 months, and transfusions were administered in the hospital outpatient clinic. Patients with mild to moderate infections were treated as outpatients, while patients with severe infections requiring parenteral treatment with multiple antibiotics were hospitalized. For the study patients, the use of medical resources was documented for a 6-month pretreatment period to establish baseline values while they were on conventional therapy, followed by a 12-month period of interferon therapy. Yearly costs are estimated, partly from the resource use documented and partly on the basis of resource consumption estimates provided by a Delphi group of experienced physicians. Unit costs for the costing are taken from a number of different sources, such as hospital rates for transfusions, wholesale prices plus a markup for drugs, and cost estimates from other studies. The present value of expected future earnings was included, employing age- and sex-specific estimates and an annual discount rate of 5%.

Over a 12-month period, 3% of the interferon patients and 28% of the controls died, primarily reflecting a change in the incidence of fatal infections, as 2% of the interferon patients had fatal infections compared to 23% of the controls. During the 6 months prior to interferon therapy, the patients required progressively increasing transfusion support, reflecting increasing severity of thrombocytopenia and anemia. Reversal of this was achieved in 73% of the interferon patients (18% of the controls), and this was paralleled by a decrease in the use of transfusions to almost none within 2–5 months after treatment was initiated. Prior to interferon treatment, the patients also had progressive exacerbation of granulocytopenia and increase in the number and severity of infections, and by the start of therapy 62% had severe granulocytopenia. The frequency of infections decreased from 31% during the first 3 months of therapy to 6% later on, and the frequency of hospital admissions decreased from 15% to 1%. The overall direct costs were estimated to be $ 5000 for the interferon patients and $ 14,000 for the controls, primarily reflecting lower costs for supportive care for the interferon patients, especially a saving in hospital admissions for severe infections. Indirect costs were reduced from $ 64,000 for the controls to $ 4500 for the interferon patients, due to the increased survival expectancy for the interferon patients.

Desch et al. (1992) used a decision analysis model to consider the question of the optimal timing of autologous BMT in patients with Hodgkin's disease who have relapsed after a first course of chemotherapy. Until recently, the only option for such relapsed patients was salvage chemotherapy with a non-cross-reactive regimen. Between 35% and 60% of the patients achieve a complete response with this strategy, but the 5-year survival rate is no higher than 25%–35%. Autologous BMT following high-dose chemotherapy seems to offer an attractive alternative to this, as some phase II trials have shown higher response rates and disease-free survival rates than have been reported in most series with salvage chemotherapy. The problem then is to determine the optimal timing of autologous BMT. In accordance with experiences with other types of tumor, autologous BMT should be administered before the development of overt drug resistance; however, there is a non-negligible transplantation-related mortality rate, ranging from 4% to 56%.

The decision analysis was based on data from the published clinical literature, which does not contain any direct comparison of the effectiveness of salvage chemotherapy and autologous BMT (ABMT). Five different strategies were considered:

1. Immediate ABMT during the first relapse
2. ABMT only if the patient achieved a complete remission with salvage chemotherapy
3. ABMT only if a patient relapsed from a salvage chemotherapy remission or did not respond to salvage chemotherapy
4. ABMT after salvage chemotherapy regardless of response
5. Salvage chemotherapy

After either ABMT or salvage chemotherapy, the patients may be in one of three clinical states, i.e., complete remission, partial remission, or toxic death. The clinical sequelae depend on the patient's state and not on the regimen, so they were identical regardless of whether the patient received ABMT or salvage chemotherapy. Survival after failing ABMT or third-line chemotherapy was not considered.

In the absence of direct clinical trials comparing the alternatives, the clinical data were taken from combined case series of salvage chemotherapy and ABMT patients, respectively. Although the regimens used in these are not identical, the data were combined by multiplying the rates from each series with its number of patients divided by the total number of patients. Some probabilities were obtained by surveying nine experienced oncologists and using the average of their estimates. Outcomes or utilities were measured in terms of discounted survival years, with arbitrary utility values assigned by the authors. As a surrogate measure of costs, a number of charges estimated from local experience or published reports were used. Four types of cost were included, in each case using convenient, rounded numbers: salvage chemotherapy (usually on an outpatient basis), ABMT (with prolonged hospital stay), early fatalities (fewer hospital days, but much more time in intensive care), and radiation (used for some patients in partial remission). Follow-up costs were assumed to be identical, while costs of possible complications were ignored because of the lack of data. Benefits were discounted, as they may occur far in the future, while the costs were not, as they occur immediately after the decision.

Considering costs alone, the regimen of salvage chemotherapy alone is by far the least expensive, but it is also one of the least effective. The least effective regimen is to administer ABMT only if the patient achieves complete remission after salvage chemotherapy. The most effective treatment strategy is to use ABMT only if a patient relapses from a complete remission after salvage chemotherapy or does not respond to salvage chemotherapy, and this is also the most cost-effective in terms of incremental costs per year of life saved compared with the strategy of salvage chemotherapy alone. The incremental cost-effectiveness ratio is $ 26,200 for the strategy of using ABMT in the second relapse, while it is $ 421,000 for a strategy of using ABMT immediately during the first relapse and $ 235,000 for the strategy of using ABMT after salvage chemotherapy regardless of the response. The rank order of the strategies is not changed by performing a number of sensitivity analyses, but the patient's prognostic category may be important if it can be estimated from clinical variables. For good-prognosis patients, ABMT in the second relapse is still the optimal strategy, but for poor-prognosis patients it is better to use chemotherapy to determine the chemosensitivity and then to use ABMT for the responders.

Norum et al. (1996) estimated the costs of treatment for Hodgkin's disease in Northern Norway and assessed the outcome of treatment in terms of quality-adjusted life-years (QALYs). By comparison with a constructed "no treatment" alternative, a kind of cost-utility analysis was performed. The "no treatment" alternative was based on the consensus reached by a panel of experts that the mean survival of untreated Hodgkin's disease patients would be 2 years with a quality-of-life score of 0.14 on a 0–1 scale. Apparently, the "no treatment" alternative is assumed not to incur any cost. This assumption will tend to inflate the cost-utility ratios calculated.

All 55 Hodgkin's disease patients treated at the only university hospital in Northern Norway between 1985 and 1993 were included in the study. The charts of these patients, comprising all stages of disease and with many different treatment regimens and modalities (chemotherapy, radiotherapy, and combinations of these), were analyzed retrospectively in terms of demographic and clinical characteristics, treatment modality, clinical outcome, and treatment costs. The resource utilization registered comprised days of hospitalization (only days needed for treatment of Hodgkin's disease), hospital hotel stays (the great geographical distances in Northern Norway often require patients to stay overnight even though hospitalization is not necessitated by the treatment), radiotherapy, cytotoxics (a standard dose is assumed for all patients), and antiemetics. In addition, travel costs of the patients are included at a fixed rate per trip. Unit prices used are gross averages (e.g., a fixed price per field of radiotherapy), provided by the financial department of the University Hospital and the national health insurance administration.

At the end of 1994, the 49 survivors were sent a questionnaire, in which they were asked to describe their present state of health and quality of life in terms of the system developed by the EuroQol group (see, e.g., Williams 1990). The system comprises a state of health description questionnaire with five dimensions (e.g., mobility, self-care) and an evaluation of the health states on a visual analogue scale from 0 to 100. For the purpose of determining the gain from treatment, it is assumed that the mean survival of patients treated for Hodgkin's disease is 20 years after diagnosis. In order to determine the gain in QALYs, the survival gain (compared with the 2 years' survival assumed for patients without treatment) is multiplied by the patients' indication of their present quality of life in the questionnaire. The mean value for the 42 patients replying (86%) was a quality-of-life score of 0.77, with only minor differences between patients in the various stages of disease.

Overall survival was 90% at 5 years and 86% at 10 years. The costs are given in British pounds, and the average health care costs for primary treatment of Hodgkin's disease were estimated to be £ 8400,[6] with no differences according to stage of disease. The average total costs were estimated at £ 12,500, with significantly higher costs for patients with more advanced disease due to a higher frequency of relapse among these. It was assumed that 65% of the patients return to the workforce for a period of 20 years, and this reduces the loss in Human Capital due to Hodgkin's disease (compared to the untreated patients). The crude gain (or reduced loss of Human Capital) was determined by first making a traditional Human Capital calculation and then taking 10% of this to allow for the arguments of the supporters of the friction cost method (see "A Brief Introduction to Economic Evaluation" and "The Economic Burden of Cancer," this volume). The production gain used in the calculations is then determined as 10% of the value found by the friction cost correction, based on the argument that the appropriate amount to use in an economic evaluation is the fraction of the overall production gain likely to end up as increased health care funding (see Olsen 1994, one of the coauthors of the study by Norum et al. 1996).

Bringing together all the different epidemiological and economic assumptions in a single model allows a calculation of cost-utility ratios in the form of incremental costs per QALY gained by treating Hodgkin's disease patients. A range of cost-utility ratios are presented, depending upon whether production gains are included (subtracted from the incremental costs of treatment)

[6] By using general (and not health care-specific) PPPs, which are published yearly, this amount corresponds to roughly US$ 13,000.

and whether future treatment benefits and costs are discounted and at what rate. A number of sensitivity analyses are also reported, the major factor influencing the value of the cost-utility ratio being the quality of life assumed for the survivors of the treatment. The largest range of values reported is from £ 550 to £ 1650 per QALY, with the highest value when both the gain in QALYs and the costs are discounted by 10%.

Concluding Remarks

The main characteristics of the economic assessments of treatments for the various hematological malignancies are summarized in Table 1.

The large majority of economic studies of hematological malignancies identified and retrieved for this survey are concerned with either AML or Hodgkin's disease, and the major focus has been on identifying all the resource items used in the management of these patients. The outcomes of treatment have not been given much consideration in these studies, and there are hardly any attempts at precise assessment of the outcomes. The principal merit of this kind of study is therefore to provide (in many cases) relatively detailed baseline information about the standard management of the various types of patients. The unit cost figures used are often suspect, but when data on resource utilization are reported separately, they may be useful for future comparative studies.

Of the full economic evaluations found, two analyze the same clinical issue, i.e., induction chemotherapy in AML patients comparing regimens containing daunorubicin or idarubicin, respectively. Despite using very different analytical approaches and sources for resource utilization and unit costs, the two studies agree in finding that idarubicin is a dominant solution for obtaining complete remission. The meaning of this unconventional use of the technical notion of domination (see "A Brief Introduction to Economic Evaluation," this volume) is in this case that the average costs per treated patient are about the same, while the frequency of complete remission is higher in the idarubicin group, implying that the average costs of obtaining a complete remission are lower in the idarubicin group. Only one of the studies includes more than this intermediate outcome (complete remission) and finds that the costs per year of life gained are also lower for the idarubicin group.

The two studies concerning BMT in AML and Hodgkin's patients are both plagued by weak efficacy data, only based on case series and without any direct comparison of the treatments in randomized controlled trials. Given the weakness of the data, both studies sensibly limit their levels of ambition to providing a set of more or less complex and elaborate sensitivity analyses. The simplest of these approaches is to determine some threshold values for the relative gain in survival from BMT, which changes the cost-effective ratio in ways that may be decisive for decision making. One of these critical points is where BMT changes from being a dominant solution to being a more effective but also more costly treatment, which requires a difficult

Table 1. Main characteristics of economic assessments dealing with treatments for patients with hematological cancers

Reference	Disease category	Treatments examined	Main characteristics of the study
Tenvall et al. (1994)	AML, all patients from diagnosis to death	Multistage model of disease and treatment process	Cost-of-illness analysis Societal perspective Model of disease and treatment process, showing the flow of a cohort of patients through the various possible stages, treatments, and end points; probability rates and transition rates selected from the literature; cost data from a recent retrospective study and assumptions; indirect costs based on national average wage figures, assumptions, and life expectancy tables More than half of the total cost-of-illness is accounted for by indirect costs, most of which are caused by premature mortality; of the direct costs, initial therapy accounts for almost 60%, maintenance therapy for 8%, and relapses 23%
Marie et al. (1992 a, b)	AML patients	Conventional induction chemotherapy	Determination of the costs of obtaining a CR Hospital perspective Retrospective examination of patient charts and notes for 15 patients in one institution to iden tify cost items; supplemented with resource utilization from large randomized controlled trial; unit costs from price lists and hospital administration Eleven patients achieved CR after one induction, four after two; the costs rise more than proportionately, due to increased need for supportive care
Brodin and Stalfelt (1993)	AML patients, all stages	Standard combination chemotherapy	Determination of the costs of managing AML patients with standard treatment Hospital perspective Retrospective examination of case notes for 54 newly diagnosed AML patients in one institution; 304 different cost items identified and regrouped; unit prices based on the prices used for internal billing, believed to reflect average cost; patient-specific costs allocated to individual patients, nonspecific costs collected and averaged Median survival and costs much lower for those not achieving CR; average cost per patient decreased with increasing age, reflecting a diminishing probability of achieving CR
Phillips et al. (1991)	AML in children	Standard therapy and intensification of therapy	Determines the impact on resources consumed and outcomes of the intensification of therapy Perspective not stated explicitly, no costing Retrospective examination of case reports from case series of patients, subdivided in less intensive (1972–1982) and more intensive therapy (1983–1987); patient follow-up till 1990; patients considered comparable; treatment much intensified, the latter group typically in clinical trials

Table 1 (continued)

Reference	Disease category	Treatments examined	Main characteristics of the study
			Clear improvements in outcomes seen, accompanied by increases in resource utilization which have not been costed; median days in hospital increased from 35 to 170, antibiotic courses from two to seven, antifungal courses from none to three, and days with parenteral nutrition from 0 to 55
Pashko et al. (1991)	AML patients	Induction therapy with cytarubine+daunorubicin or idarubicin	Cost-effectiveness analysis Third-party payer perspective Retrospective examination of patient charts for 120 patients included in a single institution randomized trial; only the costs of induction therapy included, while postremission therapy and treatment of nonresponders are excluded; unit prices used are charges (national averages) Overall rate of CR and overall survival significantly higher in the idarubicin group; total charges per treated patient about the same, but the mean charge per CR and per year of life gained significantly lower for the idarubicin group; thus idarubicin seems a dominant solution; sensitivity analyses show no changes of direction of results
Lobo et al. (1991)	AML patients	Induction therapy with idarubicin or daunorubicin	Cost-effectiveness analysis Hospital perspective, not stated explicitly Efficacy data from the results of four international randomized trials, only one of which showed a significant difference; resource utilization data (number of hospital days, transfusions, and days with antibiotics) from large randomized trial combined with detailed analysis of case notes for ten patients; unit costs determined partly by time and motion study Overall treatment costs almost the same, the higher costs of idarubicin being offset by lower costs for diagnostics and general and supportive treatment; average cost for achieving a CR significantly lower with idarubicin, indicating a dominant solution; the costs of more final outcomes are not given
Welch and Larson (1989)	AML patients	BMT vs. chemotherapy	Cost-effectiveness analysis Hospital perspective, not stated explicitly Retrospective examination of case series of consecutive patients in one institution; five cost items counted in case records and used in the analysis (hospital days, with/without intensive care, laboratory tests, surgery, and radiological examinations); estimates of costs based on charges and cost-to-charge ratios; effectiveness measured as survival after induction therapy

Table 1 (continued)

Reference	Disease category	Treatments examined	Main characteristics of the study
			If the survival gain from BMT compared to chemotherapy is 40% or higher, BMT is a dominant solution; if the gain is less, there is a trade-off between survival gain and higher costs
Ozer et al. (1989)	Hairy cell leukemia patients with progressive disease	Interferon-alfa-2b vs. conventional therapy	Cost-effectiveness analysis Hospital perspective, not stated explicitly Case series of 128 patients with progressive disease treated with interferon compared with historical controls; resource use in baseline and after starting interferon extracted from patients' case notes; other estimates for resource use provided by a Delphi group of physicians; unit costs from a number of sources, e.g., official rates and charges, previous studies Compared to the historical controls, fewer of the interferon patients died within a 12-month period, primarily due to fewer fatal infections; compared to baseline, the interferon patients achieved a fall in transfusions and a decrease in the frequency of infections; overall, both direct costs and indirect costs for the interferon patients are lower than for the controls
Desch et al. (1992)	Hodgkin's disease	ABMT in patients who relapsed after first induction	Cost-effectiveness analysis of various strategies for the timing of ABMT in relation to SC Third-party payer perspective Clinical data taken from combined case series for ABMT and SC, respectively, in addition to some probabilities elicited from physicians; survival years assigned arbitrary utility values by the authors; charges estimated from local experience or from published reports used as surrogates for cost; four cost categories included: the costs of SC, of ABMT, of early fatalities, and radiation; follow-up cost assumed identical, complications ignored because of lack of data Cost-effectiveness ratios estimated vary by more than a factor of 15; the highest cost-effectiveness ratio is found for the strategy of using ABMT immediately during first relapse, while the lowest ratio is found for giving ABMT in second relapse, which is then the optimal strategy; sensitivity analyses do not change the rank order of the strategies, but the patient's prognostic category may be important
Norum et al. (1996)	Hodgkin's disease, all stages	All treatments used in practice	Cost-utility analysis, by comparison with a hypothetical "no treatment" alternative Combined provider and patient perspective

Table 1 (continued)

Reference	Disease category	Treatments examined	Main characteristics of the study
			Retrospective analysis of charts for all Hodgkin's disease patients treated at one hospital in terms of resources used and outcomes; resources included are days of hospitalization, hotel stays (geography), radiotherapy, cytotoxics, antiemetics, and patient travel cost; unit prices are gross averages provided by hospital and regional health care authorities; utility scores provided by surviving patients using the EuroQol instrument; no treatment alternative constructed based on consensus panel of physicians; production gain calculated by modification of the friction cost method Overall survival 90% at 5 years, 86% at 10 years; average costs for primary treatment do not vary with the stage of disease, while the total treatment costs are much higher for patients with advanced disease due to more frequent relapse; a range of cost-utility ratios are presented, varying with respect to the inclusion or not of production gains and whether future costs and outcome gains are discounted or not

AML, acute myeloid leukemia; BMT, bone marrow transplantation; ABMT, autologous BMT; SC, salvage chemotherapy; CR, complete remission.

trade-off to be made. As a first approach to complex problems with a paucity of pertinent data, studies such as these merit attention and they may assist in designing future, more definitive studies, inter alia by identifying which variables are most in need of supplementary collection of reliable data.

Supportive Care I: Emesis and Infections

Introduction

Cancer treatments are generally not only damaging for the malignant cells, but also for the normal cells as well. Most cytotoxic agents, for instance, are not specific for tumor cells but also affect normal cells, particularly those of rapidly proliferating tissues such as the bone marrow, oral and gastrointestinal epithelia, and skin and hair roots. Thus the classical toxic side effects associated with chemotherapy are hair loss (alopecia), nausea and vomiting (emesis), and reduced production of various forms of blood cells in the bone marrow (myelosuppression). A major component of the myelosuppression that occurs in patients receiving chemotherapy is neutropenia, i.e., a fall below the normal range of the blood neutrophil count. Neutrophils are the predominant type of the form of white blood cells called granulocytes, whose main function is to fight *bacterial infections* and which is also the main defense mechanism against *fungal infections.*

The ability of normal tissue to withstand or to quickly regenerate from the damage caused to it during treatment is generally considered to be a central dose-limiting factor and may be a major hindrance to effective treatment. For instance, neutropenia is often dose limiting, frequently preventing a planned chemotherapy schedule from being followed in practical patient management. Either the periods between administrations of drugs are prolonged, the doses used are decreased, or the schedule is terminated altogether before all the planned cycles have been performed. Each of these changes presumably reduce the effectiveness of the therapy. On the other hand, neutropenia increases the risk of catching an infection, which is often a serious or indeed a fatal event in cancer patients. In fact, infection is the most common cause of death in cancer patients receiving chemotherapy, accounting for 40% of deaths in patients with solid tumors and up to 65% of deaths in lymphoma and leukemia patients.

"Supportive care" is the term designating treatment intended to reduce or eliminate the toxic side effects of the various antitumor treatment regimens and thereby to enable these to be carried out as scheduled more often than is usually the case in current clinical practice. Supportive care may also be used to enlarge the current toxicity-determined dose limits, a strategy which may be expected to lead to better cure rates and outcomes in general, because it is widely believed that there should be a positive dose–response relation for a number of treatment regimens (especially in combination chemotherapy). The scientific documentation for a clear dose–response relation is in most cases actually rather weak or even nonexistent; nevertheless, major research efforts continue to be directed at improving supportive care in a way that will allow an intensification of the antitumor therapy.

In this chapter and the following, four forms of supportive care will be considered, because they are of potentially great therapeutic importance, but also because they may have a major economic impact, inter alia due to the fact that the acquisition costs of the new products and procedures being launched are usually rather high. Not surprisingly, they have also attracted a great deal of interest from economic researchers engaged in economic evaluation of cancer treatment regimens.[1]

The four types of supportive care are:

1. Antiemetics
2. Antimicrobials, especially antibiotics and antifungals
3. Prevention or reduction of neutropenia by means of growth factors (the colony-stimulating factors, CSFs)
4. Bone marrow (BMT) and peripheral blood stem cell transplantation (PBSCT)

This chapter will be concerned with the two first forms of supportive care, while the two last will be treated in the following chapter.

Emesis and Antiemetic Therapy

Nausea and vomiting induced by cytotoxic drugs is a significant clinical problem. From the patient's perspective, emesis may be the most distressing treatment-related effect of cancer chemotherapy, which can also lead to anticipatory nausea and vomiting and may ultimately result in the patient's refusal to continue therapy. More commonly, disruption of scheduled chemotherapy cycles may potentially lead to suboptimal therapy or treatment failure. In itself, emesis may lead to complications such as dehydration, electrolytic imbalance, malnutrition, and aspiration pneumonia.

Ever since the first effective antiemetic agent became available, the question of costs has been raised, even granted that there is a great need to control this type of toxicity which is most disturbing and highly feared by pa-

---

[1] These are often sponsored by the manufacturers of the products concerned, who obviously have an interest in demonstrating that high acquisition costs may in many cases be offset by reductions in other cost items or may be associated with important therapeutic gains. The sponsoring of economic evaluations by parties with a clear economic interest in the outcome is a controversial issue, even more than the equally widespread practice of pharmaceutical producers sponsoring conventional clinical trials without economic end points. The most extreme position has been taken by the prestigious *New England Journal of Medicine*, which has adopted a very strict editorial policy with regard to publishing economic evaluations financed by the industry.

tients. A justification that has often been given for high antiemetic costs has been that the use of effective agents may result in shortened hospital stays. Another is that finding convenient regimens for single antiemetic doses may be a cost-effective strategy because for some antiemetics the costs of drug preparation and administration can exceed the acquisition costs.

Control of chemotherapy-induced emesis is currently becoming a standard of care. This represents a marked change that has occurred over the last 15 years. The progress in knowledge includes the recognition of several distinct emetic problems, identification of effective antiemetic agents and their appropriate doses and schedules, the testing of combination regimens with greater efficacy, and the synthesis of newer agents with an improved therapeutic index.

Studies support the hypothesis that emesis is caused by stimulation of receptors in the CNS or in the gastrointestinal tract, and some receptor areas of particular interest have been identified, especially one called the vomiting or emetic center. Another important area is the chemoreceptor trigger zone (CTZ), which is sensitive to chemical stimuli from both the blood and the cerebrospinal fluid. Cytotoxics or their metabolites may stimulate receptors (e.g., dopamine or serotonin receptors) in the CTZ, and impulses generated here may then be transmitted to the vomiting center and lead to the initiation of emesis. The first effective antiemetic identified, metoclopramide, blocks serotonin receptors (specifically the so-called 5-HT_3 receptor), but with less affinity than it has for dopamine receptors. Therefore, very high doses of metoclopramide are required for it to act as a 5-HT_3 antagonist. In recent years, several agents have been synthesized that bind with greater affinity and specificity to 5-HT_3 receptors than metoclopramide. The earliest and most well known of these is called ondansetron, but several others have been marketed subsequently or are under development.

Three distinct types of emetic problems have been identified among cancer patients, and it is important to pay attention to which type of problem is to be prevented or treated, since their causes and treatments may differ. These emetic syndromes are as follows:

1. *Acute chemotherapy-induced emesis*, which most often starts between 1 and 2 h after starting chemotherapy. Untreated, this emesis clears after several hours in many patients, while others continue to be troubled for many days.
2. *Delayed emesis*, beginning 24 h or more after chemotherapy administration. It is less severe than acute emesis and not simply a deferral of acute problems to later periods.
3. *Anticipatory emesis*, i.e., nausea or vomiting beginning before the administration of chemotherapy, which is probably a conditioned response typically occurring in patients who have experienced poor control of emesis during courses of chemotherapy in the past. Treatment-related associations (such as merely reexperiencing the hospital environment) may trigger the emesis.

In general, the chemotherapeutic agents most frequently associated with emesis also induce the most severe episodes. The most highly emetogenic cytotoxic agent is cisplatin, which causes emesis in *all* patients if effective antiemetics are not given. It results in a median of over ten episodes in patients receiving it in high doses (≥70 mg/m^2). New antiemetic agents are normally tested against chemotherapy regimens containing cisplatin. Trials show that, depending on the exact dose of cisplatin, the control rate obtained with metoclopramide varies between 42% and 51%, while the control rate obtained with ondansetron varies between 65% and 75%. In addition to these and the other new 5-HT$_3$ receptor antagonists, a number of treatment possibilities exist, e.g., phenothiazines, corticosteroids, and benzodiazepines (in particular against anticipatory emesis). Some combination regimens are also being tested, e.g., metoclopramide or ondansetron combined with dexamethasone.

Currently, many clinical trials are being conducted in order to determine the relative benefits of the various 5-HT$_3$s – ondansetron, granisetron, and tropisetron – but no definitive results are yet to be found. They seem to have more or less the same antiemetic efficacy, so other factors such as convenience (for instance, granisetron is given only once, while ondansetron is injected several times, and granisetron is more potent and has a longer half-life than ondansetron) and patient preference may be the decisive factors. The net costs of antiemetic treatment are influenced by the costs of hospitalization, as effective control can decrease or eliminate hospitalization, the costs of the agents themselves, and the costs of preparing and administering them. Another factor is that effective antiemetic therapy may have the impact of increasing the chemotherapy costs, as more patients will become able to follow their scheduled treatment.

Economic Evaluations

An estimation on the impact of chemotherapy-induced emesis on patients' functional status and the costs of managing them, based on a survey of patients from five Canadian centers, was provided by O'Brien et al. (1993). The survey patients were not restricted with respect to cancer type, chemotherapy regimen, or antiemetic drug, and both in- and outpatient regimens with moderately to highly emetogenic chemotherapy were considered. All the patients received antiemetics prophylactically, most commonly as a regime of metaclopramide+dexamethasone in various doses, sometimes with other antiemetic agents added. The 5-HT$_3$s had not yet been introduced, and the study was intended to provide background data for future studies with these new agents.

The patients' functional status was assessed by an emesis-specific functional living index, where the patients were asked to rate on a 7-point scale the impact that nausea or vomiting had on nine items of functioning, including an assessment of overall functioning. An overall standardized index score was constructed for nausea and vomiting, respectively, and the patients' scores before and after chemotherapy were compared to determine the differential impact of nausea and vomiting on their functional status. At the oncology centers, patients were followed closely by research nurses, who monitored and recorded episodes of emesis and recorded any resources used for prophylaxis or management. Outside the centers, patients were asked to register the number and degree of emetic episodes and what kinds of action they had taken. The survey data on resource consumption were combined with estimates of unit prices based on various secondary data sources, e.g., official salary scales and hospital purchase prices. Indirect costs were included, with patient and caregiver time valued based on average and minimum industrial wage rates.

A total of 78% of the patients reported at least one episode of nausea or vomiting over the survey period, and 16% reported anticipatory emesis. Episodes of emesis had a negative impact on all areas of functioning examined, primarily as reduced leisure time activities, reduced performance of household tasks, and hardship on family. All patients received antiemetic prophylaxis and therefore incurred some direct costs. The average for all patients were CAN$ 53[2] and CAN$ 63 for the patients with at least one emetic episode. The main costs to the health care system were those of increased nursing time for managing emesis and hospital admission of severe cases (about 3% of all patients). Average indirect costs for patients with one or more emetic episodes were CAN$ 121, almost all of these being due to patient and caregiver time.

No cost-utility analysis has been identified, but Plosker and Milne (1992) refer to some quality-of-life assessments and preliminary cost-effectiveness analyses, which will be described below, as well as to some efficacy studies of ondansetron in comparison to the more traditional treatments. Thus a recent meta-analysis of six randomized, controlled trials of ondansetron versus metaclopramide involving 705 patients that could be evaluated demonstrates statistically significant odds ratios in favor of ondansetron in avoiding both nausea and vomiting.

Plosker and Milne refer to a quality-of-life assessment when these treatment alternatives (both with the addition of dexamethasone) were used in breast cancer patients who had not previously received chemotherapy. Quality of life was evaluated before and after each 5-day course of chemotherapy by using the Rotterdam Symptom Checklist, with separate analyses performed for the psychological, physical, and functional activity subscales. The only statistically significant differences found were in the psychological subscales, in favor of ondansetron. Another study examined the impact of ondansetron on quality of life for a group of cancer patients whose emesis had not been controlled with standard antiemetics during previous chemotherapy regimens. The current chemotherapy regimens were claimed to be equally emetogenic as the previous ones, and the patients were asked to assess the impact of emesis on quality of life by using the emesis-specific functional living index mentioned above. The design of the study is not made entirely

[2] Approximately US$ 46 if the 1990 PPPs are used.

clear, but it seems that the patients were asked to assess their current quality of life and compare it with their recollection of the previous courses of chemotherapy, when they received traditional antiemetics. The validity of the results, showing significantly improved values on the functional index with ondansetron, is therefore highly questionable.

One of the preliminary cost-effectiveness analyses alluded to above was carried out by Buxton and O'Brien (1992), who evaluated ondansetron versus metaclopramide based on crude cost data, partly because the price of ondansetron had not been set at the time of the study. The clinical data were taken from a trial with a randomized cross-over design between two cycles of cisplatin-containing chemotherapy separated by a 3- to 4-week interval. The trial was stopped early, because an interim analysis indicated superior efficacy of ondansetron, so only 76 patients could be evaluated after having received both antiemetics. The authors do not explain why they chose this trial for the exercise. The main outcome measure was frequency of emetic episodes, and the trial showed complete or nearly complete control in 75% of the patients receiving ondansetron compared to 42% receiving metaclopramide. The incidence of adverse events such as headache, sedation, and diarrhea was low and equal across the treatments.

A decision tree with four partitioning criteria was constructed. These criteria are the probability of suffering significant emesis, the probability of suffering significant antiemetic side effects, the probability of these side effects being treated, and the probability of the side effects being resolved. This results in ten different end points for each treatment arm. Finding the costs for each end point, weighing them by their probabilities, and summing them across each treatment arm then gives the expected costs of each antiemetic regimen. The costing is not based on empirical data but on various cost assumptions, e.g., using existing guidelines for good nursing practice in the management of emesis.

The first type of analysis performed is a calculation of the threshold price for ondansetron, i.e., the price at which the expected costs of each of the two antiemetic regimens are equal. The baseline result is a threshold price ratio of ondansetron to metaclopramide of 3.2:1, i.e., the acquisition price of ondansetron may be more than three times higher than the price for metoclopramide in order to equalize the expected costs. Further, a cost-effectiveness analysis was performed, with effectiveness defined in two different ways. If effect was defined as the proportion of patients with no significant emesis, the threshold price ratio was estimated as 5.0:1, and if the effect was defined as the proportion of patients with no significant emesis *and* no significant side effects, the critical ratio was 5.1:1. These results were found to be sensitive to the assumptions made about the costs of managing emetic episodes and of treating side effects of antiemetics. Not surprisingly, there was a positive relation between the size of these costs and the critical threshold price ratio.

Another early contribution was a pilot study by Cunningham et al. (1993), based on an open, multicenter parallel group study lasting 24 h in which all patients were hospitalized. Eligible patients received their first course of highly emetogenic chemotherapy, primarily cisplatin based, and they were randomized to receive either ondansetron or metaclopramide. The number of emetic episodes and details about adverse events were registered by nursing staff, who also recorded details on all materials used in the administration of the antiemetics, materials and "rescue" medication for failures, medication against adverse events, and time spent caring for patients with emesis or adverse events. Treatment success was defined as no significant emesis *and* no adverse event. Drug prices were taken from the official drug formulary, material prices are from an official price list, and average wage rates for the medical staff were also taken from official sources. However, no information on the quantities of the various resources used are provided.

A total of 32 patients participated in the study, and the success rate was 50% with ondansetron and 22% with metaclopramide. The median number of emetic episodes in failures was one for patients on ondansetron and four for those on metaclopramide, and the rate of adverse events in the metaclopramide group was twice the rate in the ondansetron group. While the mean utilization costs were more than double for ondansetron (a ratio of 2.4:1), the costs per success with the two treatments were found to be almost equal, between £ 90 and £ 95.[3] Just looking at the acquisition prices for the drugs gives a ratio of 3.7:1 for ondansetron/metaclopramide. It should be noted that the optimal dosage of ondansetron has not yet been determined, and the doses used for this study are probably several times higher than actually needed.

A further provisional study was carried out by by Jones et al. (1992), who analyzed the impact on the budget of a hospital department of different strategies for using the 5-HT_3s granisetron and ondansetron for antiemesis. A model was constructed to represent the baseline conventional pattern of treatment for a cohort of patients receiving chemotherapy. Based upon the documented clinical benefits of using the 5-HT_3s, a series of antiemetic strategies were considered, in which a successively larger proportion of all antiemetic treatments were based on 5-HT_3s. The incremental costs of using each of these strategies compared to the baseline strategy were calculated seen from the hospital's perspective. In order to put them in a "relevant context," the incremental costs were set in relation to the total costs of chemotherapy for the department, based on figures from the hospital's accounting department. The model required assumptions about the emotegeneity of the chemotherapy given and about the relative efficacy of the two antiemetics against the various forms of emesis (acute and delayed), as there were no direct comparisons between ondansetron and granisetron at the time.

The increase in the total costs of chemotherapy varies between 3% and 10% if the 5-HT_3s are used only for acute emesis and between 12% and 34% if they are used for both acute and delayed emesis, because they have not convincingly been shown to be better than the conventional antiemetics against delayed emesis. One conclusion of the study is that about a third of all chemotherapy patients can be given 5-HT_3s prophylactically for an overall budgetary increase of

[3] Around US$ 220 if PPPs of 1990 are used for conversion.

less than 4%, which, according to the authors, is justified by the clinical benefits. No documentation for this statement is given, however.

Finally, two more definite and well-founded economic evaluations of antiemetics have appeared. Ballatori et al. (1994) conducted a retrospective cost-effectiveness analysis from the hospital perspective, reanalyzing data from a multicenter, randomized double-blind study of 289 cancer patients scheduled to receive cisplatin-containing chemotherapy in a moderate dose for the first time. The data on clinical efficacy are those from the first 24 h after administration of cisplatin, measured as complete protection from vomiting and complete protection from both nausea and vomiting. Emetic episodes occurring after the patients' discharge from hospital were not considered. Staff time estimates were based on time and motion studies, and the calculations of costs for antiemetic administration, of emetic episodes, and of adverse events related to the antiemetics were carefully documented with many details on both resource quantities and unit prices for the cost calculations provided. Further, the stability of the calculations was tested by sensitivity analyses.

The results provided are for the first cycle of chemotherapy, where the efficacy in protection from vomiting was 79% for ondansetron and 60% for metaclopramide, while the efficacy in protection from both nausea and vomiting was 69% and 50%, respectively. With regard to acquisition prices, the ratio between ondansetron and metaclopramide was about 5.2:1, while the ratio for total costs was about 3.8:1. On the ondansetron regimen, the costs remained stable during the three cycles of chemotherapy, while on the metaclopramide regimen the costs increased due to a progressive loss of efficacy. With respect to the costs of complete protection from vomiting, the ratio between ondansetron and metaclopramide is 2.4:1, while for complete protection from both nausea and vomiting it is 2.3:1. The incremental cost-effectiveness ratio is about 450,000 lire for both efficacy measures.[4] The sensitivity analyses showed that these results were rather stable.

A similar economic evaluation of ondansetron versus metaclopramide, but this time for patients receiving chemotherapy with cisplatin in a high dose, was performed by Zrobzek et al. (1994). The efficacy data were taken from a meta-analysis including both randomized comparison trials and case series and from observations of clinical outcomes for only one of the agents. The studies in the meta-analysis were combined using weighted means, which is justified by the fact that there were no significant differences between the findings of the individual studies, but the weights used are not explained. Complete response to antiemetic treatment is defined as no episodes within 24 h after administration of chemotherapy, major response as one to two episodes (set equal to 1.5 in the calculations), and failure as three or more episodes (set equal to five in the calculations). Costs are calculated based on official acquisition prices and labor time estimations by the staff and the housekeeping manager.

---

[4] I.e., about US$ 413 when converted using the PPPs of 1990.

From the meta-analysis, the weighted means showed that 44% of the ondansetron patients responded completely versus 30% of the metaclopramide patients, of which 47% were failures compared with 33% in the ondansetron group. The proportions of major responders were equal. On the basis of these data and the definitions of major response and failures, the expected number of emetic episodes is calculated to be 2 for ondansetron and 2.7 for metaclopramide. To allow for a cost-utility analysis, it was assumed that this reduction in emetic episodes plus the documented reduction in adverse events as well is worth 5 units on a quality-of-life scale running from 0 to 100. As this gain is only sustained for 24 h, the gain for ondansetron patients was calculated to be 0.00014 quality-adjusted life-years (QALYs). The incremental cost per QALY is thus determined as about US$ 168,00 for a person weighing 40 kg and as about $ 408,000 for someone weighting 70 kg. The results are considered stable, as in most cases the sensitivity analyses result in a cost per QALY of over $ 100,000. This is true even if the gain in QALYs is doubled to a value of 0.10. One reservation is that ondansetron patients vomit later than patients taking metaclopramide, which may have led to an underregistration of the number of emetic episodes in the ondansetron patients if they were allowed to leave the clinic earlier and had to take care of any emetic episodes themselves.

Another consideration worth bearing in mind when evaluating results such as these is whether incremental cost per QALY is really an appropriate end-point measure to use in such cases concerning phenomena (e.g., acute emesis) which are strictly limited in time. The results frequently turn out to be rather ridiculous numbers, while it seems intuitively plausible that the patients' quality of life is definitely seriously affected, albeit for a very limited span of time. At the moment, this can be nothing but speculation, but it seems likely that many patients would be very willing to pay to avoid such side effects.[5] In general, economists tend to prefer valuing outcomes by willingness-to-pay measures instead of utilities, and this seems to be one instance where the method of evaluation may have a considerable impact and make an important difference in the decision-making process.

In a recent paper, Plosker and Benfield (1996) reported some studies on the cost-effectiveness of another of the $5HT_3$ receptor antagonists, granisetron, which they interpreted as indicating that granisetron may be more cost-effective than ondansetron (see also Eisenberger 1994). It was not possible to procure the original papers referred to[6] before the deadline for the collection of material for this report, but it is obvious from the overview article that everything depends on the assumptions made with regard to acquisition costs, which depend on the dosages assumed and the particular price

[5] A parallel might be found in the market for dentist services, where many patients require anesthesia for the drilling of cavities, even though such anesthetics are frequently not reimbursed at all. I am not aware of any cost-utility analyses of an anesthetics/no anesthetics policy, but it seems likely that such an analysis would result in an equally absurd cost per QALY figure.

[6] Published papers are Johnson and Bosanquet (1995) and Jobet et al. (1995). In addition, some abstracts are mentioned.

which the institution pays (if the viewpoint of the analysis is that of the hospital, which is the most common). Plosker and Benfield (1996) provide a table showing the possible variations in acquisition costs depending on the assumptions made. The costs calculated (per treatment episode) vary from ondansetron being one third cheaper than granisetron to ondansetron being five times more expensive.

Most direct clinical comparisons between ondansetron and granisetron show that there is no statistically significant difference in their efficacy in preventing acute episodes of emesis and that their effectiveness in preventing delayed vomiting is equally limited. Accordingly, Jobet et al. (1995) used a cost-minimization approach, comparing the direct costs per patient treated, which are shown to be about 20% lower for granisetron with the baseline assumptions. A later revision of the model, occasioned by changes in list prices and in the recommended dosage for ondansetron, resulted in there being no difference in the direct costs. Johnson and Bosanquet (1995) used data from two randomized clinical trials for a retrospective evaluation calculating the direct costs, comprising acquisition costs of antiemetic drugs, intravenous administration, and attending to and treating breakthrough vomiting. The baseline result, with efficacy data from both trials, was that granisetron was more cost-effective than ondansetron. This result was not sensitive to a number of changes in the variables in one-way sensitivity analyses, but when the dosage of ondansetron was reduced to the one currently recommended, the difference in costs disappeared.

A cost-utility analysis of granisetron compared with ondansetron or other antiemetic regimens has not yet been published. From the very close resemblance in the therapeutic profiles of granisetron and ondansetron, however, it is to be expected that the cost per QALY for granisetron would also be very high and probably not much different from that for ondansetron. The remarks made above about the inappropriateness of cost per QALY as an outcome measure apply equally to granisetron, of course.

Concluding Remarks

Table 1 summarizes the economic assessments of antiemetic treatments described and their main characteristics.

The course of events in the area of economic assessments of new antiemetics seems to be almost exemplary, a typical example of what may be observed when new pharmaceutical agents with a more or less justified claim of superior activity are launched at significantly higher acquisition prices than the available alternatives.

Initially, some preliminary cost-effectiveness analyses appear, comparing the new type of agents (in this case ondansetron, the first of the 5-HT_3s) with the standard treatment (metaclopramide). These preliminary assessments, which are summarized and discussed in Cox and Hirsch (1993), seem partly to be intended to assist in the price-setting procedure of the manufacturer of the innovation by finding a sort of threshold price which will equal-

Table 1. Main characteristics of economic assessments dealing with antiemetic treatments

Reference	Disease category	Treatments examined	Main characteristics of the study
O'Brien et al (1993)	All kinds of cancer patients receiving chemotherapy	Antiemetics (before introduction of 5-HT_3s) against chemotherapy-induced emesis	Cost-identification study, aimed at providing baseline data for future studies of the impact of introducing new drugs such as the 5-HT_3s Provider perspective, i.e., hospital Prospective survey of all cancer patients receiving chemotherapy in five hospitals; monitoring of all emetic episodes and the associated consumption of resources; unit prices used were official salary scales and hospital purchase prices; indirect costs included; patient assessment of impact on their functional status 78% of patients experienced at least one episode of emesis; main direct cost caused by the nursing time to manage episodes
Buxton and O'Brien (1992)	Cancer patients receiving cisplatin-based chemotherapy	Ondansetron vs. metaclopramide	Preliminary cost-effectiveness analysis Hospital perspective, not stated explicitly Clinical data from trial with a randomized cross-over design with control of emesis as the main end point; no empirical cost data, but assumptions, e.g., guidelines for good nursing practice; no price for ondansetron available at the time One aim is to determine a critical threshold acquisition price for ondansetron, i.e., the price equalizing the expected costs of the antiemetics; the result is found to be sensitive to assumptions about the costs of managing emetic episodes and of treating side effects of antiemetics
Cunningham et al. (1993)	Patients receiving first course of highly emetogenic chemotherapy	Ondansetron vs. metaclopramide	Preliminary cost-effectiveness analysis Hospital perspective Clinical data from open, parallel group study, with no significant emesis and no adverse event as success criterion; resource utilization recorded by nursing staff; prices used from official sources (e.g., official drug formulary) Success rate of 50% for ondansetron (on average one emetic episode in the failures) and 22% for metaclopramide (four episodes in failures); acquisition cost of ondansetron almost four times higher, but the expected cost of a success is about equal
Jones et al. (1992)	A hypothetical cohort of cancer patients given chemotherapy	Ondansetron vs. granisetron	Cost-identification study, analyzing the impact on hospital budget of various strategies with respect to use of antiemetics Hospital perspective

Table 1 (continued)

Reference	Disease category	Treatments examined	Main characteristics of the study
			Model representing baseline for conventional pattern of treatment is constructed; new strategies considered consist in basing successively larger proportions of all antiemetic treatments on 5-HT_3s; incremental costs of such strategies calculated, assumptions about emetogeneity of chemotherapy and about relative efficacy of the two 5-HT_3s ondansetron and granisetron The costs of chemotherapy increases by 3%–10% if the 5-HT_3s are used only for acute emesis, and by 12%–34% if they are used for both acute and delayed emesis
Ballatori et al. (1994)	Cancer patients in first course of chemotherapy with low-dose cisplatin	Ondansetron vs. metaclopramide	Cost-effectiveness analysis Hospital perspective Retrospective analysis of data from randomized double-blind study of 289 cancer patients, with efficacy in protection from vomiting and from nausea and vomiting as main end points; staff time estimates from time and motion studies, many details on resource quantities and unit prices used are given; careful sensitivity analyses Ondansetron most efficacious for both end points and with highly varying cost ratios depending on the exact question posed, e.g., the expected cost of complete protection from vomiting by ondansetron is about 2.3 times the cost with metaclopramide; results are shown to be rather stable
Zrobzek et al. (1994)	Cancer patients in chemotherapy with high-dose cisplatin	Ondansetron vs. metaclopramide	Cost-effectiveness and cost-utility analysis Hospital perspective Efficacy data from an unpublished meta-analysis including both randomized studies and case series; cost calculations based on official acquisition prices and labor time estimates by staff and housekeeping manager; the impact on quality of life is assumed, measured in Δ QALYs Expected number of emetic episodes calculated to be 2 for ondansetron, 2.7 for metaclopramide; the consequent gain in QALYs is assumed to be 5 units (on a 0–100 scale) sustained for only 24 h, i.e., Δ QALYs is 0.00014, and the ensuing cost-utility ratio is very high

5-HT_3, serotonin blocker; QALY, quality-adjusted life-year.

ize the costs of obtaining a success with each of the treatments; they are based on weak data with respect to both relative efficacy and costs. Without claiming more for the studies than the weak data allow, these studies seem to justify the high acquisition price of the innovation, by showing that this is offset by greater efficacy and lower derived costs, e.g., costs caused by adverse events. In this case, the studies tend to show that the acquisition price for ondansetron may be three to four times higher than that for metaclopramide without resulting in higher costs for achieving a successful outcome in antiemetic treatment.

Later on, better-founded economic assessments appear based on much more reliable data, and these tend to moderate the initial claims concerning the value for money of the new agent, despite its high acquisition price. Thus a careful retrospective cost-effectiveness analysis based on data from a randomized controlled trial of the two antiemetic treatments used in moderately emetogenic chemotherapy estimated the costs of complete protection from emetic episodes to be more than twice as high with ondansetron. The difference in relation to the preliminary studies is partly due to a significant modification of the relative gain in efficacy assumed for ondansetron. This modification of the relative treatment efficacies is also seen in the second of the more mature economic assessments, this time based on an unpublished meta-analysis including data from various types of studies, including randomized controlled trials and case series.

Subsequently, some analogue compounds are launched on the market (in this case other 5-HT_3s, e.g., granisetron) followed by more or less elaborate comparisons of the latter compared with the original innovation, while the standard regimen is often left out of the subsequent comparisons. In this case, direct randomized controlled trials comparing ondansetron and granisetron show quite similar activity and efficacy. The economic assessments thus take the form of cost-minimization analyses, but the results of these seem to be very dependent on the assumptions chosen, especially about the optimal dose of ondansetron, which seems not to have been definitively determined.

Another issue of one of the studies in this section is the appropriate choice of outcome measure for economic assessments of treatments aimed at preventing or diminishing the frequency or severity of events which are extremely unpleasant but last for only a very short time. Although economists usually favor the use of unidimensional utility measures such as QALYs in order to ensure comparability between many diverse outcomes, the use of other outcome measures should be encouraged when analyzing treatments with this aim. Otherwise, the exceptionally high cost-utility ratios resulting from the estimation, which are primarily caused by the very brief duration of the desired effect rather than by differences in costs, may easily lead to erroneous conclusions.

Infections in the Cancer Patient and Treatment with Antimicrobials

Infection is of major concern in all treatment of malignant disease. There are well-established associations between malignancy, immunosuppression, and infectious morbidity and mortality, with bacteria and fungi being the most commonly encountered microorganisms, while viral and parasitic infections may also be involved as primary or secondary complications. The types of infections and the responsible pathogens have been well characterized and may often be predicted, because they are related to specific predisposing factors, such as immune deficits caused by the particular disease or granulocytopenia caused by aggressive antineoplastic therapy, especially cytotoxic chemotherapy.

The malignancies associated with specific immune deficits that predispose to infections with particular microorganisms include the lymphomas, in which the patients have abnormalities of the immune system that increase their risk of viral infection, e.g., herpes simplex, and fungal infections, e.g., cryptococcus. Patients with acute leukemia are most often subject to infections with gram-negative bacteria because of the quantitative and/or functional granulocytopenia caused by the disease.

Of greater concern for this chapter, however, are the deficiencies of host defense mechanisms caused by therapeutic interventions such as cytotoxic chemotherapy, BMT, irradiation, or corticosteroids. The granulocytopenia caused by aggressive cytotoxic chemotherapy is the primary risk factor for severe bacterial infections. Identified predisposing factors for invasive fungal infections include prolonged hospitalization, especially due to profound granulocytopenia, previous exposure to antimicrobials, corticosteroids, invasive procedures requiring central venous catheters, and total parenteral nutrition. In patients undergoing allogeneic BMT, the suppression of T-cell defenses to avoid rejection of the transplant makes them highly susceptible to viral infections.

The major cellular defenses against bacteria and fungi are the granulocytes, and the degree of granulocytopenia, whether a consequence of the disease itself or of therapeutic interventions, is directly related to the incidence of serious infections with these pathogens. A remarkable increase in the incidence of serious infections is seen once the patient's granulocyte count falls below 500 cells/µl. Patients with counts below 100 cells/µl are at the highest risk. It is also evident that the duration of neutropenia is another major risk factor, making the extent and duration of neutropenia the most clearly identified risk factors for serious bacterial and fungal infections. Leukemia patients are more likely to develop infections than patients with solid tumors because neutropenia can persist for up to 4 weeks in leukemia patients, compared with only a few days in patients with solid tumors.

More than 80% of the documented infections in cancer patients have been found to arise from organisms that are endogenous to the gut or skin microflora of the patients, almost half of which are acquired during hospital stay. The most frequent isolates are gram-negative and gram-positive bacteria and fungi of the genera *Candida* and *Aspergillus*. A series of EORTC trials from 1973 to 1990 have documented a rather constant incidence of bacteremia in febrile granulocytopenic patients of around 23%, with a marked increase in the incidence of gram-positive bacteria and a fall in the incidence of gram-negative bacteria. This change in the incidence patterns is observed worldwide. The sources contributing to infecting the hospitalized patient are transmission from staff to patients and between patients, contamination of food, air, water, and equipment such as catheters, respirators, and humidifiers, and surgical and medical procedures. Poor hand-washing routines among physicians and others caring for seriously ill cancer patients are considered to be particularly important transmission mechanisms.

Evaluation and Management of Febrile Cancer Patients

Fever is common in cancer patients, and there are many potential noninfectious causes, such as certain cytotoxic drugs (e.g., bleomycin and cytosine arabinoside), blood products, allergic reactions, and the disease process itself. Frequently, however, fevers in cancer patients (especially neutropenic) are caused by infections. Even after extensive evaluation, an infectious cause is only found in up to 30%–40% of febrile neutropenic patients, and about 85% of these are due to bacteria (see the above-mentioned series of EORTC trials over a number of years, which consistently identified bacteria in 23%–25% of febrile neutropenic patients).

Detection and management of these infections is complicated by two important factors:

1. Neutropenia alters the patient's inflammatory response, so that classical signs and symptoms of infections (e.g., pyuria, pain, erythema, swelling) may be blunted or lacking altogether.
2. An undetected and untreated infection may be rapidly fatal in this type of patient.

As there are no reliable methods that allow the physicians to determine clinically whether a febrile neutropenic episode is caused by an infection or other reasons, it has become standard practice that all neutropenic cancer patients developing fever must be treated promptly with an empirical antibiotic regimen, without awaiting the results of microbiologic cultures. There is no definite threshold for the temperature or the neutrophil count, and the direction and rate of change is considered more important than the absolute count. A common suggestion for the absolute values that define an episode of febrile neutropenia is a temperature of 38.5 °C or above (or three consecutive elevations above 38 °C taken at least 4 h apart) and a neutrophil count less than 500 cells/μl.

The criteria for empirical antibiotic management are that the regimen must be broad, must achieve high bactericidal levels, and must be as nontoxic and easy to administer as possible. Therapy begins as soon as the patient develops signs and symptoms of infection, and response is evaluated 3–5 days after starting treatment. If the patient responds, the antibiotics should be continued for at least another 7 days, and if the patient remains febrile, the initial regimen should be modified on the basis of culture and sensitivity results and the patient's clinical state. The single most important advance in the management of febrile neutropenic patients is this policy of prompt initiation of broad-spectrum antibiotic treatment. Before this, the mortality rate of patients with some gram-negative infections was about 80%. Since the change in policy, the survival rate for febrile neutropenic patients has been over 90%.

Traditionally, a combination of two or more antibiotics has been used in order to obtain sufficient coverage, but as no particular combination has been proven to be clearly superior, the usual recommendation has been for any given institution to make its own choice based on the local epidemiology of the various bacteria. A standard combination antibiotic therapy for febrile neutropenia consists of a first-generation cephalosporin, an aminoglycoside, and an antipseudomonal penicillin. Today, third-generation cephalosporins and carbapenems offer a single-agent alternative, which is attractive, because they are easier to administer, less toxic, and less costly. Unlike many of the earlier aminoglycoside-containing regimens, which carried a significant risk of nephrotoxicity and ototoxicity and required frequent monitoring of serum drug concentration, the newer antibiotics available for monotherapy do not require monitoring of serum levels and they have minimal toxicity. These advantages, combined with reduced time requirements for preparation and administration, would be expected to be associated with an economic advantage.

There is still considerable controversy regarding the use of single-agent antibiotic therapy, especially the third-generation cephalosporin ceftazidime, against febrile neutropenia. Several investigators believe that ceftazidime is a safe and effective alternative to combination treatment, while others insist that, although the initial response to ceftazidime may be acceptable, treatment modification is required with sufficient frequency to warrant initial therapy with a combination regimen instead.[7] Based on several trials showing equal response to ceftazidime and combination regimens but fewer side effects in the ceftazidime group, many centers use ceftazidime as the standard of care for initial management of febrile neutropenia.

Other promising monotherapy drugs, e.g., imipenem and meropenem, are under evaluation against this new standard. Imipenem has the broadest spectrum of all available antibiotics; however, the need for antibiotic changes has not been less in the imipenem group compared with the ceftazidime group in direct comparisons. Such comparative trials have further showed equal efficacy, but also a significantly higher incidence of sometimes serious toxic side effects in the imipenem group. While for this reason imipenem is less often used as standard therapy, an important role for the agent is considered to be as a "backup" antibiotic, which can be used when bacteria strains resistant to ceftazidime occur. This may happen increasingly often, as there is widespread overuse of third-generation cephalosporins.

Given the changing pattern of incidence of bacteria, it is also a matter of controversy whether the empirical antimicrobial therapy should routinely in-

---

[7] Uniformly, the need for modification of therapy has been found to be higher in patients with identified pathogens than in patients with fever of unknown origin.

clude antibiotics active against gram-positive bacteria, such as vancomycin and teicoplanin. The argument against universal administration of these agents is that most gram-positive infections are of rather low virulence, so that a policy of withholding vancomycin until identification of the pathogen may be considered safe. Several studies support this viewpoint, as they show no survival benefit of routine use of vancomycin.

Growing experience with early empirical broad-spectrum antibiotics has made it increasingly clear that neutropenic patients should generally be classified into at least two risk categories on the basis of the anticipated duration of their neutropenia (see Freifeld and Pizzo 1995). If the patients can be differentiated into one of these groups, either prospectively or as soon as possible after hospital admission for fever and neutropenia, this might have great importance for the general management of neutropenic cancer patients. "Low-risk" neutropenic patients have durations of neutropenia less than 7 days, and they are likely to have minimal or even no sites of infection and no high-risk comorbidities. They seem to do well with a wide variety of therapeutic regimens. "High-risk" neutropenic patients, in contrast, are anticipated to remain neutropenic for more than 7–10 days, and other high-risk factors identified are medical comorbidities, poor performance status, extended hospitalization, early onset of febrile neutropenia after administration of chemotherapy, and uncontrolled malignant disease. High-risk patients are much more subject to secondary infections, and frequently they require the addition of further antibiotic agents to the original regimen. If the fever still persists, they will often also be treated empirically with antifungals.

A differentiation between different risk groups would allow a more targeted approach to the management of febrile neutropenia. However, there is currently little prospectively collected and validated information with regard to risk factors that predict the risk of infection after chemotherapy for patients that are about to begin a first or a new course of chemotherapy (ASCO 1994). Inferences from the literature suggests that patients with compromised bone marrow reserve due to extensive prior chemotherapy or poor performance status and more advanced cancer may have a higher risk for chemotherapy-induced infection. There is also some indication that patients with a previous history of febrile neutropenia may be at higher risk of developing a recurrent fever when they receive the same doses of chemotherapy again.

The recent introduction of several potent antibacterials in an oral form has led to reassessment of routine intravenous antibiotic therapy of various serious infections. Severely ill patients receiving initial empirical intravenous antibiotic therapy may be switched to appropriate oral therapy once the pathogen has been identified and the clinical condition has begun to improve, usually after about 3 days of treatment. For low-risk patients, there are clinical trials with outpatient intravenous or oral antibiotic therapy with promising results.

The potential advantages of oral therapy compared to intravenous therapy include the fact that minimal expertise is required for their administration, eliminating or reducing the labor cost for preparation and administration and the utensils necessary for intravenous administration. In addition, the acquisition costs of the drugs themselves are usually lower for the oral form. Oral medications imply a greater flexibility in clinical care, possibly with earlier discharge or avoidance of hospitalization altogether. Even hospitalized patients will need less nursing if intravenous medication is avoided, and they will not be exposed to the risks of line infections and other complications of intravenous administration. The patients will probably be more comfortable and enjoy greater independence, and the possibility of earlier discharge will reduce the patients' exposure to nosocomial pathogens, which are responsible for the majority of the infections.

However, this is still an area of ongoing research, with other trials showing that large proportions of patients originally assigned to outpatient therapy later required readmission due to unresolved infections or persistence of fever. It is thus clear that, even with the currently available criteria for classification of low-risk patients, it is not possible to predict the complications arising in a significant proportion (about one fourth) of these patients. A policy of treating febrile neutropenic patients with oral antibiotics on an outpatient basis will certainly require good patient compliance and close contact with the patients on the part of the health care personnel involved.

Oral antibiotic therapy, usually with oral fluoroquinolones, is of course limited to patients who can swallow pills, and this is often a problem in cancer patients. Trials are being carried out with the purpose of simplifying intravenous antibiotic schedules so that they need only be administered once daily. There are as yet no data from large randomized trials comparing inpatient versus outpatient administration of intravenous antibiotics, but the existing data indicate that patients with a rising granulocyte count, a short anticipated duration of neutropenia, and improvement in the signs of infection (if any) may be good candidates for a policy of early discharge from hospital to finish their course of antibiotics as outpatients. However, stopping antibiotic therapy too early in patients that remain granulocytopenic may lead to serious deterioration of their clinical state, especially if they are persistently febrile or suffering from an undiscovered infectious process. More studies to establish the safety and efficacy of early discontinuation of antibiotics compared to a full course of therapy are thus needed.

Several strategies for prophylactic antibiotic regimens have been explored in a large number of clinical trials. So far, no single strategy has stood out as singularly effective, and each has its advantages and problems. A large number of clinical trials aiming at investigating various measures to prevent or reduce infections identify careful hand-washing practices among physicians and other personnel groups as the most important. Other measures to prevent the acquisition of new microorganisms include maintenance of a cooked diet during periods of granulocytopenia and various techniques of isolating the patient from potentially harmful factors. The most comprehensive such effort is the total protective environment, in which a sterile environment is created in a clean-air room. Such a policy does reduce the number of infections in patients with very low granulocyte counts, but does not offer a survival advantage because of the improvements in treating established infections. Currently, modifications of the total protective environment are used, but only for patients undergoing allogeneic BMT and patients with an anticipated duration of severe granulocytopenia of 1 month or more.

Prophylaxis with antibiotics aims at reducing the load of endogenous pathogens, the main source of which is the patient's gastrointestinal tract. Regimens aimed at reducing the total gastrointestinal flora of bacteria are not recommended, while policies of "selective decontamination" are being actively investigated. The results of many follow-up clinical trials of such policies are conflicting, however, possibly because of poor and varying study designs, nonuniform patient groupings, and failure to report or document compliance with the prophylactic regimens. The potential for reduction in infectious morbidity and mortality by antibiotic prophylaxis must be balanced against the risk of prolongation of granulocytopenia (which can be caused by antibiotics) and the possible emergence of resistant organisms. Successful use of this approach requires close monitoring to properly adjust the antimicrobial regimen for resistant or newly emerging species, and this surveillance is expensive and time-consuming.

Another means of prophylaxis against infections is to administer CSFs immediately after administration of chemotherapy in order to reduce the incidence and shorten the duration of the subsequent neutropenia. Several randomized trials have documented that the anticipated effect in these intermediate end points can be obtained, but no study has demonstrated a survival benefit as a result of decreased infectious mortality, neither have the CSFs been found consistently to reduce the incidence of documented infections in neutropenic patients, and a policy of general prophylaxis of infections by means of CSFs is not recommended (see the ASCO guidelines for the use of the CSFs referred to in the following chapter; ASCO 1994, 1996). Another possibility is to use immunoglobulins, especially in connection with allogeneic BMT, in which they have been shown to significantly reduce the incidence and severity of acute graft-versus-host disease (GVHD) and to significantly decrease the frequency of sepsis and local infections.

Patients with prolonged periods of profound neutropenia after intensive chemotherapy or ablative irradiation are at increased risk of acquiring *invasive fungal infections*. Diagnosing invasive fungal disease in immunocompromised patients is very difficult (e.g., because thrombocytopenia makes biopsy a high-risk procedure), and there is as yet no reliable test available to allow accurate diagnosis early in the development, e.g., by detecting specific antibodies. Invasive fungal infection is therefore often an autopsy detection, and several reports indicate that it is an increasing cause of morbidity and mortality in granulocytopenic patients. In hematological cancers, invasive fungal infections have been documented in 10%–40% of patient autopsies. The lack of accurate diagnostic tests and the fact that withholding therapy while awaiting a definite diagnosis may allow dissemination of the disease provide the rationale for the empirical use of antifungal therapy in patients with febrile granulocytopenia that remain microbiologically unidentified and do not respond to broad-spectrum antibiotic therapy after 4–7 days. Several retrospective and prospective studies support the empirical institution of antifungal therapy by documenting that early institution of therapy improves the outcome in terms of deaths caused by invasive mycoses.

The traditional antifungal regimen is amphotericin B, which, however, has severe side effects such as fever, chills, nausea, and vomiting, and less commonly, hypotension, bronchospasms and seizures, and nephrotoxicities of various kinds. The recommended doses of amphotericin B are not based on controlled clinical trials and depend on the site of infection. Alternatives to amphotericin B are badly needed and eagerly sought after, but for patients with serious fungal infections the treatment options are currently few, and amphotericin B is still evaluated as the most reliable. For empirical antifungal therapy, fluconazole and liposomal formulations of amphotericin B are currently considered promising alternatives to amphotericin B, while ketoconazole is no longer seen as an acceptable substitute because of lack of efficacy against deep mycoses. For patients with an established fungal infection, amphotericin B in higher doses is still mandatory.

Antifungal prophylaxis has also been studied extensively because of an increasing incidence of fungal infections in immunocompromised patients. The most frequently evaluated agents for antifungal prophylaxis have been nystatin, amphotericin B, miconazole, clomitrazole, and ketonazole. The data are hard to interpret because the studies suffer from divergent patient criteria, disparate dosage regimens, nonuniform response criteria, and lack of appropriate controls. Another problem is the inherent difficulty in the definitive diagnosis of fungal infections. With these problems in mind, some tentative conclusions may be formulated:

1. After an adequate dose of antifungal agent has been administered, there has been a consistent decrease in fungal colonization, but this has not clearly resulted in a decreased incidence of invasive mycotic disease, although a decrease in superficial infections has been found in some studies.
2. Several studies employing prophylactic and empirical antifungal regimens have reported a shift in the colonization pattern of fungal organisms, mostly toward more resistant species. The potential benefits of prophylactic antifungal therapy must thus be balanced against the toxicities, epidemiologic considerations, and relative efficacy of the regimens employed. Widespread antifungal chemoprophylaxis is currently not recommended.

Economic Evaluations of Antibiotic Treatments

Quite a large number of economic evaluations have been carried out in the field of antibiotic treatments of infections, especially focusing on the therapeutic and economic impact of replacing (as much as possible and as soon as possible) intravenous administration of antibiotics with an oral form of the same or another drug. Most of these studies do not, however, select and describe the patients according to their original diagnosis, but describe only the site and the severity of infections. It is therefore difficult to find more than a few articles evaluating the costs and effects of various treatments of cancer patients with more or less serious infections, but the results of many studies without identification of the patients' primary diagnosis may also be relevant for cancer patients (see, e.g., Eisenberg et al. 1987). Given the information provided by these articles, however, there is no way of telling with any certainty whether such inferences are valid and relevant.

Sequential antibiotic therapy (SAT) is the term sometimes used to refer to the practice of limiting the use of intravenous antibiotics to the early stages of infection and then converting to oral agents for the duration of treatment. A strategy of SAT would be expected to offer a number of benefits for both the patient and the hospital. In hospital, the use of oral instead of intravenous drugs increases patient comfort and mobility, and there is less risk of inflammation of the vein and line-related infections. Earlier discharge from hospital also decreases the risks of incurring other nosocomial infections, and earlier return to family and possibly to work or other activities may be expected to provide enhanced quality of life. For the hospital, much of the time of pharmacists and nurses are tied up in the preparation and delivery of intravenous antibiotics, and by reducing the use of intravenous drugs, these large amounts of personnel resources may be freed for other purposes.

On the other hand, there is a perceived higher risk of therapeutic failure with oral treatment, as poor compliance with the planned oral regimen could lead to relapse of infection and possibly to readmission. Inadequate or incomplete treatment of infections may also lead to the development of microbial resistance, which is a serious and growing problem that may be very difficult to monitor adequately outside the closely supervised hospital setting. Even with compliant patients, therapeutic failures may occur, e.g., because of interactions with other drugs that the patients are taking concurrently and that decrease the bioavailability of the oral antibiotics. For these and other reasons, many clinicians are much more comfortable using intravenous rather than oral drugs in treating serious infection and hesitate in adopting an SAT strategy.

One good example of the above-mentioned type of article, and the only one which will be discussed here, is the overview article by Balfour and Faulds (1993) on the use of oral ciprofloxacin in the treatment of serious infections in patients with nonidentified primary diagnoses. They distinguish a number of factors which should be considered as direct costs of treating serious infections. Associated directly with the intravenous antimicrobial therapy are costs for the acquisition of the drugs and for preparing and administering them. Personnel, such as the pharmacist, technician, and nursing staff, are involved and they use various ancillary materials, such as gloves, needles, syringes, intravenous administration set and accessories, heparin flush, and intravenous delivery solution. Delivery costs may be substantially affected by route and frequency of administration, with bolus injections costing considerably less to deliver than infusions. For drugs with a narrow safety margin, such as the aminoglycosides, it may be necessary to monitor plasma drug concentrations closely, with the frequency of antibiotic assays being determined by the degree of severity of the disease.

In addition, costs may arise from treatment failure and adverse events, e.g., necessitating additional medical consultations and drug therapy and perhaps prolonging hospitalization or even requiring treatment in an intensive care unit. In addition, there are the costs of hospitalization, as intravenous antimicrobial treatment is usually given in hospital. The new treatment strategy considered is to switch patients with serious infections from various intravenous treatments to oral ciprofloxacin after 3 days of parenteral treatment, while patients with less serious infections may be given oral ciprofloxacin from the outset of treatment. The existing economic evaluations of such a shift in strategy invariably apply a health care provider perspective only (although rarely stated explicitly), while a wider, societal perspective would seem to be indicated for evaluating a treatment strategy such as this one, as it is most likely to shift costs from the hospital to the patient and the community.

In three economic evaluations conducted alongside randomized clinical trials, the reductions in antibiotic costs from this switch varied from 43% to 83%. All of these evaluations only comprise direct costs, but they differ widely with respect to which cost factors are included, and there are also some variations in the sources for unit costs quoted, e.g., for the drugs themselves (average wholesale prices versus actual hospital acquisition prices). Only one of these evaluations included the costs of laboratory tests necessary for monitoring the serum antibacterial concentrations for patients receiving certain intravenous antibiotics such as aminoglycosides and costs associated with treatment failures and adverse effects, without, however, presenting these cost elements separately. The clinical trials, in which a number of different parenteral antibiotic regimens were used according to the clinicians' discretion, all found that the rates of clinical and bacteriological response and total duration of the antibiotic therapy were similar in oral and parenteral treatment groups, so the economic evaluations are performed as cost-minimization analyses.

Intravenous antibiotics do not necessarily require hospitalization, however, but can sometimes be administered in the patient's own home. Seen from the hospital perspective, this means that a bed will become available for another patient, and it will also reduce the time spent by personnel involved in the delivery and administration of intravenous antibiotics. On the other hand, if the hospital is made responsible for providing the patients with the necessary materials, this may entail some extra costs. It will probably also be necessary to use some personnel resources for training and supervising the relatives of the patients in the necessary techniques for administering the intravenous infusions.

Wiernikowski et al. (1991) provided a fairly preliminary economic evaluation of a pilot study of such a home intravenous antibiotic program in pediatric oncology. Analyzed from the hospital's point of view, the costs of the home program were determined to be about one third of the costs of administering the antibiotics on an inpatient basis. However, the calculations are very crude, using for instance the average total daily hospital costs, unmodified, multiplied with an observed average length of stay for hospital treatment of neutropenic episodes to calculate the costs of inpatient treatment.

Dranitsaris et al. (1995) examined whether the clinical advantages of antibiotic monotherapy with a drug such as ceftazidime compared with combination therapy including aminoglycosides also results in improved cost-effectiveness. The clinical advantages are relative lack of nephro- and ototoxicities compared to aminoglycosides, reduced preparation and administration time, and the absence of a need to monitor serum drug concentration. Combination therapies analyzed were cephalosporin+aminoglycoside+antipseudominal penicillin (CAP) and (aminoglycoside+antipseudominal penicillin (AP). A meta-analysis was performed of clinical studies from 1966 to 1993 comparing any of the three regimens (ceftazidime, CAP, or AP) to determine estimates of their relative effectiveness and incidence of adverse drug reactions. The criteria for inclusion in the meta-analysis were that the trials should be properly randomized and that they should be concerned with cancer patients with febrile neutropenia. The estimated rates were used in constructing a decision-making model to determine the relative cost-effectiveness of the regimens.

The clinical outcomes were assumed to be assessed on day 4 after therapy start, and responders were assumed to continue unmodified therapy for a further 7 days. For treatment failures, i.e., where the microorganism was not eradicated after 4 days or persistent fever necessitated a modification of the therapy, three different scenarios were examined, with varying assumptions about what antibiotics to add and further actions to take. All costs were calculated from the hospital perspective, and current standard practice at the authors' institution was used to determine the frequency of various tests over a standard treatment period of 14 days. The sources for the various unit prices used are given, but their validity and consistency is difficult to judge, as they range from local pharmacy and nursing workload measurement statistics to average daily hospitalization costs calculated at the provincial level (Ontario, Canada). Cost-effectiveness ratios were found by dividing the expected costs of each regimen (costs of response plus costs of failure) by the response rates found in the meta-analysis.

The pooled response rates for the regimens were 75% for CAP, 64% for ceftazidime, and 59% for AP, but the differences were not found to be statistically significant, as the confidence intervals were fairly wide (there were only six trials in the meta-analysis). The most costly adverse reaction was nephrotoxicity (up to 4 extra hospital days), which occurred in about 6% of the patients treated with CAP and AP and in 0% in the ceftazidime groups. If equal effectiveness of the regimens is assumed, ceftazidime turns out to be the cheapest. When average cost-effectiveness ratios, as mentioned above, were calculated, however, the CAP regimen turned out to have the lowest ratio no matter which of the three scenarios in the case of therapy failure was assumed, while AP invariably had the highest and the ceftazidime regimen was in between. The average cost-effectiveness ratios for CAP were between CAN$ 11,000 and 12,000.[8] The average ratios were found to be between CAN$ 12,000 and 14,000, so CAP would seem to be a dominant solution with the given data.

A preliminary cost-effectiveness analysis of giving prophylactic intravenous immunoglobulin to patients with chronic lymphocytic leukemia (CLL) was published by Weeks et al. (1991). The intention of the article was merely to report an approximate study, basing a decision analysis on existing and easily available data, in order to see whether it seemed to be indicated to initiate a full-blown study with prospective data collection. The efficacy data were taken from a randomized clinical trial in which CLL patients particularly susceptible to infections were randomized to prophylactic immunoglobulin or to placebo every 3 weeks for 1 year. A statistically significant difference was found, with 23 bacterial infections in the 41 treated patients and 42 infections in the controls. After stratification into trivial and major infections, however, the difference was no longer significant. No difference in mortality was observed. For those patients who had an infection, the expected number of infections per patient was estimated as 1.4 in the treatment arm and 2.25 in the placebo arm.

It was assumed that a trivial infection means 5 days of hospitalization, while a major infection means 15 days in hospital. Estimates of resource consumption were based on the authors' judgment (and subjected to extensive sensitivity analyses). The costs of treatment, adverse reactions, and infections were derived from actual cost data provided by two Boston hospitals. Estimates of quality of life or the utilities for the patients in the various relevant health states were obtained from a group of ten experienced oncologists using a standard gamble approach. Mean estimates for a day spent in the different states were 0.87 for CLL without infection, 0.86 with trivial infection, 0.46 with major infection, and 0.66 when receiving prophylactic immunoglobulin and having no infection.

Assuming in the baseline case that the infusions with immunoglobulin cause the patients no inconvenience at all, treatment for 1 year was estimated to produce an expected gain of 0.0023 QALYs (i.e., 0.8 quality-adjusted days) per patient per year of treatment. The marginal costs of the treatment, i.e., the additional costs of treating one patient less any saving on that patient's other health care costs, were estimated to be just under $ 14,000, resulting in a cost per QALY of approximately $ 6 million. If the inconvenience of the infusions is taken into account, the prophylactic treatment may result in a loss of quality-adjusted life expectancy. For the individual patient, the result depends on his or her relative utilities for the baseline state and the superimposed infection. Sensitivity analyses show that all estimates would have to be

[8] The authors indicated an exchange rate as of November 1993 of CAN$ 1 = US$ 0.76, so these ratios are around US$ 9000.

changed in the direction most favorable for immunoglobulin and to a clinically unrealistic degree if the cost-effectiveness ratio should become considerably more favorable for the prophylactic treatment. No further (and resource-consuming) data collection and analysis seems indicated.

Finally, an economic assessment of alternative antifungal therapies will be reported. The cancer populations particularly at risk of severe disseminated fungal infections are patients who are immunocompromised as a result of intensive chemotherapy and BMT recipients. The signs and symptoms of invasive fungal infections are often nonspecific, and in many cases the indication for antifungal treatment is fever that does not respond to antibacterial or antiviral treatment. As mentioned above, amphotericin B has for a long time been the drug of choice in these patients, despite its quite frequent and serious side effects. Recent studies have shown that amphotericin B encapsulated in liposomes is less toxic, and such preparations have been shown to be effective in treating patients with severe mycoses who have failed to respond to conventional amphotericin B or who develop nephrotoxicity following this treatment.

In a retrospective examination and costing of patient charts for a small case series of patients from one institution, Persson et al. (1992) examined the relative costs and effects of liposomal and conventional amphotericin B. The case series comprised all patients admitted to the institution with a confirmed diagnosis of systemic mycoses, except those dying within 2 days of diagnosis. A third of the patients had received BMT, while the rest were liver and kidney transplantation patients. The first 29 patients were treated with conventional amphotericin B between 1981 and 1989, and the other 29 patients were treated with the liposomal formulation between 1989 and 1991. To counter criticisms based on the problems inherent in historical comparisons, it is claimed that the department concerned obtained no major improvements in patient or graft survival during the study period.

Data on the treatment and the consumption of health care resources for the two populations were collected from the patient records at the hospital. The registration comprised the period from the date of diagnosis of the mycosis until discharge from the hospital or death. Only direct health care costs were calculated, with unit prices coming partly from an internal price list from the hospital (cost per treatment day for various types of transplantation patients) and partly from a separate calculation for each individual patient of costs of some expensive drugs, according to the official price list for pharmaceuticals in Sweden.

The effectiveness of the antifungal treatments was measured by the proportion of patients discharged from the hospital alive, i.e., 12 out of 29 for the conventional and 20 out of 29 for the liposomal amphotericin B group. The calculation was actually done for the individual transplantation groups, which resulted in very small numbers of patients and hence very uncertain estimates. Thus, out of the total of 19 BMT patients, one out of eight patients in the conventional group and seven out of 11 in the liposomal group were discharged alive. The difference in the proportion of patients being discharged alive was then multiplied by expected survival rates for patients surviving the various types of transplantation in order to estimate the gain in expected survival time, which was ascribed to liposomal amphotericin B. The expected survival rates were found by extrapolations from observed survival rates, based on the assumption that the conditional survival probabilities would remain constant outside the observation period.

The treatment time with the antifungal drug was similar, i.e., on average 21 days, in the two treatment populations, while the number of days of hospitalization from the onset of mycosis until discharge from hospital was much longer in the liposomal group, i.e., 54 days on average versus 39 days for the conventional group. This results in additional treatment costs for the liposomal group, i.e., in total about SKr 270,000[9] for the BMT group, somewhat more for the liver transplantation group, and less than half of this amount for the kidney/pancreas transplantation group. These additional costs were divided by the estimated gain in survival, i.e., 1.78 years for the BMT group (for a total estimated life expectancy of 3.5 years), in order to determine the estimated additional cost per life-year gained, which becomes SKr 152,000 for the BMT group or about US$ 20,000 (both costs and life-years gained were discounted by 5%). With the very small number of patients in the study, these estimates are of course extremely unstable. The effectiveness measure used must also be considered as dubious. In an historical comparison, many changes other than the change in antifungals used may have contributed to the improvement observed in the proportion of transplantation patients with a diagnosis of systemic mycosis being discharged alive from the hospital.

Concluding Remarks

The main characteristics of the economic assessments of anti-infection treatments in cancer patients are summarized in Table 2 below.

It is commonly expected that antibiotic treatment with single agents such as the carbapenems or third-generation cephalosporins instead of the traditional combination regimens would offer a clear economic advantage. These agents require less time for preparation and administration, and they are less toxic than many of the earlier aminoglycoside-containing regimens, which require frequent monitoring of the patients' serum drug concentration because of significant risks of nephrotoxicity and ototoxicity.

The only study of this issue explicitly referring to cancer patients with febrile neutropenia which was identified and retrieved for this survey does not corroborate this common sense hypothesis, however. The efficacy data of the study are taken from an unpublished meta-analysis, and this might be problematical, even though the finding of no statistically significant differences between the regimens compared is uncontroversial. The costing methods

[9] The 1990 PPPs were US$ 1 = SKr 7.51, making this amount equal to about US$ 36,000.

Table 2. Main characteristics of economic assessments dealing with anti-infective treatments in cancer patients

Reference	Disease category	Treatments examined	Main characteristics of the study
Dranitsaris et al. (1995)	Cancer patients with febrile neutropenia	Antibiotic monotherapy (ceftazidem) vs. combination therapies (various)	Cost-effectiveness analysis Hospital perspective Clinical efficacy and adverse event data from unpublished meta-analysis of randomized studies; different clinical scenarios (e.g., in the case of no resolution of fever) assumed; resource utilization and unit price data mainly from the authors' institution, but also based on calculations from regional level; calculation of average cost-effectiveness ratios No statistically significant difference in response ratios found, and most adverse reactions in combination groups; if equal effectiveness is assumed, ceftazidime is less costly, but average cost-effectiveness ratio lowest for combination antibiotic therapy (cephalosporin+aminoglycoside +anti-pseudominal penicillin)
Weeks et al. (1991)	Patients with CLL	Prophylactic intravenous immunoglobulin	Preliminary cost-utility analysis based on available data to assess need for further data collection and analysis Hospital perspective Retrospective decision model with efficacy data from randomized trial of prophylactic immunoglobulin vs. placebo in CLL patients; resource utilization data based on assumptions, unit costs are cost data from two hospitals; estimates of quality of life (utilities) obtained from group of oncologists Statistically significant reduction in number of infections in the immunoglobulin group (although not after stratification into trivial and major infections) and no difference in survival; this is translated into a gain of only 0.0023 QALYs, which implies a very high cost-utility ratio; the results are shown to be rather stable
Persson et al. (1992)	Patients with systemic mycoses, some of them cancer patients after BMT	Conventional vs. liposomal amphotericin B	Preliminary cost-effectiveness analysis Hospital perspective Retrospective examination and costing of case records for a small number of patients in one institution; historical comparison of patients treated with conventional vs. liposomal amphotericin B; effectiveness measured as proportion of patients discharged alive; this proportion is multiplied by expected survival time to find gain in expected survival time

Table 2 (continued)

Reference	Disease category	Treatments examined	Main characteristics of the study
			Significant gain in success with liposomal drug (but very small number of patients, so estimates are unstable); days of antifungal treatment similar, much longer hospitalization in liposomal group, so liposomal costs are much higher; cost-effectiveness ratios are determined for each of the three types of patients included in the study

BMT, bone marrow transplantation; CLL, chronic lymphocytic leukemia; QALY, quality-adjusted life-year.

used seem to be relatively sound (despite too few details being given), and assuming equal effectiveness, ceftazidime (a third-generation cephalosporin) turns out to be the less costly, although not as clearly as perhaps expected. However, the authors then use the exact efficacy rates found in the meta-analysis in order to calculate average cost-effectiveness ratios. By this methodological twist, a combination turns out to be the most effective and least costly. The safe conclusion seems to be that the expected clear cost advantage for monotherapy is not found, which is quite surprising and warrants further examination.

The study of the use of prophylactic immunoglobulin to prevent infections in CLL patients is a good example of the usefulness of carrying out a preliminary analysis on the basis of data immediately at hand. The available resources for carrying out economic assessments are limited, and the likely gain in knowledge compared to the expected costs of achieving it should always be an important consideration.[10] In this case, the results of the preliminary analysis were very clear and convincing, and it is likely that the results will commonly be more equivocal. Even then, a preliminary analysis may be useful in pointing out the main questions of concern, which should then be the focus of further data collection efforts.

[10] In other words, the decision about whether to carry out an economic evaluation in order to clarify a particular economic issue or problem should itself be subject to a kind of economic evaluation of the likely costs and benefits (value of the gain in information) achievable by the assessment. It may be impossible by purely logical means to avoid such a chain of reasoning leading to an infinite regress (because each decision may in turn be claimed to require an economic assessment), so we recommend the use of common sense instead of pure logic.

Supportive Care II: Hematological Support

Introduction

The present chapter is concerned with bone marrow dysfunction in cancer patients and the consequent need for skilled use of hematological support. The bone marrow dysfunction may be a consequence of the disease, e.g., in leukemia patients, or it may be an effect of treatment by cytotoxics or irradiation. In diseases affecting the bone marrow, treatment is directed at curing the patient's bone marrow or replacing it with bone marrow from a donor. In malignancies not directly involving the bone marrow, the most important dose-limiting factor of many forms of treatment, especially chemotherapy regimens, is their myeloablative and immunosuppressive effect, making the patients susceptible to infections by many different microorganisms. If there is a positive dose–response relationship for the treatment concerned, this factor may also have a serious impact on the treatment results obtainable.

The various possible uses of so-called recombinant human hematopoietic growth factors are the main focus of this chapter. The clinical use of these growth factors has been made possible in practice by the invention and widespread practical use of new biochemical techniques (so-called recombinant DNA technology), which allow the production of large quantities. The best-known growth factors are the colony-stimulating factors (CSFs). These are glycoprotein hormones that control the proliferation, differentiation, and maturation of hematopoietic progenitor cells (i.e., cells that subsequently develop into the various types of blood cells). Granulocyte CSF (G-CSF) is a specific and late-acting agent that predominantly stimulates the proliferation of granulocytes and their development into mature neutrophils. It also affects the function of mature neutrophils by stimulating their release from the bone marrow into the peripheral blood and by increasing their activity in fighting infections. Granulocyte–macrophage CSF (GM-CSF) is less specific than G-CSF and acts at several stages in the proliferation and differentiation of the progenitor cells being created in the bone marrow.

Both CSFs may be useful in the prophylaxis and treatment of febrile neutropenia in patients receiving standard-dose chemotherapy, but currently G-CSF is considered the most interesting for this indication, as GM-CSF may itself induce fever and other adverse effects, while adding no benefits compared to G-CSF. The use of CSFs against febrile neutropenia in leukemia patients has been cautioned by the fear that the growth factors might also accelerate the growth of leukemia cells. Another important possible use of the CSFs is as hematological support of chemotherapy. In high-dose chemotherapy accompanied by bone marrow rescue with stem cell transplantation, the CSFs may be used to accelerate the patient's hematological recovery and thereby reduce the risk of infections. Another interesting effect of the CSFs is that they can be used to condition the donor of transplantable cells, either the patients themselves or another person, by mobilizing progenitor cells in the peripheral blood and thereby increasing the possibility of peripheral blood stem cell transplantations (PBSCT).

Febrile Neutropenia and Colony-Stimulating Factors

Despite hospitalization and antibiotic therapy, there is a certain infectious mortality resulting from febrile neutropenia. The mortality rates reported vary somewhat, but the order of magnitude is generally 5%–10%. The rate may be somewhat higher in patients who have been treated with intensified high-dose chemotherapy. In addition to this, febrile neutropenia may also lead to prolonged hospitalization exceeding 1 week, during which the patients will be subjected to numerous diagnostic procedures and intravenous antibiotic therapy with its associated potential complications. In addition, episodes of febrile neutropenia will also typically lead to subsequent delays in delivery of chemotherapy or in dose reductions, which may render the chemotherapy less effective than possible. Accordingly, avoiding febrile neutropenia or reducing the number of such episodes would be expected to enhance patient survival chances and quality of life, reduce the costs of hospitalization, and improve the delivery of chemotherapy.

Numerous clinical studies of the efficacy of the CSFs in the prophylaxis and treatment of febrile neutropenia have been carried out to date (see, e.g., Mayordomo 1995a, b). The following brief overview is based upon the guidelines issued by the American Society of Clinical Oncologists (ASCO) in the end of 1994 and updated in 1996, which contain a detailed description and analysis of the available data from clinical trials, according to the various possible uses of the CSFs (ASCO 1994, 1996). It is important to distinguish carefully between the different indications for use, because the quality of the evidence[1] of their efficacy varies considerably.

Primary prophylaxis is the administration of CSFs to patients from the very first course of chemotherapy, without awaiting evidence of whether the patients develop febrile neutropenia or not. The value of primary administra-

[1] In the above-mentioned publications, the available evidence is systematically graded and weighted according to the recommendations made by Sackett (1989) and Cook et al. (1992). According to these, the best-level evidence comes from a single high-powered randomized, controlled trial or from a meta-analysis of multiple, well-designed controlled studies, while the worst is to be found in case series and single clinical examples.

tion depends on the degree of myelosuppressiveness of the chemotherapy regimen. For regimens with an expected incidence of febrile neutropenia of 40% or more, several trials have shown that the use of CSFs may reduce the incidence by approximately 50%, with a higher quality of the evidence for the G-CSFs than for the GM-CSFs. For less myelosuppressive chemotherapy regimens, the value of primary prophylaxis is not clearly established, and neither is there any conclusive data supporting such use of the CSFs for patients considered to be at higher than normal risk for chemotherapy-induced infections. The evidence only shows a reduction in the incidence of febrile neutropenia and a faster neutrophil recovery. In none of the randomized CSF trials was there a difference in infectious mortality, response rates, or survival between the CSF- and placebo-treated patients.

In secondary prophylaxis, the administration of CSFs is limited to patients who have had a prior episode of febrile neutropenia. The rationale for this strategy is to direct the use of CSFs to a more restricted subset of patients who are most likely to benefit, thus sparing the many patients who may not need CSFs the costs and inconvenience of therapy. There has as yet not been a prospective, randomized trial of the possible effect of secondary prophylaxis with either of the CSFs in decreasing the likelihood of febrile neutropenia in subsequent cycles for patients who have had an episode in an earlier cycle of chemotherapy. There is some evidence, but not of the highest quality, to suggest that secondary administration of either of the CSFs can reduce the duration of neutropenia and the risk of febrile neutropenia. The guidelines state that secondary prophylaxis may be considered even in patients in whom fever has not developed but prolonged neutropenia has caused considerable dose reductions or delays in administration. However, unless there is clear clinical evidence for the importance of maintaining chemotherapy dose intensity, the physicians are advised to consider dose reduction as an attractive alternative.

The CSFs are also widely used as a therapy, especially for patients with febrile neutropenia, but there is even some interest in using it in patients with established neutropenia but no fever (yet). Apart from restricting and targeting their use even more to patients with documented neutropenia or febrile neutropenia, this strategy may be justified by the theoretical possibility that CSF-stimulated neutrophils may be more effective in protecting against fever or clearing infection and/or that CSF-treated patients may have a shorter duration of neutropenia with a consequent reduction in the risk of infection. For the afebrile patients, there is no evidence of a shortening of neutropenia or of clinical benefit. For patients with febrile neutropenia, five randomized trials give conflicting evidence, with the variations in outcomes apparently due to differences in patient characteristics, study design, and data analysis. The evidence indicates no reduction in infectious mortality, and for most patients only little improvement in quality of life.

However, some hypotheses, which of course need confirmatory evidence from prospective trials, have been derived from these studies, indicating that patients with protracted neutropenia or evidence of tissue infection may benefit from the addition of CSFs to the usual antibiotic regimen. This may include patients with pneumonia and with invasive fungal infections, both of which have a poor prognosis. Data from one large center show that five sixths of the 3% of patients who died of febrile neutropenia had pneumonia. On the other hand, studies showing the safety of hospital discharge as soon as the patient is afebrile and the neutrophil count is rising and the success of outpatient antibiotic therapy for patients with uncomplicated febrile neutropenia imply that a general strategy of giving CSFs to all patients with (febrile) neutropenia is not very likely to be beneficial.

Patients with acute myeloid leukemia (AML) deserve separate mention, as virtually all AML patients receiving induction therapy and most of them receiving intensive consolidation therapy develop fever that requires intravenous antibiotics and hospitalization. CSFs cannot be expected to eliminate severe neutropenia in these patients because of the nature of the underlying disease and the intensity of the chemotherapy regimens, but they may shorten the duration of neutropenia and thus decrease the incidence of serious bacterial infections and fungal infections, with consequent reductions in hospitalization time and in empirical antimicrobial therapy; in addition, they may also increase the likelihood of complete remission in first induction and improve the delivery of subsequent consolidation therapy. The available randomized trial data show high-quality evidence of accelerated neutrophil recovery in AML patients treated with CSFs while in induction therapy, but the effect on other and more interesting outcomes is less clear. None of the trials showed reductions in the length of hospital stay, while one study showed a significant reduction in the rate of serious infections and prolonged relapse-free survival in a high-risk elderly population treated with GM-CSF. These results were, however, not corroborated by another study, so it is judged that firm recommendations on this use of CSFs cannot yet be given (ASCO 1994).

There is little justification for using the CSFs to increase dose intensity moderately (to levels not requiring progenitor cell support) outside clinical trials (ASCO 1994). The clinical evidence for a dose response beyond the doses used in standard regimens has been limited. Most of the evidence comes from retrospective analyses of delivered dose or dose intensity as a fraction of that specified in the regimen, but this kind of evidence cannot exclude the possibility that toxicity leading to deviations from the scheduled regimen is a marker for patients with a bad prognosis and that higher than normally scheduled doses will have no incremental benefit. There are, however, some prospective studies in which patients intentionally given lower than standard chemotherapy doses suffered from decreased disease control and worsened survival. In addition, a few randomized studies show improved disease control from higher than conventional dose intensity, but altogether the ASCO panel considers the evidence to be insufficient, although promising.

Economic Evaluations

Before taking up the studies of the use of CSFs, a study concerning another aspect of the hematological support of leukemia patients, namely blood transfusions, will be described.

A cost analysis of a very restricted part of the induction therapy for AML patients was published by Blumberg et al. (1995), who assessed the impact of using blood group-identical platelets and leukodepleted platelets and red blood cells for transfusions. Another example is Balducci et al. (1993), which will not be treated further, however, as the data are very weak. The background for the study is that recent data from randomized clinical trials have shown that use of blood group (A, B, or O)-identical platelet transfusions and white cell depletion of platelet and red blood cell transfusions by filtration (leukodepletion) may lead to a reduction in refractoriness to platelet transfusions and a reduction in transfusion needs, respectively. Other possible benefits of leukodepleted transfusions are reductions in transmission of white cell-associated viruses and transfusion-induced immunosuppression.

The study is based on a retrospective examination of the charts of all the adult patients treated in the hematology department of the authors' institution between 1985 and 1992. It is claimed that the institution's policy with regard to criteria for the use of blood components was unchanged during this period,[2] while the transfusion techniques changed from no matching of blood groups and no filtering in the beginning to matching but no filtering and finally, from early 1990, to both matching and filtering for all patients. Data on patient charges and platelet and red blood cell transfusions were retrieved from the hospital and laboratory computer records, and no patients were excluded from the analysis for any reason. Hospital accounting information on the relationship between charges and costs in 1992 was used to estimate the amount of dollars that were saved (or lost) for patients receiving the regimen with blood-group matching and filtering. All costs and resource utilization figures were calculated both on a per hospital day basis and on a per hospital admission basis to avoid the possibility of variability between patients and treatments leading to understated differences in intensity, length, or success of treatment.

Both lymphoid and myeloid acute leukemias were included in order to have a larger number of patients (a total of 120) for the analysis. No matter which of the three transfusion regimens mentioned above was used, all groups of patients received a similar number of transfusions and had identical lengths of hospital stay, but compared to the unmatched (blood group) and unfiltered group of patients, the matched and filtered group received significantly fewer platelet transfusions (83 vs. 146, on average) and the need

[2] However, the authors do mention that, by the chosen methodology, they cannot rule out the possibility that some of the results were due to some gradual and perhaps not (or barely) noticed changes in the practices of the institution due to the increasing pressure for cost containment.

for support services also decreased, as measured by the number of blood gas and chemistry charges issued, by dollar charges for all ancillary services, and by dollar charges for all subcategories except respiratory therapy. With regard to platelet transfusions, a reduction of about US$ 3300 was seen, while the purchase cost for the filters was $ 875 per patient.

A similar analysis was performed for relapsed lymphoma patients receiving autologous BMT, who were divided into two cohorts according to regimen, the first receiving matched but unfiltered transfusions and the other receiving both matched and filtered transfusions. In all cases where there was a significant difference between the two cohorts, a large reduction in charges or in resource utilization was seen for the group receiving the matched and filtered regimen, i.e., there is a significant reduction in mean length of hospital stays, use of platelet concentrates, red blood cells, total hospital charges, total ancillary service charges, blood bank charges, and pharmacy charges. Purchase costs of about $ 640 per filter were offset by savings in blood component purchase costs of about $ 4000, and total hospital charges were about $ 46,400 less per patient, which is translated into a reduction in actual net costs of around $ 23,000, as the authors assume that variable costs are approximately 50% of the hospital charges in their institution. The use of resources and charges per day did not vary between the two groups, which suggests that the patients differed not in their need for support services but in how long this need lasted, reflected in length of stay.

To provide a background for future studies of the economic impact of the CSFs, Sagmeister et al. (1992) published an assessment of all the costs of a febrile neutropenic event (FNE) in patients undergoing chemotherapy, including institutional and international differences. FNE is defined as the simultaneous occurrence of a neutrophil count below 1000 cells/ml and fever over 38.2 °C. The cost assessment was based on a specific collection of structured data sets in four hospitals in Germany and three hospitals in Switzerland. The data on frequencies of events and the typical services provided according to differing management strategies were obtained by interviews with oncologists and administrators and by a group survey method equivalent to the Delphi technique. By this method, the reliability of the responses is believed to be increased, as the respondents are given feedback from their peers. As cost data, the approximations believed to be the best available were used, e.g., calculated costs for patient days in hospitals, prices for antibiotics, official fees for medical procedures performed, and services delivered. It was assumed that G-CSF would be used for primary prevention, i.e., would be given to all patients undergoing chemotherapy, and data on the efficacy of G-CSF in reducing the incidence of FNE was taken from early clinical studies (which need to be corroborated).

The median cost of an FNE was calculated to be ECU 4100 in Germany (range, 2200–10,000) and ECU 4500 in Switzerland (range, 1400–7900).[3] It is clear that

[3] With the purchasing power parities (PPPs) of 1990, these medians are slightly under and over US$ 4000, respectively.

the differences between institutions within each country are much larger than the differences between the countries. The largest interinstitutional variability (1:25) was observed for patients without FNE, while for patients with FNE the variability was smaller, but still impressive, of the order 1:5. When the data were differentiated according to tumor type (solid tumors vs. acute leukemias), the variability within the groups was reduced to the order of 1:3. The costs of FNE were much lower in patients with solid tumors, but the incidence of these was much higher. Other important factors causing the large variations in costs are differences in discharge policies (average length of stay) and differences in placing patients in critical care units. It is claimed that using the G-CSFs for primary prevention will reduce the costs for the institutions by between ECU 600 and 1200 per chemotherapy cycle, depending on the efficacy assumed for G-CSF and on the pattern of disease incidence in the specific institutions.

Another calculation of the costs of a neutropenic episode was given by Montero et al. (1994), based on a retrospective evaluation of the clinical histories of patients admitted in 1991 to a specific oncology ward with neutropenia induced by chemotherapy or radiotherapy. Patients with fever but with a normal neutrophil count were excluded. An estimate of the costs of recovery for these 16 patients was made, taking into account length of stay in hospital, number of days in isolation, analytical tests performed, type and costs of therapy administered, blood transfusions given, health assistance received, etc. Unit costs were either based on official sources, such as price lists for laboratory tests and drugs, or on assumptions. For instance, the costs of a stay in an isolation unit were taken to be double the costs of a normal hospital day, based on the reasoning that isolation always makes it impossible to admit another patient into the same room.

A total of 11 out of the 16 patients were only admitted once, and the rest two or three times, except for one patient requiring seven admissions. The mean period of hospitalization was 12 days (range, 6–25 days), and the patients were assumed to require the attention of each of the various types of staff members (doctors, nurses, and nurse auxiliaries) for an average of 25 min per day. The average costs per admission due to neutropenia were calculated to be around 330,000 pesetas.[4] This is reduced by some 10% if the patient is not placed in an isolation room.

An equivalent calculation, but limited to patients with hematological cancers, was published by Leese et al. (1994) in a study based on a previous survey carried out by Leese (1993). Clinical data from the medical records of 46 patients with hematological malignancies admitted in 1991 to a single general district hospital with febrile neutropenia were retrospectively collected. FNE was defined as sustained temperature in excess of 37.5 °C simultaneously with a neutrophil count of less than 1000 cells/ml. Cost figures were provided by the hospital's accounting department; however, apart from the statement that drug prices were equal to the hospital's purchase price, no real information is given about the derivation of the prices. Resolution of an

[4] Approximately US$ 4000 if converted by the PPPs of 1990.

FNE was defined as a temperature of less than 37.5 °C for at least 48 h, but the treatment costs were calculated for the days from the onset of fever up to the point of discharge from the hospital. Using this principle is believed to better reflect the true costs of treating patients with neutropenia, who might have significantly delayed morbidity despite resolution of fever.

The average length of hospital stay was 17 days (median, 15 days), and the median cost per FNE over the 46 episodes was £ 2068,[5] ranging from £ 418 to £ 7023. For these calculations, an inpatient cost per day of £ 82.5 was used, while the cost per day in the intensive care unit was set at £ 1035. For all episodes, inpatient costs accounted for 58% of the total costs, drug treatment for 26%, and diagnostics 16%. A differentiation according to diagnosis (distinguishing between AML, non-Hodgkin's disease, and Hodgkin's lymphoma) did not reveal any significant differences.

The use of G-CSFs in small cell lung cancer (SCLC) patients with febrile neutropenia has attracted much interest, and several economic assessments of this issue have been published. Three of these are based on efficacy data from the clinical trial by Crawford et al. (1991), which was a pivotal study in the registration of the G-CSF filgrastim. The patients had SCLC, stratified according to performance status and the presence or absence of bone marrow involvement and were randomized between prophylactic G-CSF or placebo. The chemotherapy regimen consisted of cyclophosphamide+doxorubicin+ etoposide, up to six cycles, from day 1 to 3, with 21 days between cycles (provided that sufficient hematological recovery had been achieved and that tumor progression had not occurred). On day 4 of each cycle, patients began receiving daily subcutaneous injections of the study medication, G-CSF or placebo, and injections were continued until the absolute neutrophil count rose to more than 10,000 cells/µl. Patients were monitored closely, and if their body temperature rose above 38.2 °C with an associated neutrophil count of less than 1000 cells/µl, the patient was hospitalized and treated with standard intravenous antibiotic therapy while continuing daily injections with the blinded study medication. For patients experiencing febrile neutropenia in a cycle, the randomization code was broken and the patient removed from the blinded portion of the study. The hospitalization rates in the first cycle, in which the patients were balanced with respect to the initial stratification criteria, were 0.26 for the filgrastim group and 0.55 for the placebo group.

Glaspy et al. (1993) used the hospitalization data for patients from three of the study sites involved in the trial by Crawford and coworkers in order to assess the costs associated with the use of filgrastim seen from the third-party payer's perspective (see also Glaspy and Jakway 1993). Itemized hospital bills and physician charges were obtained from the three centers or associated community hospitals, while charges for radiological procedures required by the protocol and charges associated with inpatient chemotherapy were excluded. Data were collected for all the chemotherapy cycles, but the cost analysis focused on the first cycle, as patients were removed from each

[5] About US$ 4900 when using the PPPs of 1990 for conversion.

treatment arm after each cycle. Filgrastim was not marketed at the time of study, so a "reasonable" price had to be estimated. Other costs associated with its use were monitoring of the patients with additional blood counts, injection supplies, and education in self-injection (time of physician or nurse). An economic model was constructed in which the net costs of filgrastim were found by subtracting the total resources used by the filgrastim group from the total resources used by the placebo group.

Three health care financing perspectives were analyzed, i.e., a charge model, a Medicare model, and a cost model, recognizing that patients and third-party insurers pay for health services using different payment mechanisms. In the charge model, invoiced charges were used; in the Medicare model, the diagnosis-related groups (DRGs) paid by Medicare were used; and in the cost model, true costs were estimated by multiplying each hospital's charges with individual cost-to-charge ratios, according to Medicare sources. Charge data were collected for 68 patients from the three hospitals, and for these patients the rates of hospitalization in the first cycle were 14% for filgrastim and 69% for placebo. The mean length of stay was 3.6 days for filgrastim patients, with mean charges of $ 4258, while for the placebo patients it was 7.3 days and $ 8469 in charges. The mean expected charges were $ 596 for the filgrastim group and $ 5843 for the placebo group.

The estimated impact of filgrastim varied depending on the model employed. The charge model used the hospitalization data from the larger clinical trial (and not just the 68 patients), and this yielded a net saving of $ 1250 per cycle (including the assumed cost of filgrastim). The Medicare model resulted in net incremental costs per cycle of about $ 600. The number of hospitalizations was reduced, but because of the fixed DRG payment mechanism employed, this did not reduce the cost to Medicare of the hospitalizations that occurred. In the cost model, filgrastim resulted in an additional cost of about $ 140 per cycle. The same patterns are seen in the sensitivity analysis, which indicates that the results are robust.

Lyman et al. (1993) used the baseline probabilities for hospitalization risk, survival etc. from the trial by Crawford and coworkers in a decision model with the purpose of determining the cost-effectiveness of using G-CSFs for primary prophylaxis or for therapeutic purposes. The costs included are the total costs of hospitalizations for FNE and the total costs of G-CSF per chemotherapy cycle. The cost figures used to calculate the costs of hospitalization and G-CSF administration were based on daily charges available from a specific cancer center. Items such as diagnostic and monitoring tests, cultures, and consultations were excluded. The costs of hospitalization for FNE included charges for room, antibiotics, fluids and tubing, and professional fees. The costs of G-CSFs included charges for the agent and for its administration. Excess costs were calculated as the additional costs associated with hospitalization for FNE and/or treatment with G-CSF above the costs for individuals not hospitalized for FNE and not treated with G-CSF.

The baseline value for the expected excess costs in the case of no therapy with G-CSF, i.e., the costs of FNE, was estimated as $ 5500. If G-CSFs were used for primary prophylaxis, the expected excess costs became \$ 4750, while they were \$ 6875 if G-CSF was used therapeutically for patients hospitalized with FNE. If the excluded costs for additional diagnostic and monitoring tests etc. were to be included, the prophylactic use of G-CSF would probably seem to be even more favorable. After extensive one-way and multivariate sensitivity analyses, including Monte Carlo simulations, it is concluded that routine therapeutic use of G-CSF after admission with FNE is never supported by the cost data, while its use for primary prophylaxis may reduce the costs significantly in certain clinical settings. This is especially true for patients with a high risk of developing infection or infection-related complications because of a risk of FNE higher than 40% or previous hospitalization for FNE. For patients with an intermediate risk of FNE (20%–40%), primary prophylaxis with G-CSF may be cost saving, provided the daily hospital costs are higher than \$ 1500, hospitalizations for FNE last for more than 15 days, or the daily costs of G-CSFs are less than \$ 150. With a risk of FNE below 20%, primary prophylaxis will not be cost saving.

Nichols et al. (1994) combined data from the trial by Crawford and coworkers with data on the incidence of FNE and days of hospitalization from a retrospective, unselected case series of 137 SCLC patients at a single university hospital between 1987 and 1992, none of whom were treated with G-CSF. The guidelines for hospitalization with FNE were fever of ≥38.5 °C and an absolute neutrophil count of 500 cells/ml or lower. Guidelines for discharge were that patients had been afebrile for at least 24 h and that the neutrophil count was rising. Data on the effect of G-CSF were taken from the trial by Crawford and colleagues, assuming that the administration of G-CSF would have reduced the total number of days in hospital by 45%. Average charges for G-CSFs and for an FNE were estimated by reviewing the charges for two series of patients treated at the hospital, giving an estimate of about \$ 2000 for G-CSF per cycle of chemotherapy and about \$ 1200 per day of hospitalization of a patient with neutropenic fever. The cost impact of various strategies of G-CSF use was considered.

Overall, 18% of the patients in the case series were hospitalized with FNE. Of these, two thirds were hospitalized in connection with the first cycle of chemotherapy. Seven treatment-related deaths occurred, of which six were judged to be related to FNE. Over a total of 583 cycles of chemotherapy for these patients, there were 26 hospital admissions for FNE, resulting in a total of 155 hospital days. It was calculated that if G-CSF had been used prophylactically, the total charges would have been about \$ 1.3 million, i.e., the sum of the charges for administering G-CSF in all cycles of chemotherapy and charges for hospitalizations for FNE occurring despite this general prophylaxis. A strategy of secondary prophylaxis, where G-CSF is used in all cycles of chemotherapy following an FNE, resulted in total charges of about \$ 276,000. Reducing the doses of chemotherapy instead of using G-CSFs was calculated to result in charges of about \$ 193,000.

With the assumptions used, the charges for G-CSF would have to be about \$ 150 per cycle of chemotherapy if a strategy of primary prophylaxis should be revenue neutral compared to a strategy of reducing the doses of chemotherapy if FNE occurs. This is less than a tenth of the charges actually estimated for patients at the same hospital. One of the main explanations for the very low threshold value for the charges for G-CSFs, i.e., the value of charges which is required to make a strategy of primary prophylaxis revenue neutral, even if it is assumed that G-CSFs are 100% effective in preventing hospitalizations due to FNE, is that the incidence of FNE in the case series was low (compared to an incidence of 77% in the placebo arm of the trial by Crawford and coworkers).

Drummond and Davies (1994) attempted to assess the impact of the G-CSF lenograstim on health care costs, based on the results of a clinical trial that examined whether the prophylactic use of G-CSF would permit a significant increase in the dose intensity of chemotherapy in patients with good-prognosis SCLC. A total of 65 patients with at most one adverse prognostic factor were randomized to chemotherapy (vincristine + ifosfamide + carbopla-tin + etoposide) with or without adjuvant G-CSF. The intervals between cycles of chemotherapy were not fixed in advance, but were determined by the attainment of certain threshold levels for white blood cell and platelet counts. The primary perspective of the cost analysis was that of the government, and the principal source of data was the clinical trial database. The general approach to costing was to use unit cost estimates pertaining to a tertiary referral center for SCLC and, if such estimates were not available, to use national average unit prices. The derivation of unit prices is described in some detail, and they seem to be a mixture of precise estimates of real costs and less precise, but convenient estimates. The costs of G-CSF is set to zero in the calculations, as no official market price existed at the time of the analysis. In principle, an intention to treat principle was used for the cost analysis, but data were not available for patients who withdrew from the clinical trial.

The results of the clinical trial were that the cumulative dose-intensity index was significantly higher in the G-CSF group. Nonsignificant differences in favor of the G-CSF group were that fewer had one or more documented infections and that there was a trend towards better survival at the end of the 2-year follow-up period. On the other hand, there was a nonsignificant higher short-term mortality rate in this group, probably due to the toxicity of the more intensive chemotherapy regimen they were receiving. There were no differences in the average length of hospital stay, in the time spent in a general ward or in intensive care units, or in the length of inpatient stay for chemotherapy or any other purposes. There were fewer admissions in the G-CSF group for treatment of (suspected) infections, but more for transfusions and anemia therapy. There was a trend towards higher utilization of blood products and nonscheduled laboratory investigations for the G-CSF group, but no differences with respect to the number of days of anti-infective therapy or the number of days with chemotherapy or protocol-determined examinations and services.

Overall, the average costs for the G-CSF group were higher, i.e., £ 9700 vs. £ 9000,[6] even though the costs of the G-CSFs themselves were not included.

[6] About US$ 22,000 if converted by the PPPs of 1990.

The main factors behind this not statistically significant difference were higher costs for inpatient care, blood products, and laboratory investigations, offset to some extent by lower costs for anti-infectives and prophylactic medication. The results were not very sensitive to variations in unit prices, but this was the only form of sensitivity analysis performed.

Souêtre and Qing (1994) performed a cost analysis from the hospital perspective of the use of the G-CSF lenograstim for primary prophylaxis of chemotherapy-induced neutropenia in patients with non-Hodgkin's lymphoma. Clinical and resource utilization data were collected in parallel with a French multicenter, randomized, double-blind trial, in which 162 patients were randomized to chemotherapy with or without G-CSF. For both groups, a fixed 56-day assessment period was chosen (the minimum time period necessary to receive four full cycles of chemotherapy), because it was believed that an unequal incidence of infection would lead to an unequal period of administration of the full course of chemotherapy. The economic analysis is based on the intention to treat principle. For patients that withdrew prematurely, data on infections and rehospitalization after their withdrawal were collected retrospectively, while it was assumed that their remaining resource utilization was the same as for the patients continuing in the trial.

Clinical outcomes considered were the proportion of patients with a documented infection, the rate of dose optimization (completion of four cycles of chemotherapy), the average number of chemotherapy cycles per patient, and chemotherapy delays (days of delay for each cycle). The economic outcomes were number of hospital days (e.g., total, days in intensive care units), drug therapy (number of days of chemotherapy, lenograstim, antibiotics), and number of blood products administered. Unit costs were found by a number of methods, such as finding a standard hospitalization cost by using the weighted average of the per diem prices for 11 hospitals and using a standard tariff list for a number of other services. The study drug, lenograstim, was not included in the cost calculations, as there was no official price at the time of the study.

There was no significant difference between the proportion of patients in the two groups that experienced infections, while the percentage of patients that completed the four cycles of chemotherapy was significantly higher in the lenograstim group (49% vs. 7% in the placebo group). There was a significant difference in the number of cycles of chemotherapy completed (3.4 vs. 2.7 in the placebo group), and the mean number of days of delay was 0.5 for lenograstim patients and 2.5 for the placebo group. The average consumption of all types of resources considered was higher for the placebo group, significantly so for number of days on inpatient intravenous antibiotics, and the average total cost for the placebo group was also higher than for the G-CSF group (FF 122,831 vs. 115,534). From this apparent saving of roughly FF 7000,[7] the costs of the lenograstim therapy should of course be deducted, but no such attempt is found in the paper. However, it is not very

[7] About US$ 1600 when converted by the 1990 PPPs.

likely that the net cost saving found for the lenograstim group would be sustained if these costs were included.

Mapelli et al. (1994) performed what they consider primarily to be a cost-identification analysis from the perspective of the national health service of the economic impact of using the G-CSF lenograstim as an adjunct to chemotherapy of inflammatory breast cancer. Costs were calculated by applying Italian and German unit costs to resource utilization data derived from a French clinical trial with the primary aim of assessing the effect of adjuvant lenograstim on neutrophil recovery and infections during high-dose chemotherapy. In the multicenter trial, 61 patients received lenograstim on an outpatient basis (subcutaneous injections), while 59 received placebo. The chemotherapy was administered in four cycles, with 4 days in hospital and 3-week intervals. Patients were observed for the minimum time needed to complete a full course of chemotherapy, i.e., 84 days, and patients withdrawn earlier were analyzed on an intention to treat basis, with data on resource utilization after withdrawal being collected retrospectively. As for resource use for participants still in the trial, only days of hospitalization, days of chemotherapy, and days of antibiotic therapy were measured. Laboratory and diagnostic tests were excluded from the analysis with the reasoning that they were mandated by the trial protocol.

Unit costs were derived from a number of sources. For instance, hospitalization days in Germany were costed by an average of the usual daily allowances for a number of hospitals (with great variations observed), while for Italy the total costs per inpatient day were calculated from personnel costs, hotel costs, and overheads (calculated as 5% of the sum of the others). The costs of chemotherapy, antibiotics, and blood products were calculated directly from the patient case report forms. The costs of lenograstim and the costs of home nursing visits to administer it were ignored, as the drug was not marketed at an official price at the time of the study.

A total of 49% of the patients in the lenograstim group and 72% in the placebo group presented with a documented infection, although only less than a third of all these were microbiologically confirmed. However, there was no difference in the rate of complete response after four cycles of chemotherapy. There was a nonsignificant trend towards more delays of chemotherapy in the placebo group, they spent more time in hospital for reasons other than administration of chemotherapy (9.8 vs. 7.4 days, nonsignificant), the rate of withdrawals in this group was significantly higher (20% vs. 5%), and they received antibiotics for significantly more days (4.8 days). There were no differences in blood products utilization. Overall, the number of days on antibiotics was a third less in the lenograstim group than in the placebo group, and they had 24% less days of hospitalization for any reason other than administration of chemotherapy. The costs of chemotherapy were higher in the lenograstim group because they had fewer chemotherapy delays and hence benefited from 1.2 more days of chemotherapy on average (the time frame of the follow-up was fixed in advance to a certain number of days). Overall, the total direct costs for the lenograstim group were calculated to be about a third less than for the placebo group in both Italy and Germany.

There has been considerably less interest in the economics of the GM-CSFs, with only two papers identified and retrieved for this survey, both concerned with its use in connection with BMT for patients with hematological cancers. Gulati and Bennett (1992) used a randomized trial of 24 patients with relapsed Hodgkin's disease, all of whom had previously received either chemotherapy or radiotherapy, receiving either GM-CSF or placebo within 24 h after BMT and continuing this therapy for 30 days or until the neutrophil reached at least 1000 cells/µl and remained stable. All care was given in either an intensive care unit or in a BMT unit, and before initiation of the study clinical guidelines about the use of in-hospital resources were set up in order to ensure that decisions influencing important study end points were made consistently from patient to patient. Thus prophylactic antibiotic treatment was given twice daily for 1 week before the BMT, and platelet transfusions were to be given when the platelet count was less than 2000 cells/µl. For patients with neutropenic fever (temperature elevation to 37.5 °C or higher), empirical antibiotic treatment was given, and if the temperature elevation persisted despite this for more than 48 h, an antifungal (amphotericin B) was added on an empirical basis. Guidelines for hospital discharge were also fixed in advance.

Resource use for each patient was determined by reviewing medical records and hospital bills. The categories considered were hospital accommodation, laboratory tests, radiologic and diagnostic tests, antimicrobial therapy, blood products, physician consultations, respiratory, physical, and occupational therapy, and medically indicated surgical and invasive procedures. So-called normative prices or charges for each type of resource consumed were derived from various sources, e.g., by interviewing physicians and other providers to obtain estimates of anticipated fees. For others, such as pharmaceuticals and laboratory tests, available prices from price lists were multiplied by charge-to-price ratios, varying according to price range. The resulting charges were justified by their conformity with the charges used in other studies in the field of cancer. The use of GM-CSF was not costed in the baseline analysis, because the specific product used was not yet registered and marketed, but in sensitivity analyses the price of another, already marketed GM-CSF was used.

The analysis was carried out despite a claim that the patients in the two groups were not completely equivalent with regard to previously received therapy, which might influence their probability of profiting from the BMT. The possible bias was believed to be unfavorable to the GM-CSF patients. These patients had a significant advantage compared to the placebo group with respect to the period on the study drug (17 vs. 27 days), the period before the absolute neutrophil count returned to 1000 cells/µl (16 vs. 27 days), and the duration of platelet transfusion dependency (13 vs. 21 days). There were no differences in disease-free survival after 32 months of follow-up; all 24 patients had neutropenic fever and required systemic antibiotic therapy, and both groups had similar rates of laboratory-confirmed bacteremia, fungemia, pulmonary infections, and pneumonia. The GM-CSF patients had significantly fewer days of hospitalization, reflecting an insignificant trend towards lower use of all the types of resources considered. The calculated mean total charges for the GM-CSF and the placebo group were US$ 43,600 (no costs for the GM-CSF included) and $ 61,900, respectively. In sensitivity analyses, it was shown that GM-CSF would be cost saving with a price of up to $ 1200 per day. For comparison, the current price of an analogous GM-CSF product was given as $ 300 per day, and with this price the average saving per patient would be about $ 16,000.

Luce et al. (1994) examined the health care utilization pattern and the resulting bills for patients with lymphoid cancer who received GM-CSF or placebo prophylactically before undergoing autologous BMT. The clinical data were taken from a randomized, double-blind trial, and the economic analysis was conducted retrospectively (but in a blinded fashion) based on data from 41 patients coming from one institution, with one patient (placebo) being excluded as a cost outlier. The study medication was administered as a 2-h intravenous infusion on consecutive days from the day of the BMT to 20 days after. No patients received subsequent courses of GM-CSF within 100 days after the BMT. The duration of illness was defined as beginning the day after the infusion of the study drug until 100 days postinfusion or until the patient was discharged or until death. The utilization of medical resources was measured, using duration of hospitalization, including all readmissions, inpatient and outpatient use of hospital services in the period following infusion of the study drug, and physician services. The costs were calculated by generating bills for all types of resources consumed, so charges were used no matter what the patients' insurance or financial status. For GM-CSF a predicted price is used, as the study drug was donated; later, the drug was marketed at approximately the predicted price. A number of missing values were imputed.

In order to "ensure that early death should not contribute to positive economic analysis," ten patients (one quarter) were excluded from the analysis. The main result reported was a marginally significant reduction of about 20% for the GM-CSF group in initial hospitalization charges, mainly due to a shortening of the initial hospital stay by almost 7 days (20%), while there were no differences in the charges per day of the initial hospitalization nor in the rate of rehospitalization. The total amount of charges were about $ 12,000 lower for the GM-CSF group, but this difference was not found to be statistically significant. By far the most important components in the reduction of charges for the GM-CSF patients were a reduction in room charges and in charges for intravenous medication (including alimentation and antibiotics), which is consistent with the reduction in inpatient days being the underlying factor.

Recently, Uyl-de-Groot et al. (1996a) published a simplified economic model for hospitals with the aim of determining all the relevant direct hospital costs in relation to chemotherapy-induced fever and its treatment and possibly prophylaxis. The perspective of the study was that of the hospital, and three different categories of treatment choices were considered:

1. G-CSFs administered to patients receiving intensive chemotherapy
2. G-CSFs given prophylactically during and after standard chemotherapy cycles on an outpatient basis
3. G-CSFs given in combination with antibiotics in patients with solid tumors or non-Hodgkin's disease receiving standard chemotherapy on an outpatient basis in order to shorten the period of fever and neutropenia

Baseline values for the clinical probabilities, e.g., the probability of developing fever and neutropenia and the number of days with antibiotics or/and G-CSF, were taken from a literature review. Although the sources used are indicated, there is almost no discussion of the often divergent results, and the choices made are not motivated. The same remarks apply to the data given for unit costs, which are allegedly derived from earlier Dutch studies on the cost-effectiveness of cancer treatments, but which appear rather to be estimated round figures, probably in the neighborhood of the results of the studies mentioned.

The results of the calculations, comprising baseline values and a number of sensitivity analyses, e.g., determining threshold values of key variables, will not be detailed here. In general, they show that the administration of G-CSFs may actually lead to savings in the costs of daily hospital practice and that their prophylactic use in patients receiving intensive chemotherapy and their use for secondary prophylaxis in patients receiving standard chemotherapy is generally cost saving compared to an alternative with conventional antibiotic therapy. This, however, depends on the daily hospital costs and length of stay assumed. If, for instance, standard chemotherapy is administered in regional hospitals, which is often the case, where the daily costs are lower than for hospitals providing intensive hematological care, as assumed in the calculations, the use of G-CSFs does not result in savings. In general, the results seem to be sensitive to changes in the assumptions, but the simple model seems to be a useful tool which can be used by local hospital administrations in order to get a rough idea about the economic impact of various treatment regimens, provided that they have some relevant local data to fill in.

Concluding Remarks

The economic assessments of the various uses of the CSFs described in the foregoing are summarized in Table 1.

When looking at the many studies concerned with determining the costs of FNEs, it might be tempting to interpret the near equivalence of the results of a number of these calculations as an indication of convergence towards a "true" value (see also Faulds 1996; Faulds et al. 1992; Frampton and Faulds 1996). However, this would no doubt be a misinterpretation, given the differences in the range of cost items included and in the methods used for valua-

Table 1. Main characteristics of economic assessments dealing with the use of colony-stimulating factors (CSFs)

Reference	Disease category	Treatments examined	Main characteristics of the study
Sagmeister et al. (1992)	Patients with FNE	Typical management strategies in Germany and Switzerland	Cost-determination study Perspective not stated explicitly Data on frequency of events and typical procedures provided obtained by interviews with oncologists; cost assessment based on specific collection of structured data sets for limited number of institutions; unit prices are calculated costs for hospital stays, official fees for services and procedures, official drug prices Median costs are 10% lower in Germany; interinstitutional variability within countries is much larger than variations between countries; important factors behind the large variations are differences in discharge policies and differences in placing patients in critical care units
Montero et al. (1994)	Oncology patients with FNE	All treatments administered	Cost-determination study Perspective not explicitly given Retrospective investigation of clinical records of 16 patients admitted with FNE induced by chemo- or radiotherapy; estimate of costs of recovery, based on data on resource use from the clinical records; unit costs from official sources (e.g., prices for laboratory tests) or assumptions Range observed of the various resource items quite wide, and cost distribution very skewed, with mean costs much higher than the median
Leese et al. (1994)	Patients with hematological malignancies and FNE	All treatments considered	Cost-determination study Perspective not explicitly stated Resource utilization data from inspection of medical records of 46 patients admitted to a single hospital; cost figures from the hospital's accounting department, but little information about their derivation except for drug prices (hospital's purchase price) Results are expressed as median costs, with an almost 20-fold range; overall, inpatient hospital stays account for 58% of the costs, drug treatment (antibiotics) for 26%, and diagnostics 16%; no differences according to diagnosis
Glaspy et al. (1993)	SCLC patients with FNE	Use of G-CSFs	Impact on costs of using G-CSFs Third-party payer perspective (Medicare) Retrospective examination of hospitalization data for 68 patients in three institutions participating in clinical trial; cost analysis focused on first cycle of chemotherapy; three health care financing perspectives examined: charge model, Medicare model, and cost-to-charge ratio

Table 1 (continued)

Reference	Disease category	Treatments examined	Main characteristics of the study
			In first cycle, 14% hospitalized for FNE in G-CSF group, 68% in placebo group, and mean length of stay about half in the G-CSF group; mean expected charges for G-CSF patients are about 10% of the mean for the placebo group; impact of G-CSF depends on the financing model employed, and the results vary between a saving in net costs and significantly increased costs
Lyman et al. (1993)	SCLC patients with FNE	Use of G-CSFs for primary prophylaxis or for therapy	Cost-minimization analysis Third-party payer perspective Baseline probabilities for hospitalization risk, survival etc. from randomized clinical trial; cost figures used are based on daily charges from a cancer center Expected costs with prophylactic use of G-CSF slightly lower than baseline expected costs of FNE, which again are lower than costs of using G-CSF therapeutically; after extensive sensitivity analysis and simulations, it is concluded that prophylactic use of G-CSF will be cost saving if the risk of FNE is higher than 40%, and potentially cost saving with a risk of FNE of 20%–40%, provided hospital costs are over a certain threshold
Nichols et al. (1994)	SCLC patients with FNE	Primary vs. secondary prophylaxis of FNE with G-CSF	Cost-minimization analysis Third-party payer perspective Combines efficacy data from randomized trial of G-CSF with data on incidence of FNE and days of hospitalization from an unselected case series of patients not treated with G-CSF; assumes that G-CSF would have reduced hospital days by 45%; average charges for a FNE and for use of G-CSFs estimated by examining charges for series of patients Overall, 18% incidence of FNE in the case series; the lowest cost strategy is found to be to reduce the doses of chemotherapy; the costs of primary prophylaxis with G-CSF (including the costs of FNEs that occur despite prophylaxis) is about six times higher, while secondary prophylaxis with G-CSF is 50% more costly than reduction of doses of chemotherapy
Uyl-de-Groot et al. (1996a)	FNE in all types of cancer patients	Various types of strategies, e.g., G-CSF for prophylaxis of patients in intensive chemotherapy or treatment with G-CSF to shorten FNE	Cost-identification study Hospital perspective Model with clinical probabilities taken from a (selective) literature review; unit cost data taken from other Dutch studies of cost-effectiveness of various cancer treatments In general, the results show that G-CSFs may lead to hospital cost savings; compared to conventional antibiotic therapy, prophylaxis with G-CSFs in patients in intensive chemotherapy and their use for secondary prophylaxis in patients receiving standard chemotherapy will lead to cost savings; the result is not stable against changes in assumptions about daily costs and length of stay, however

Table 1 (continued)

Reference	Disease category	Treatments examined	Main characteristics of the study
Drummond and Davies (1994)	Patients with good-prognosis SCLC	High-dose chemotherapy with G-CSF support	Cost-minimization analysis Public sector perspective Integrated in clinical trial of adjuvant G-CSF vs. nothing, 65 patients; unit cost estimates from a referral center for SCLC and national average unit prices; no cost of G-CSF is included (not yet marketed at the time of the study) There were nonsignificant differences in favor of the G-CSF with respect to number of patients with infections and a trend towards better survival; average costs about 10% higher for the G-CSF group, because of higher costs for inpatient care, blood products, and laboratory investigations, while costs of anti-infectives were lower
Souêtre and Qing (1994)	Patients with non-Hodgkin's lymphoma	High-dose chemotherapy with G-CSF support	Cost-effectiveness analysis Hospital perspective Clinical and resource utilization data collected in parallel with a randomized clinical trial, 162 patients; fixed 8-week assessment period (time required for four cycles of chemotherapy); clinical outcomes considered were number of infections and number of patients receiving chemotherapy as intended; economic outcomes were number of hospital days, drug therapy, and number of blood products; unit costs from standard lists of tariffs and from averaging cost data from 11 hospitals; no costs of G-CSF included (not marketed at the time of study) No significant difference in the proportion of patients with infections, but significantly more G-CSF patients received the chemotherapy as intended; average costs a little higher for the placebo group (5%), and their use of all types of resources considered were higher, significantly so for number of days on inpatient antibiotics
Mapelli et al. (1994)	Patients with inflammatory breast cancer	High-dose chemotherapy with G-CSF support	Cost-identification study National health service perspective Resource utilization date derived from a clinical trial aiming at assessing the impact of G-CSF on number of infections and neutrophil count; period of observation is 12 weeks, corresponding to a full course of chemotherapy; number of days in hospital, days on chemotherapy, and days of antibiotic therapy measured; unit costs (for Germany and Italy, respectively) derived from a number of sources, no costs of G-CSF included (not marketed at the time of study) Significantly fewer patients in the G-CSF group had documented infections; the total direct costs for the G-CSF group were found to be about a third smaller in both countries, with higher costs of chemotherapy (delivered as intended more frequently) and fewer days of hospitalization (for any reason) and antibiotic therapy

Table 1 (continued)

Reference	Disease category	Treatments examined	Main characteristics of the study
Gulati and Bennett (1992)	Patients with relapsed Hodgkin's disease	BMT with GM-CSF support	Cost-identification study Perspective not explicitly stated Resource use data from retrospective review of charts and hospital bills for 24 patients in randomized trial, which included objective clinical guidelines for resource use; extensive recording of resource categories; unit costs from physician interviews and published charges multiplied by cost-to-charge ratios; no cost of GM-CSF included (not marketed at the time of study) No differences in survival after 32 months of follow-up; all patients had FNE and required antibiotic therapy; GM-CSF patients were on study drug for fewer days, had faster recovery of neutrophil count and less need for platelet transfusions; significantly fewer days of hospitalization for the GM-CSF group and total costs calculated are about a third lower
Luce et al. (1994)	Patients with lymphoid cancer	Prophylactic GM-CSF before autologous BMT	Cost-identification study Third-party payer perspective Clinical data from randomized clinical trial; cost data for 41 patients in this trial, coming from one institution; retrospective (blinded) recording of resource utilization, including all services provided; source of cost data are the billings for the patients, and charges are used as unit costs; for GM-CSF, a predicted price is used Initial hospitalization charges are 20% lower for the GM-CSF group (marginally significant), mainly because of a 20% shorter initial hospital stay; charges per day are equal, as are the rates of rehospitalization; this shortening of initial hospital stay (and associated intravenous medication) is the main factor explaining smaller overall charges for the GM-CSF group (not significant)

FNE, febrile neutropenic episode; SCLC, small cell lung cancer; G-CSF, granulocyte CSF; GM-CSF, granulocyte-macrophage CSF; BMT, bone marrow transplantation.

tion of the costs. Another significant variation to notice is in the definition of FNEs, which must also often be considered as far removed from the criteria used in ordinary clinical practice. The assumed incidence of some of the studies analyzing the impact of prevention of FNE by CSFs must be considered to be very much higher than what is usually seen in clinical practice.

Several of the papers assessing the costs and benefits of CSFs are unusual in *not* including the costs of the CSF drugs in the calculations. The reasons given for this important exclusion are that the study drug was provided free of charge by the manufacturer, that it was not yet marketed at the time of study, or something similar. Such exclusions do not render these assessments invalid (provided that the exclusion is appropriately emphasized, which is not always the case), but the main purpose and interest of such studies would seem to be to serve as a guidance for decisions on the part of the manufacturer or perhaps on the part of a public price control authority, although this is less commonly the impression.

The theoretically very promising clinical potential of the CSFs has not yet been clearly and convincingly corroborated by results of randomized and controlled clinical trials (see also Fox 1994; Jönsson and Karlsson 1993; Le Coroller et al. 1994). There is as yet no evidence from randomized controlled trials that the CSFs can improve overall or disease-free survival in patients treated with standard chemotherapy doses. A reduction in the number and duration of FNEs has been documented, allowing more patients in the CSF arm of trials to receive the scheduled doses, but this has not resulted in demonstrable effects on survival. Multiple studies of adjuvant therapy with CSF to allow intensification of chemotherapy have shown that this is feasible, but there is as yet little data to support the expectation of improved survival, even in cancers believed to be sensitive to dose intensification.

With respect to the use of CSFs to prevent or treat FNEs, the ASCO guidelines (ASCO 1994, 1996) state that, for treatments with a high incidence of FNE (generally ≥40%), there is first-class evidence for the justification of primary prophylaxis with CSF. In addition, they refer to a cost-effectiveness modeling study showing that primary prophylaxis will result in a cost saving if the incidence of FNE is 40% or higher. There is no direct reference to the study by Lyman et al. (1993), but the figures given and the description in general indicates that this is indeed the study to which the guidelines refer. In this way, a particular study is (rather arbitrarily it seems) selected and elevated to a level of authority which is not justified either by the study design or by the quality of the data employed.

Either of the other two studies on the question for the same group of SCLC patients could with equal justification have been singled out, and this would have resulted in quite different threshold values in the recommendations. The study by Uyl-de-Groot et al. (1996a), examining various types of strategies for using CSFs to prevent or treat FNE in patients with all types of cancer, which is based on clinical data from a literature review (unpublished) and estimates of actual unit costs instead of charges, provides much more equivocal results. The sensitivity analyses performed show that the results are far from robust against changes in assumptions about daily hospital costs and length of stay. At baseline, compared to conventional antibiotic therapy, cost savings may be obtained by using CSFs for prophylaxis in patients receiving intensified chemotherapy or by using them for secondary prophylaxis for patients receiving standard chemotherapy. These results are quite different from those obtained by Lyman et al. (1993). It is also important to notice that reduction of chemotherapy doses remains a valid and less costly alternative in many treatment contexts.

The studies reported here on the use of CSFs to support patients given high-dose chemotherapy vary somewhat with respect to the impact on the frequency of infections and on costs, while they agree on leaving out the costs of CSFs and in using intermediate outcome measures such as proportion of patients receiving the intended schedules and doses of chemotherapy. There are no significant survival differences documented, and patient quality of life is not a variable considered in any of these studies. Neither is the impact on total average costs of including the costs of CSFs investigated, even as a rough estimate or in the form of a threshold estimate. This approach should definitely not be recommended, especially taking into account the fact that a essential purpose of carrying out economic evaluations is to provide information that may be generalized outside the specific setting of the study. Even within a particular setting in such a study (e.g., hospital, region), however, it should not be expected that drug manufacturers will continue to provide drugs free of charge.

In a recent reappraisal of the established "pharmacoeconomic" results concerning the use of the G-CSF filgrastim for the prophylaxis and treatment of chemotherapy-induced neutropenia and fever, some very interesting and pertinent data are referred to (Frampton and Faulds 1996). According to the survey, a recent review of the prescription patterns for G-CSFs in 30 academic health centers in the United States showed that they were used for appropriate indications in about 70% of the cases, while the correct dosages (according to the manufacturers' recommendations) were only given in about 50% of cases. These data on the inappropriate use of G-CSFs, which apparently do not even include cases of inappropriate nonuse of the drugs, are remarkable, not least because they were collected in academic centers, which would be assumed to be above average in the quality (understood as adherence to the norms of *evidence-based medicine*) of their prescription patterns. In addition, one might speculate that the relatively high acquisition costs of the G-CSFs, which in many institutions is the main argument for not using them (routinely), would lead to exceptional care being taken in prescribing them, leaving one to wonder about the quality of prescription for other drugs with less focus on the acquisition costs.

Transplantation of Blood Progenitor or Stem Cells

Bone Marrow Transplantation

The term BMT refers to two distinct types of therapy. Allogeneic BMT includes procedures used primarily to treat diseases of the bone marrow and involves the collection and transplantation of marrow from a donor other than the patient. The aim of allogeneic BMT is to destroy the patient's diseased marrow with either cytotoxics or radiation, thereby curing the disease. After this, the donor's marrow is infused into the patient. Autologous BMTs are directed at a wider number of diseases and involve marrow obtained from the patient. Autologous BMT may involve therapy that is directed at many different types of cells and not necessarily diseased bone marrow. However, the intensity of therapy is such that the marrow cells would be killed as a consequence of the therapy. Therefore, marrow from the patient is harvested before the start of the therapy and then reinfused into the patient once therapy against the disease has been completed. For this reason, this form of therapy is frequently referred to as "high-dose chemotherapy with bone marrow rescue."

The rate at which allogeneic BMT can be performed is limited by the ability to find a suitable marrow donor. The most likely place to find donors is among siblings of the patient, yet even here the likelihood that any individual sibling will be an ideal human leukocyte antigen (HLA)-matched donor is only one in four. In situations in which an HLA-matched sibling donor cannot be found, the search is expanded to include other family members, mismatched siblings, and HLA-matched unrelated donors through donor registries. Compared with autologous BMT, allogeneic BMTs are generally more established but more complex and expensive. Allogeneic BMT is standard therapy for CML, acute leukemias, lymphomas, multiple myeloma, neuroblastoma, and a number of noncancerous conditions.

Autologous BMT has primarily been tried in diseases which do not involve the bone marrow, thereby taking advantage of the possibility of increasing the dose of chemotherapy or irradiation far beyond the tolerability limit set by the bone marrow. The rationale for this high-dose treatment is a presumably positive dose–response relation. Gradually, experiments with autologous BMT have also been performed on patients with diseases involving the bone marrow. This is especially relevant in situations in which no suitable donor for an allogeneic BMT can be found, as autologous BMT may then be tried as an alternative. The bone marrow of the patient is aspirated after a period of intensive treatment with cytotoxics or radiation, but this treatment is restricted by the requirement not to kill all cells in the marrow, because repopulation and remission should be allowed. This method entails a certain risk that malignant cells will survive in the aspirated marrow and therefore cause a relapse of the disease after reinfusion, so a number of methods to *purge* the aspirated marrow, i.e., to remove or destroy any residual malignant cells, were developed during the 1970s and 1980s. A great amount of experimental work remains to be carried out in order to clarify the importance of the various purifying methods.

After identifying a suitable donor for an allogeneic BMT, the next step is a pretreatment conditioning, the aim of which is to kill all malignant cells in the body. The patient is therefore given the most intensive cytotoxic and radiation treatment possible without resulting in too much damage to organs other than the bone marrow. The primary dose-limiting organs are the lungs and the alimentary canal. The most frequent pretreatment is cyclophosphamide for 2 days followed by whole-body irradiation, sometimes fractionated (although this is controversial). The patient is also given drugs to suppress the immune system so that his or her body will not reject the transplanted marrow. In this phase, many side effects occur, e.g., emesis, diarrhea, low blood counts, and damage to vital organs, and because the patient's immune system is severely weakened, he or she is susceptible to infections from bacteria, viruses, fungi, parasites, and other pathogens. For this reason, the patient is usually placed in protective isolation, given antibiotics to fight infection, and sometimes provided with G-CSF to stimulate cell growth.

The BMT itself follows soon after the pretreatment conditioning, and the donated marrow is infused through an intravenous catheter. The marrow travels through the blood stream to the bone marrow cavities, where the donated marrow begins to manufacture new blood cells in a process called engraftment. This usually occurs 2–4 weeks after the BMT. This is followed by the prevention and treatment of complications in the months immediately after the marrow infusion, the most common being graft rejection or failure to engraft, graft-versus-host disease (GVHD), infection, and recurrence of the original disease. GVHD should be considered to be at least partly caused by immunocompetent T cells in the donated marrow attacking the host and resulting in a well-known syndrome of diarrhea, weight loss, and skin damage. It is usually classified from grade 0 (no evidence of GVHD) to grade IV, the latter being a life-threatening condition. The serious acute attacks may involve all the patient's skin, intestines, and liver. GVHD, usually in a milder form, may also be a chronic condition.

Closely associated with GVHD is an interesting phenomenon usually called the graft-versus-leukemia effect. This mechanism is presumably due to cytotoxic T cells that, in association with GVHD, react against even weak transplantation antigens found on leukemic cells that are hereby eliminated. It has been shown that leukemic patients have a greater probability of remaining in remission if they have had GVHD, especially in the chronic form. Consequently, patients who have received marrow from an identical twin have the highest relapse risk, followed by those receiving donated marrow cleaned of T cells. The lowest relapse has been seen in patients receiving donated marrow not cleaned of T cells and who have had both acute and chronic GVHD. However, because of the lethality of acute severe GVHD, the lowest relapse rate was not associated with the best survival, which is seen in patients with moderate acute and chronic GVHD who have received donated marrow not cleaned of T cells (see SBU 1991, i.e., the report on BMT from the Swedish Board of Medical Technology Assessment).

The techniques for autologous BMT of malignancies involving the bone marrow are in many respects the same as for allogeneic BMT of malignant hematologies. The principles of pretreatment are the same, and the aim is to eliminate the tumor and afterwards save the patient by BMT; however, there are two important distinctions between allogeneic and autologous bone marrow. Autologous bone marrow can contain malignant cells even if the patient is in remission at the time of bone marrow harvest, and one cannot be sure that the bone marrow is free from malignant cells even if these cannot be identified by conventional cytological or immunological methods. The other difference is that the immunological complications of allogeneic BMT, caused by incompatibility of HLA or other immunological systems, cannot occur in autologous BMT. The methods for avoiding relapse or immunological complications, respectively, therefore diverge.

In the phase with a seriously reduced number of white blood cells, the so-called leukopenic phase immediately after BMT, the predominating infection problem is serious bacterial septicemia. After 3–4 weeks, the growth of the (re)infused marrow in the bone marrow usually leads to a rising number of white blood cells, and after some further time the level may become normal. Despite this, the patient may still suffer from immunoincompetence and therefore be susceptible to infections with bacteria and viruses. A drastically reduced immune function usually lasts for the first 5 months after BMT, whether it is allogeneic or autologous. In addition, antibody function is reduced for a long time after BMT, while the levels of the immunoglobulins IgG and IgM return to normal fairly early after the transplantation. Recipients of autologous grafts do not develop GVHD and have a faster immune recovery and thus a much lower risk of developing late bacterial infections than patients receiving allogeneic grafts. The same remarks seem to apply to most viral infections, especially to symptomatic cytomegalovirus (CMV), prophylactic strategies against which are only applied to recipients of allogeneic grafts.

Strategies for infection prophylaxis include isolation of patients in laminal airflow rooms, barrier nursing, the use of sterile food, and the use of agents such as intravenous immunoglobulin, antimicrobial agents, and CSFs.

In addition to procedure-related death, BMT is associated with significant risks for physical and psychosocial morbidity. A variety of late physical effects of BMT are recognized, including pulmonary problems, cataracts, infertility, relapse of the original disease, chronic GVHD, and development of a secondary malignancy. Late psychosocial effects include occupational disability, sexual dysfunction, psychological distress, and low self-esteem. The severity of the reactions to BMT generally increases with age, so treatment is rarely considered for patients aged 55 or older. Thus, while allogeneic BMT is considered standard treatment for the other three most frequent leukemias, BMT is not a common therapy for CLL, because this disease almost always occurs after middle age (see GAO 1994).

All three leukemias which are treated with allogeneic BMT progress through various phases, and these are crucial in determining the appropriateness of BMT. In general, the earlier in the progression of the disease a transplantation is performed, the better the prognosis for the patient, but the higher the probability that the procedure will not be necessary. However, in the early phases of acute leukemia, it is often difficult to distinguish between patients who will be cured by conventional chemotherapy and those who will eventually require a BMT. Given the procedure-related mortality risk of around 5%–10% for BMT, it is difficult to determine exactly when the risk of the procedure outweighs the dangers from the disease, and this point will be different for each of the diseases. The pertinent points to consider in balancing the short-term benefits of chemotherapy (low treatment-related mortality rate but high risk of relapse) and the long-term benefits of BMT (greater likelihood for those surviving the immediate risk of the treatment) for each of these diseases are described in some detail in the chapter on "Hematological malignancies".

Allogeneic BMT is the preferred option for leukemia patients with a suitable donor, but, as mentioned above, autologous BMT is considered a reasonable alternative for patients without an HLA-matched donor. It is also used against a number of solid tumors, especially those for which it is believed that increasing the dose intensity of chemotherapy will improve the outcomes considerably. As stated by Hillner et al. (1994), however,

"... evidence supporting the efficacy of autologous BMT from randomized trials is lacking, either because it is not feasible to perform such studies or because there is a general reluctance on the part of the investigators to randomize patients. Therefore presumptions about the superiority of autologous BMT compared with traditional approaches do not lend themselves to formal clinical or economic evaluation... For patients with many solid tumors, autologous BMT will not add any additional benefit, if the management is withheld until the patient has failed multiple courses of different chemotherapeutic agents and, subsequently, developed extensive drug resistance. As a result, autologous BMT has been moved forward in the therapeutic sequence, but appropriate studies proving the usefulness of this approach compared with standard therapies has yet to be assessed in clinical trials."

A recent EORTC trial (Zittoun et al. 1995) randomized more than 900 AML patients in first remission between intensive chemotherapy, allogeneic BMT, and autologous BMT and found no significant difference in overall survival, while both types of BMT resulted in significantly better disease-free survival. In Hodgkin's disease, a very small randomized trial with relapsed or refractory patients showed a marked improvement in disease-free survival in patients receiving high-dose chemotherapy with autologous BMT. This treatment is now requested by these patients as standard therapy, and it will most likely be very difficult to recruit patients for future trials aiming at refuting or corroborating the preliminary results (see Hillner et al. 1994). The subgroup of patients that have been most extensively treated with autologous BMT comprises poor-prognosis non-Hodgkin's lymphoma patients who do not obtain complete remission or who relapse after a remission. Several randomized trials, also trying to determine the optimal timing, are under way, but there are no currently completed trials in which autologous BMT has been proven to be superior to standard salvage chemotherapy.

In solid tumors, noncomparative phase II studies have been used to identify combinations of therapy that produce encouraging response rates and acceptable toxicity. Randomized comparisons are lacking, and inherent in the phase II studies are limitations in their generalizability because of patient selection and influences from previous treatment, regardless of the dose and regimen used. High-dose chemotherapy with autologous BMT has been used for testis cancer, ovarian cancer, and SCLC, but randomized trial data are not available for any of these diseases. For breast cancer, there is considerable controversy about the use of autologous BMT. Randomized comparisons of chemotherapy doses in metastatic disease neither support nor refute the idea of a steep dose–response relationship within the doses possible without

BMT. When used late in the course of the disease for patients failing multiple prior treatments for metastatic disease, high-dose chemotherapy with autologous BMT produced few remissions of only short duration. However, when used as consolidation therapy for patients who responded to induction therapy, a complete remission rate of up to 60% may be obtained, but the likely duration of this has not yet been determined.

Peripheral Blood Stem Cell Transplantation

In recent years, there has been considerable interest in PBSCT as a substitute to autologous BMT (see, e.g., Reiffers 1993). In the 1970s, studies in animals and humans demonstrated hematopoietic stem or progenitor cells in the peripheral blood. It was subsequently observed that, after moderate to high doses of chemotherapy, there was a rebound increase in the number of these hematopoietic stem cells for a few days. With the introduction of the CSFs in clinical trials, it was revealed that administration of these factors in combination with chemotherapy may increase the number of circulating progenitor cells up to 100-fold, to a number far exceeding the yield from bone marrow harvesting. PBSCT was originally suggested as a replacement for BMT, as it was thought that the contamination by tumor cells might be less in the leukopharesed products obtained from the peripheral blood than in the bone marrow cells harvested. Other advantages are that the peripheral blood stem cells can also be harvested without general anesthesia, and the technique can potentially be used in patients who have inadequate bone marrow for harvesting, e.g., because of previous irradiation.

The main advantage of PBSCT, however, is the rapidity of the hematopoietic recovery. For BMT patients, this recovery is usually obtained in 20–30 days, depending on factors such as the number of chemotherapy courses given before BMT, the regimen used, and the number of precursors in the transplant product (see, e.g., Rimm 1991). With PBSCT, the time to granulocytic recovery is faster, while the time to platelet recovery is similar in leukemia, but faster after PBSCT than BMT in most other diseases such as lymphomas and solid tumors. This more accelerated recovery is thought to be due to the infusion of larger numbers of progenitors, which are more mature than their bone marrow counterparts. The progenitor cells harvested by PBSCT therefore develop into differentiated and functional blood cells more quickly. The period of neutropenia and thrombocytopenia may be reduced to less than 2 weeks, leading to shorter hospital stays and lower procedural costs. The more rapid hematological recovery with PBSCT has also reduced the mortality associated with autografting to 2%. The use of high-dose chemotherapy and whole-body irradiation is thereby allowed in conditions in which the risk of a bone marrow autograft is considered to be too high, and the age limit for autografting has been extended to beyond 70 years (Hoyalake and Franklin 1994).

Not surprisingly, PBSCT has attracted considerable interest, also as the subject of economic evaluations (see, e.g., Uyl-de-Groot 1996b), where the two types of autologous stem cells transplantations are compared and the possible and optimal role of the CSFs in either type of procedure is being determined. Concerning the use of the CSFs, the updated ASCO guidelines (ASCO 1996) state that it has been sufficiently documented that CSFs can shorten the period of neutropenia and reduce infectious complications in patients undergoing high-dose chemotherapy with BMT. In addition, the CSFs have been shown to be effective in mobilizing autologous peripheral blood stem cells for transplantation, and trials have also demonstrated their value when administered after the transplantation. Evidence, although less convincing, also suggests clinical benefits of CSFs when administered after allogeneic BMT, and in this case they may possibly be of value in priming donor progenitor cells.

The impact of PBSCT has so far mainly been assessed in the hematological malignancies, but it is expected that its use will increase considerably in the future treatment of solid tumors of the breast, ovaries, testis, and lung. By focusing so much attention on these two alternatives for autografting, however, the fact that the efficacy and cost-effectiveness of autologous BMT is far from settled in the first place is ignored, which make its use as a comparator for PBSCT more than dubious. On the other hand, Hillner et al. (1994), as cited above, described the process whereby BMT has very quickly and without adequate evidence of superior efficacy become considered as standard treatment in certain diseases. Thus it will probably be very difficult to design new clinical trials questioning this perception and especially to recruit patients for such trials.

Finally, it should be kept in mind that autologous progenitor cell transplantations rest on several assumptions, the central of these being that there is a direct, proportional relationship between dose and response. Accordingly, the resistance of a given malignancy to chemotherapy is seen as primarily caused by administration of inadequate doses because of dose-limiting factors (primarily the need to preserve the bone marrow) and not a qualitative problem, such as the presence of a resistant clone of cells. Currently, a two to threefold increase in dose intensity is obtained by some of the more common techniques for hematological support. However, there is some evidence that the relationship between dose intensity of chemotherapy and its tumoricidal effect may be logarithmic rather than linear, which suggests that much greater increases in dose intensity may be required for total killing of all the tumor cells.

Economic Evaluations

Uyl-de-Groot et al. (1995) considered the economic consequences of introducing autologous BMT in one country, the Netherlands, in terms of the additional resources required to finance it for patients with non-Hodgkin's lymphomas and with AML. The non-Hodgkin's lymphoma group consisted of patients with intermediate or high-grade malignancy who had had a previous complete remission and thereafter a first or second relapse. They received two reinduction courses of chemotherapy and obtained partial or complete response. A total of 50 patients were studied, 25 receiving BMT and 25 conventional therapy, the schedules of which differed somewhat with respect to the combination of cytotoxics and inpatient/outpatient modalities. The four most common treatment schedules were analyzed. AML patients in first or second remission were studied, 20 receiving autologous BMT and ten receiving conventional therapy. Current treatment patterns and protocols for the above-mentioned patient groups were defined by a panel of hematologists.

The cost analysis was performed in five university hospitals and one cancer center, with a follow-up period of up to 2 years. Types of resource utilization considered were days in hospital, outpatient visits, medical procedures (laboratory services, diagnostics), medication (cytotoxics, antiemetics, and antibiotics), and blood transfusions. The resource consumption was registered using special forms and should reflect full costs, including overheads. For all types of costs, cost price studies reflecting real resource use were carried out, but these calculations are not further explained in the paper by Uyl-de-Groot et al. 1995. The additional costs of introducing autologous BMT were calculated by subtracting the costs of conventional therapy from the costs of the treatment strategies with autologous BMT. The probable economic consequences on a national level were estimated by taking information about incidence, remission, and relapse rates for the various patient groups into account.

The total costs of autologous BMT in the non-Hodgkin's lymphoma patients were calculated to be about US$ 40,000,[8] of which one fifth was incurred because of the preparations in the pretransplantation phase; the rest occurred in the transplantation phase, of which about 50% were due to hospitalization. The additional costs of autologous BMT for these patients vary between $ 27,000 and $ 37,000, depending on which of the four treatment schedules was chosen for the comparison. The pretransplantation costs for the AML patients are about the same as for the non-Hodgkin's lymphoma patients, as the bone marrow in both cases is unpurged, while the transplantation phase costs are around a third higher for the AML patients (about $ 43,000) because they stayed longer in hospital and needed more antibiotics and blood transfusions. The total costs of autologous BMT for the AML patients were about $ 51,000, which was about $ 44,000 more than the costs for conventional treatment. The costs of hospitalization were about 50% higher for the AML patients, all of whom were hospitalized (for an average of 35 days). Comparing their calculations with the results of other studies, the authors conclude that the cost differences in the various studies can mostly be explained by differences in the management of patients, e.g., in the use of intensive care units, which in some cases were used routinely regardless of the patients' condition.

Brice et al. (1995) investigate the effect on the costs of autologous BMT of using the G-CSF lenograstim as a support in order to reduce the period of leukopenia. The costs for 16 patients entered by the authors' center in a multicen-

[8] Authors' own conversion to US$, with no further explanation given.

ter trial were calculated, and the mean costs of BMT for the lenograstim group (n=10) were compared with the mean for the placebo group (n=6). All patients (who had lymphomas or solid tumors) were initially treated with chemotherapy and three of them also with radiotherapy. Patient conditioning before autologous BMT was adapted to each individual malignancy, and lenograstim (or placebo) was given from day 1 after the BMT until the total white blood cell count remained at more than 1000 cells/µl for 3 consecutive days. Costs relating to the autologous BMT were calculated for each individual patient on the basis of actual resource utilization data supplied by the hospital administration and using tariffs as of September 1990. Although some elaborate details are given on some parts of the cost calculation, e.g., the division of laboratory costs into various types such as virology and bacteriology, the costing procedures actually used are not very clear. The cost of lenograstim was not included, because it was provided free of charge by the producer.

The mean duration of leukopenia was 16 days in the patients who received G-CSF compared to 22 days in the placebo group. The mean duration of hospitalization was 28 and 33 days, respectively. The mean total costs of autologous BMT were estimated at FF 142,000 versus 166,000, respectively,[9] with the difference being attributed to different costs of hospitalization, as the drug expenditure was identical in both groups. Lenograstim did not lead to a reduction in the number of febrile episodes, but it decreased the duration of antibiotic therapy. The mean costs of autologous BMT were FF 121,000 for patients with a duration of neutropenia of 14 days or less versus FF 178,000 for patients with neutropenia for more than 14 days. Based on the recommended daily dose of lenograstim, the average costs of the drug were estimated to be FF 10,500, without any details given on the basis for this calculation. Including this figure reduces the reduction in the average total costs of BMT to about FF 13,000.

Souêtre et al. (1996) reported a cost-minimization analysis of the use of G-CSF compared to no G-CSF in lymphoma patients undergoing autologous BMT. The study design was a retrospective analysis of patient charts for a follow-up period of 100 days after the date of autologous BMT. A total of 55 patients selected at random from four French hematology centers were included based on their underlying lymphomas (Hodgkin's lymphoma, non-Hodgkin's lymphoma, or lymphocytic leukemia) and lack of previous participation in clinical trials. Patients were matched according to tumor and age at inclusion. The clinical and economic data were collected using a standardized case report form by investigators blinded to the treatments.

Clinical end points were incidence of documented infections and incidence and duration of neutropenia, anemia, and thrombocytopenia. Resource utilization data comprised length of inpatients stays, type of ward, use of antibiotics and G-CSFs, cytotoxics, blood products, and laboratory tests. No outpatient data were available. The economic analysis was performed from the hospital perspective, based on a combination of average cost per day estimates and standard cost figures for specific services and procedures. In an

[9] Equivalent to about US$ 31,600 or 37,000 when converted by the PPPs of 1990.

attempt to reduce overestimates due to double counting, a particular costing methodology was developed, with a distinction between "standard days," i.e., days with no change in intensity of care related to an intervention, and days with specific care. The costs of standard days of hospitalization were found by multiplying the number of days with standard basic care by the per diem cost for standard days. For days of specific care after interventions, the costs of specific procedures were used. The interventions considered were chemotherapy alone and chemotherapy plus radiotherapy.

The clinical data showed no statistically significant differences in the incidence of infections, while the average duration of infections was significantly shorter in the G-CSF group. The incidence of anemia and thrombocytopenia was the same.

A comparison of each individual resource utilization item shows that the average quantity used of each item (except platelet transfusions) was smaller for the G-CSF group than for the group treated with conventional care. The modest differences combined with the small number of patients implies, however, that the only statistically significant difference was in the number of days the patients were kept in hospital in connection with the autologous BMT. Changing the resources used into cost figures reflects the same pattern, but the costs of chemotherapy and blood products were higher for the G-CSF group. The costs of the G-CSFs themselves must be added to this, of course, so the difference in average total costs of the groups is a marginal $ 1300 in favor of the G-CSF group, i.e., about 3% of the average total costs. Sensitivity analyses are not directly reported, but it is claimed that the results were shown to be relatively robust to changes in the estimates of costs per day.

Uyl-de-Groot et al. (1994) compared the costs of autologous BMT, with or without mobilization by G-CSF, with the costs of peripheral blood progenitor cell transplantation (PBPCT) mobilized by G-CSF, seen from the hospital perspective. No account was taken of outcomes such as possible differences in patient quality of life or the considerable mortality and morbidity rates associated with BMT. The basis for the calculations was a retrospective study of detailed records for 63 patients receiving one of these treatments in a setting which is not specified. The patients were not equally distributed across the treatment groups with respect to diagnosis (mainly malignant lymphomas and various solid tumors), but all were treated with similar high-dose chemotherapy, the costs of which were disregarded in the analysis. PBPCT with mobilization was performed on an outpatient basis, and in cases where the patients had two reinfusions, the average costs were used. The procedures followed in the management of all the patients are described in much detail.

Costs are considered separately for the pretransplantation and the transplantation period. Pretransplantation included harvest of bone marrow or peripheral stem cells, cryopreservation and cultures, diagnostics, laboratory tests, hospitalization, day-care department medication, blood transfusions, and the insertion of a Hickman catheter. Transplantation costs included days in hospital, laboratory services, diagnostics (mainly X-rays and ECGs), medication (e.g., antiemetics, antibiotics), and blood transfusions. The costs were registered using special forms, and cost price studies determining unit prices reflecting the real use of resources were carried out for all types of costs. However, the information provided with regard to the determination of these unit prices is very limited, except for drugs, where wholesale prices were used, and laboratory examinations and other diagnostics, where an official Dutch system for determining unit prices was used.[10]

Hematological recovery was significantly accelerated with PBPCT compared with G-CSF-mobilized autologous BMT and compared with the control group (BMT alone), for whom recovery was slowest. This relation holds for all parameters with relation to hematological recovery, and it seems to be reflected in the measurements of average resource utilization. In all dimensions of costs reported, the consumption of resources was distinctly lower for the PBPCT group than for the two BMT groups, i.e., fewer hospital days, fewer days in a protected environment, fewer transfusions of red blood cells and platelets, and fewer days on G-CSF (than the BMT+G-CSF group). The average total treatment costs were correspondingly lower, i.e., $ 21,800 for the PBPCT group, $ 32,400 for the BMT+G-CSF group, and $ 30,600 for the BMT group. When costs are broken down into a number of items, it appears that the pretransplantation costs were highest for the PBPCT group, whose main advantage accordingly lies in much lower transplantation costs than the other two, especially for hospitalization, but also for other items such as diagnostics, laboratory services, transfusions, and medication.

An attempt to integrate an assessment of patients' quality of life in the analysis was presented by Beard et al. (1991), based on a retrospective examination of the case notes for 41 patients who had received a BMT, either autologous or allogeneic. For each patient, an estimate of life expectancy without BMT was noted, based on published survival data for each disease and state of disease. The time from BMT to the time of analysis or second BMT or death was recorded, together with an assessment of the patient's quality of life during that period. Each patient's degree of disability and distress in the period after BMT was assessed by an examination of their case notes and interviews with staff from the hematology unit, where necessary. This assessment was used to grade their quality of life according to the Rosser-Kind index, which combines various levels of disability and distress and assigns utility values to each such combination.

Data for utilization of resources, such as inpatient days, outpatient visits, blood products, drugs, pathology, and radiology tests, were also recorded from the individual case notes. The costing concerns the period from patient admission for BMT to the time of analysis (June 1990) or the patient's death. For inpatient days, an official unit price was used, while for outpatient visits an arbitrary amount was set. The source of unit costs for the other resources is not provided. The costing extended over a 10-year period, but all costs

[10] Results are expressed directly in US$ by using a conversion factor for 1992 of US$ 1 divided by 1.8 guilder (while the PPPs of 1990 and 1993, respectively, were 2.17 and 2.13, respectively).

were assessed in 1990 terms. However, no explanation is provided concerning the way this is accomplished.

The average total costs per BMT were estimated at NZ$ 27,000,[11] but very few details are given on the various cost items. Quality of life was markedly impaired by the BMT itself, but in most patients this impairment lasted only 3–4 weeks and in nearly all patients the quality of life was excellent 3 months or more following BMT. Severe GVHD occurred in two patients, and this was the only sustained reduction in quality of life observed. An average gain of 2.04 quality-adjusted life-years (QALYs) per patient was calculated (using only data for 29 of the patients, for unstated reasons), based on the actual survival and the estimated survival had no BMT been given. This results in a cost per QALY of NZ$ 13,300. By further assuming that patients alive at 2 years after BMT will also be alive 10 years after and have excellent quality of life during this whole period, the authors estimate a predicted cost per QALY of NZ$ 3900.

Bennett et al. (1995) examined a case series of patients with lymphoid malignancies from a single university oncological center who received autologous BMT or PBSCT as a support for high-dose chemotherapy. The aim was to determine whether a learning effect can be observed over a 5-year period from 1987 to 1991, resulting in improved outcomes and/or reduced costs. The case series included all patients who received the procedures concerned, and an attempt was made to analyze the changes while controlling for differences in patient characteristics by multiple regression analysis. Variables included for patient characteristics are histological subtype, previous chemotherapy regimens, size of mass, some laboratory values, age, sex, race, disposition at discharge, specific resource use, payer status, and costs of care. The analysis of cost data was restricted to patients surviving hospitalization, with the individual patient as the unit of analysis and using actual cost data instead of charges.

A total of 178 autotransplants for the treatment of Hodgkin's disease were performed during this period, with a steady decrease over time in the mortality rate. In the regression analysis for the outcome, the only significant factor associated with in-hospital death was the experience of the transplant team, and the best-fitting model showed a decrease in the mortality rate from 20% in 1987 to 5% in 1991. The mean costs (calculated in 1991 prices) decreased from $ 96,000 to $ 55,000, most of this reduction being due to a shortening of in-hospital stay from 51 to 32 days. In the cost regression equation, the most significant factors associated with lower costs of care included the number of previous cases and the patients' sex (men). The same tendencies with respect to costs and mortality were found by examining a similar case series of 149 patients with non-Hodgkin's lymphoma undergoing similar treatment regimens.

Concluding Remarks

The economic assessments of BMT and PBPCT described in the foregoing section are summarized in Table 2.

[11] Around US$ 21,000 if converted by PPPs of 1990.

Table 2. Main characteristics of economic assessments dealing with stem cell transplantations

Reference	Disease category	Treatments examined	Main characteristics of the study
Uyl-de-Groot (1995)	Patients with non-Hodgkin's lymphoma and AML	Autologous BMT	Assesses the increase in costs on a national basis of introducing autologous BMT for these patients Hospital perspective Investigation of management and resource utilization for 30–50 patients with each disease, receiving conventional care and autologous BMT, respectively; for all types of costs, unit costs are based on real cost studies, including overheads; additional costs of BMT found by subtracting the costs of conventional care; economic implications at national level found by extrapolation with national incidence data plus data on remission and relapse Pretransplantation costs about the same for both non-Hodgkin's lymphoma and BMT (unpurged bone marrow used), but the transplantation phase costs are higher for AML, because these patients stay longer in hospital and need more antibiotics; in both cases, comparison with conventional care leads to increased costs of the order of \$ 30,000–40,000
Brice et al. (1995)	Patients with solid tumors or lymphomas	G-CSF as support in autologous BMT	Impact on costs of using G-CSF support Third-party payer perspective Costs assessed for 16 patients enrolled by the authors' center in multicenter trial; costs calculated for each individual patient on the basis of actual resource utilization data from the hospital administration; official tariffs used as unit prices; cost of G-CSF not included (donated by the producer) No difference in incidence of FNE; the mean duration of leukopenia and of hospitalization is shorter in the G-CSF group and the total costs associated with BMT are about 17% lower than in the placebo group; the cost reduction is reduced to 10% if an estimated cost of G-CSF is included
Souêtre et al. (1996)	Patients with lymphoma or leukemia	G-CSF vs. no support for autologous BMT	Cost-minimization analysis Hospital perspective Retrospective examination of patient charts for a period of 100 days after ABMT; 55 patients collected randomly from four centers; combination of estimates of average per day costs and analysis of costs of specific procedures No significant difference in incidence of infection, but shorter duration in G-CSF group; a comparison of each individual resource use item shows lower use in G-CSF group, except for platelets, but only significant for hospital days in connection with autologous BMT; converted into cost, the difference becomes a cost saving for the G-CSF group of 3% of the average total costs

Table 2 (continued)

Reference	Disease category	Treatments examined	Main characteristics of the study
Uyl-de-Groot et al. (1994)	Patients with malignant lymphomas and various solid tumors	Autologous BMT vs. G-CSF-mobilized autologous BMT vs. PBPCT as support for high-dose chemotherapy	Cost comparison, outcomes not considered Hospital perspective Retrospective examination of detailed patient charts for 63 patients receiving one of these supportive treatments; costs of chemotherapy disregarded; unit prices based on studies of the real costs of the resources, including overheads Hematological recovery significantly faster with PBPCT than in the two BMT groups; in all items of costs reported, resource consumption distinctly lower for the PBPCT than for the two BMT groups and average total treatment costs correspondingly lower; pretransplantation costs higher in the PBPCT group, but costs in the transplantation phase much lower than in the BMT groups
Beard et al. (1991)	Patients with various diseases, having received BMT	Allogeneic or autologous BMT vs. conventional therapy	Cost-utility analysis Hospital perspective, not stated explicitly Retrospective examination of case notes for 41 patients after BMT; for each patient, estimate of life expectancy without BMT based on published survival data for each specific (stage of) disease; patients' degree of disability and distress after BMT noted, used to calculate QALYs according to the Rosser-Kind index; utilization of resources noted from patient charts; unit costs come from official unit prices and other sources, not stated; costing extends over a 10-year period Quality of life markedly impaired after BMT, but most patients had excellent quality of life 3 months after; based on actual survival and estimated survival without BMT and correcting for quality of life by means of the QALYs estimated, an average gain in QALYs is calculated and compared with the average total costs calculated for BMT; assuming that patients alive at 2 years after BMT will also be alive at 10 years, a final cost-utility ratio is calculated
Bennett et al. (1995)	Malignant lymphomas	Autologous BMT or PBSCT as support for high-dose chemotherapy	Can a learning effect be observed over a 5-year period, resulting in lower cost/better outcomes? Hospital perspective, not explicitly stated Examination of case series of all patients concerned in single center; changes analyzed while controlling for differences in patient characteristics by multiple regression analysis; analysis of cost data restricted to patients surviving hospitalization; unit costs are real cost data, using cost-to-charge ratios

Table 2 (continued)

Reference	Disease category	Treatments examined	Main characteristics of the study
			For a series of 178 autotransplants for Hodgkin's disease, a steady decrease over time in mortality is observed, from 20% to 5%; only significant factor in regression analysis is experience of the transplant team; costs have been reduced by over 40%, mainly due to 40% reduction in hospital stay; explaining factors for cost reduction are experience and patient sex (men); similar results in series of 149 non-Hodgkin's lymphomas

AML, acute myeloid leukemia; BMT, bone marrow transplantation; G-CSF, granulocyte colony-stimulating factor; PBPCT, peripheral blood progenitor cell transplantation; PBSCT, peripheral blood stem cell transplantation; FNE, febrile neutropenic episode; QALY, quality-adjusted life-year.

Despite its weak design, the study by Bennett et al. (1995) underlines the fact that learning effects may have an important impact on the outcome of economic evaluations, e.g., by increasing the efficacy of a new intervention, by decreasing its costs, or perhaps even both at the same time. Taking a potential learning effect into consideration would therefore increase the policy relevance of economic assessments, but it is contentious how this might be achieved in practice.

There is general agreement that economic evaluation should be carried out at a very early stage in the diffusion process of a new intervention in order to have any actual impact on its more or less widespread adoption in practice. If, so the argument goes, an economic assessment of a new intervention compared to the standard regimen is not carried out until a point in time at which the intervention has already been widely adopted, it is very unlikely that the assessment will have much impact on the use of the innovation, unless an unfavorable outcome of the economic evaluation is backed by some restrictions on its use. The comment by Desch et al. (1992) concerning BMT in patients with Hodgkin's disease (see the chapter on "Hematological Malignancies") is a case in point.

On the other hand, by carrying out the assessment at a very early stage, the potential learning effects cannot be taken into consideration unless one is willing to base the analysis of such effects on assumptions. One way around this problem is to adhere to a principle often evoked and enjoying widespread approval, according to which any particular evaluation of a specific economic issue should not be considered final and the economics of the issue ought to be reconsidered regularly, especially after the appearance of relevant new information. Examples of the practical use of this research strategy are extremely rare, however, possibly because of the problems of designing phase IV trials in a way that eliminates or diminishes the threat of (selection) bias in observational studies.

A result deserving specific mention is the apparent success of PBPCT compared with BMT as support for intensified, high-dose chemotherapy. PBPCT seems to be a dominant solution, with lower risks, higher efficacy, and lower costs. The results of the study included in this survey are thus corroborated by other studies published after the cut-off point for inclusion in this survey and in preliminary analyses of studies still in progress.

Palliative Care

Palliative care has been defined in many somewhat diverging ways. Recently, the World Health Organization (WHO) has adopted a definition, according to which palliative care is "the active, total care of a person whose condition is not responsive to curative treatment" (WHO 1990). This definition seems very concise and useful, stressing that such care should not be restricted to patients with malignant disease and that terminal care is only one aspect of palliative care, albeit a very important one. The concept embraces optimal symptom control and quality of life as well as appropriate rehabilitation.

Normally, the intention of palliative care in cancer patients will be to relieve symptoms from progressive malignant disease or to prevent or delay anticipated problems. The intention will not usually be to prolong life, although this may be achieved in certain cases, when the pattern of metastases is immediately life-threatening, such as extensive diffuse pulmonary infiltration or fulminating liver disease. For a specific type of palliative care, e.g., palliative chemotherapy, to be considered, its anticipated benefits should always outweigh the expected costs in terms of patient suffering from toxic side effects. The quality of life of patients undergoing palliative care should be considered in terms of patients' reports of their symptoms from cancer, adverse physical effects of treatment, level of physical functioning, psychological and social well-being etc. Until now, few clinical trials have assessed the quality of life of patients undergoing palliative care, but more studies of this kind are now being started in the hope of contributing to the determination of rational health care strategies (Ahmedzai 1997).

Rigorous assessment of the relative value for money or cost-effectiveness of various forms of palliative care is made difficult by the ethical and methodological difficulties of conducting randomized clinical trials with dying patients (see, e.g., Whinney et al. 1994). For instance, very few randomized trials comparing hospital services with home-based or hospice services have been successfully conducted and reported. Many patients and their relatives refuse to participate in randomized trials, and referring physicians may also be reluctant to participate and offer their patients the possibility of being included in a trial. There is a high rate of attrition, with patients dying before comparison points, and an expected low compliance in completing questionnaires because of patients' and care-givers' exhaustion and emotional strain. In assessing more complex interventions, such as a complete service package allowing dying cancer patients to stay in their own home with extensive medical and nursing support, it may be very difficult to avoid dilution of the possible experimental effect by control patients being "exposed" to some of the elements of the intervention package. It may also be difficult to determine the degree to which an effect or lack of effect is due to the experience, training, personal qualities, and commitment of the team members, because the interventions are usually performed and assessed on a rather small scale.

The economic assessments of palliative care in cancer patients identified and retrieved for this report focus on only two aspects of palliative care, i.e., pain management and the endeavors to establish alternatives to the usual acute care hospitals or home care for cancer patients in the terminal phase. The following account of the clinical issues will accordingly be limited to these two aspects.

Several studies focusing on patient and physician attitudes to pain management in cancer indicate that cancer pain is the most feared consequence of cancer, with about 70% of patients interviewed answering that they would consider suicide if their cancer pain became intolerable. Numerous surveys have shown that about half the patients in active treatment and up to 90% of patients with advanced disease have moderate to severe pain. The prevalence of cancer pain is influenced by several factors, one of which is the primary tumor type. Patients with bone tumor and with breast and prostate cancer have a much higher incidence of pain (60%–80%) than patients with hematological malignancies. The stage of disease is also important, with only 15% of patients with nonmetastatic disease reporting pain. A greater incidence of pain is seen for certain types of tumor, because they occur in sites proximal to neural structures or have a higher tendency to metastasize to the bones. Patient characteristics such as anxiety or depression also influence the experiencing and reporting of pain.

There are several barriers to appropriate pain management of cancer patients, including fear of addiction, lack of knowledge about analgesics and overconcern about tolerance development, lack of understanding of the pathophysiology of cancer pain, and low priority given to pain management (see, e.g., Schug and Large 1993). Patients are believed frequently to underreport the amount of pain they experience or to fail to report inadequate pain relief, and communication about the experiencing of pain between patients and physicians is generally reported to be poor. Another obstacle to adequate treatment is limited availability and lack of use of alternatives to systemic analgesics, e.g., nerve blockers or palliative neurosurgery.

Recent advances in the scientific understanding of the anatomy, physiology, psychology, and pharmacology of pain perception have led to great improvements in the management of cancer-related pain. They provide the scientific rationale for using new, improved methods of treatment, including more effective use of standard analgesic drugs, development of new drugs, use of new methods and routes of drug administration, and use of selective anesthetic and neurosurgical approaches to controlling pain. *N*-Methyl-D-aspartate (NMDA) receptor antagonists are promising new drugs that have shown the potential to obtain fine control of severe and refractory pain, even of types of pain with a poor response to morphine. There are as yet no randomized controlled trials with these agents, e.g., ketamine, but several case reports and larger case series of their use in palliative care have been published (see Ahmedzai 1997).

In determining the optimal strategy of pain management in the individual patient, the first step is obviously to identify the cause and type of the pain. This is done on the basis of history taking and review of patient records, physical examination, laboratory data, and imaging studies.

There are three major types of cancer pain:

1. *Somatic pain* results when nociceptors (i.e., receptors for pain, which are activated by injury) are activated in cutaneous or deep tissues and is typically characterized as a dull or aching, but well-located pain. An example is metastatic bone pain.
2. *Visceral pain* is the result of nociceptors being activated by infiltration, compression, extension, or stretching of the thoracic, abdominal, or pelvic viscera (i.e., any large interior organ in the body's three large cavities). It is poorly localized, often described as deep, squeezing, and pressure-like, and typically occurs in patients with intraperitoneal[1] metastases.
3. *Neuropathic pain* results from injury to the nervous system, caused by compression or infiltration of peripheral nerves or the spinal cord by the tumor or by chemical injury to peripheral nerves or the spinal cord caused by chemotherapy, radiotherapy, or surgery. Such pains are often severe and are described as burning or as pain associated with an area of abnormal sensation, intermittently with electric shock-like sensations. The most common cause is progressive disease, but such pain can also be caused by all modalities of cancer treatment or by factors not directly related to either the disease or its treatment.

Most cancer patients have somatic and visceral pain, while neuropathic pain is believed to represent 15%–20% of the significant pain problems.

The choice of treatment should also be determined by the severity of the pain and by the patient's preferences. The issue of severity is normally considered to have been definitively settled by the WHO in the mid-1980s in a set of guidelines entitled "Cancer Pain Relief." The guidelines are usually referred to as an analgesic ladder, with the first step being *mild pain*, which may often be treated with nonsteroidal anti-inflammatory drugs (NSAIDs) alone. *Moderate pain* (persisting or increasing) experienced by patients receiving a regimen recommended for mild pain should be treated by a weak opioid (e.g., codeine, propoxyphene) combined with an analgesic such as aspirin or paracetamol. Most cancer patients with *severe pain* are treated with a strong opioid (of which morphine is the prototype), possibly combined with adjuvant analgesics (e.g., tricyclic antidepressants, corticosteroids, local anesthetics) if adequate pain relief is not obtained otherwise. The proportion

[1] The peritoneum is the membrane that encloses organs such as the liver, stomach, colon, and intestine.

of patients obtaining adequate pain relief by basing therapy decisions on this analgesic ladder has not as yet been assessed in controlled studies, but a large, open-label prospective study has shown that following the guidelines resulted in good pain relief in 76% of the patients, satisfactory relief in 12%, and inadequate relief in 12%.

A possible strategy for pain management following the guidelines could be the following: After a thorough diagnostic evaluation, a plan for managing the disease and cancer pain is developed. If the anticancer therapy is effective, pain relief will usually follow, making further pain management superfluous. However, in some cases the anticancer treatment may add to pain, e.g., postsurgical pain. Actual pain treatment starts with nonopioid drugs (e.g., NSAIDs) alone or in combination, but with more severe pain, stronger analgesics (e.g., an opioid such as morphine) may be required, alone or in combination (e.g., an opioid plus a nonopioid). If effective, no further therapy is required, but if severe persistent pain does not respond to this therapy or if the side effects of the drugs are not tolerated, changing the analgesics should be the first consideration. If systemic analgesics produce excessive side effects such as confusion or sedation, epidural or intrathecal opioids may be considered. If the pain is localized, a neural blockade is indicated, and various anesthetic approaches may also be tried. Concurrently with the medical and surgical approaches, psychological support therapies should be integrated from the start of treatment, and complementary therapies such as acupuncture and relaxation training may also be tried.

Much of the current research in pain management is concerned with eliminating or reducing the common side effects of opioids, such as chronic constipation, nausea and vomiting, sedation, and pruritus, which were earlier assumed to be inevitable. This is done by synthesizing new opioids or by developing different formulations of older agents. One interesting example of the latter strategy is transdermal drug delivery of fentanyl, one of the first synthetic opioids and 70 times more potent than morphine. When applied to the skin, it penetrates quickly and effectively, and one transdermal fentanyl patch may be used for 72 h, delivering predictable amounts of the drug. This delivery system is already widely used in the United States and is predicted to become increasingly used in Europe as well (Ahmedzai 1997). New data on reduced side effects with transdermal delivery may also mean a fall in treatment costs. Other new treatments include calcitonin (a hormone) for short-term management of metastatic bone pain and bisphosphonates (e.g., clodronate) to relieve metastatic bone pain and prevent bone fractures. For patients refractory to standard treatment, the NMDA receptor antagonists mentioned above are promising, in addition to nerve blockers and epidural infusion of corticosteroids.

A number of supportive care and continuing care programs have been developed to manage patients with terminal illness, both in the hospital and in the patient's home. In these patients, treatment is focused on symptom control and palliative comfort care. The development of such programs, dating back to the opening of the first hospice in the United States in 1974, may be seen as a reaction against the neglect of the basic needs of terminally ill patients, which the normal acute care hospitals have often been accused of. Because of the predominant focus on curative interventions in these institutions, some physicians considered it necessary to perform prolonged and extensive diagnostic investigations before relieving the bothersome symptoms of dying patients. On the one hand, such patients were often offered no treatment of symptoms because they were dying, while on the other hand, many institutions chose to offer these patients therapy for every complaint, which was often misdirected because an adequate search for causes and remedies was not performed.

Patients with end-stage cancer may spend weeks to years suffering the poorly understood symptoms that normally accompany progression of the malignancy. There is a great variability in pain intensity and opioid usage as patients approach death, but a pain-free state may be an unrealistic goal in patients with advanced cancer. Other common symptoms in end-stage patients are confusion, anorexia, difficulty in breathing, difficulty in swallowing, and nausea. The ability to control and manage such and other physical complaints besides severe pain is extremely limited in patients who exhibit complicated and multiple signs and symptoms and who are furthermore not capable of enduring extensive examinations aiming at a definite diagnosis. Similar tumor pathology will produce variable symptoms in different patients, and cancer patients may be distressed by normal bodily sensations or minor symptoms may become exaggerated if recurrence of the cancer is feared.

No matter what the setting (home, hospital, hospice, nursing home), terminally ill cancer patients appear to share a common three-step decline during the terminal phase before death (approximately 15 weeks, 2 months, and 2 weeks before death, respectively). The last few weeks of life are frequently dramatic and marked by increased dependency, weakness, confusion, and inability to manage simple personal tasks such as bathing and continence. A total of 75% of a series of dying cancer patients had three or more separate complaints near death, and some had many more distinct symptoms (see Brescia 1993), while only 5% of these patients had symptoms such as diarrhea, itch, hallucinations, or panic attacks. Escalating and uncontrollable symptoms within the last 2–3 days before death are often seen, with difficulties in breathing being the most common. In rare cases, total sedation may be required to ease the patient's suffering from unmanageable symptoms.

Despite the difficulties in keeping terminally ill patients at home, most patients express a preference for dying at home, and this is the background for the conception of the idea of hospices and its rapid development into a veritable movement, at least in the United States, the United Kingdom, and some other nations such as Australia. A hospice is a program of supportive services for terminally ill patients *and* their families, provided either at home or in designated inpatient settings. Hospices are claimed to provide better pain relief than conventional care and to improve the quality of life of terminally ill patients and their families, while maximizing time spent in the home environment and minimizing aggressive and possibly traumatizing intervention. Hospices prepare patients and their families emotionally and spiritually for death and thereby anticipate better adjustment during the final phase of life and in the bereavement period. Finally, hospices have often been expected to cost less than conventional terminal care or to provide additional services (in particular, the support of the relatives) with the same total costs.

In the United States, the hospice movement developed rapidly from its initiation as a sort of mission led by a few particularly dedicated individuals in the mid-1970s into a major movement encompassing more than a thousand organizations a decade later. As a result of interest from the authorities, the National Hospice Study was initiated in collaboration between the Health Care Financing Administration (the national administrative body overseeing the Medicare and Medicaid programs run by the individual states), the scientific community, and private foundations. The study was intended to assess whether hospices attain their stated goals and to provide the authorities with a database for policy formulation.

The following three research questions were posed:

1. What is the difference between hospice and conventional care?
2. What is the differential impact of hospice and conventional care on the quality of life of patients and their families?
3. What is the impact of hospice on the health care costs incurred by terminally ill cancer patients?

The results of this study, which are reported later in this chapter, did not indicate any significant superiority for hospices over conventional care, whether in terms of patient quality of life, family outcome, or costs, except that there was a reduction in costs for hospices without inpatient facilities compared to conventional care. Since then, not much has been published and the hospice movement seems to have lost some steam, even though it has spread to a number of other countries.

In any case, formal assessments of palliative care services are fraught with difficulties (see, e.g., McQuay and Moore 1994). Random allocation to different programs will often be considered unethical, so an observational study design with its inherent problems caused by the potential for self selection bias will normally be required. In addition to this, there are difficulties in collecting clinical and quality-of-life data and other outcome measurements from dying patients. The many diversities between palliative care programs and facilities necessitate a clear definition and clarification of the study design, but the cumbersome and complex outcome measurements will frequently make it very difficult to interpret the results. For an enumeration and discussion of some of the difficulties involved in economic assessments of palliative care, the reader is referred to Rubens (1990, 1993).

Economic Evaluations of Pain Management

Bloor et al. (1994) aimed at estimating the direct costs of current medical practice in managing severe cancer pain for a typical patient in both hospital and ambulatory settings. In both settings, the costs of oral and subcutaneous therapy were compared, resulting in estimates for four different types of patients, requiring either oral or parenteral therapy, administered either in the hospital or on an outpatient basis. The calculations were largely based on assumptions about the personnel time required for administering and monitoring therapy, about the typical doses of morphine used, and about the necessary number of general practitioner and community nurse visits. These assumptions were in turn based on information from a strictly limited number of hospital consultants, nurse managers, and hospice clinicians. The responses obtained were rather variable, and as a comparison of the mean values with the results of an equivalent Canadian study using a work sampling methodology suggested an overestimation by the expert panel, extensive sensitivity analyses were carried out. The costs of treating side effects of opioid analgesics were disregarded, because the incidence of side effects is believed not to depend on the route of administration.

As unit costs, the hospital acquisition prices for drugs, supplies, and equipment were used, while the costs of personnel time were calculated by using the median salary for the relevant personnel groups plus an additional 20% in order to reflect the employer's cost (e.g., for national insurance). The baseline results for the daily direct costs of managing severe cancer pain varied between about £ 3 for oral ambulant therapy to around £ 22 for parenteral therapy given in the hospital.[2] Oral therapy in hospital and outpatient parenteral therapy lie in between, at around £ 13–15. The sensitivity analyses performed show some remarkable changes in the level of the estimated costs, but the rank order between the various types of settings was not influenced by these.

Accordingly, and not surprisingly, oral administration of analgesics, which is standard clinical practice, is also preferable when considering the direct costs of therapy. The problem is, however, that a significant proportion of the patients cannot be treated in this way. For instance, it has been estimated that more than 50% of patients with advanced cancer will eventually be unable to tolerate oral morphine because of problems with swallowing, persistent nausea and vomiting, bowel obstruction, intolerance to oral opioids, incident pain, and poor compliance. Ensuring adequate pain management for these patients requires that alternative routes of administration are used.

The authors consider the potential cost savings by using transdermal administration of opioid analgesics with a dose that lasts for approximately 3 days. This has been shown in clinical trials to successfully control pain in cancer patients. For in-hospital patients, costs of supplies and equipment will

---

[2] Converted by the purchasing power parity (PPP) value for 1992 (the general, not the health care-specific one), the costs of the most expensive therapy amount to about US$ 35.

obviously be completely averted when compared to parenteral therapy, and compared to oral administration personnel costs should be greatly reduced due to the single 3-day dose. For ambulant patients, it is presumed that transdermal therapy may reduce the necessity of the frequent control visits by community nurses and general practitioners to the same level as for outpatients on oral therapy, which will lead to substantial savings on personnel costs compared to subcutaneous therapy. The possible disadvantages of transdermal therapy, which the authors do not attempt to quantify, are that additional analgesics and patient monitoring may be required during an initial dose titration and stabilization period and possibly also to control breakthrough pain once the patients are stabilized.

Moulin (1992) aimed to assess the treatment outcome for a retrospective series of 60 cancer patients who required continuous subcutaneous infusion of opioids.[3] Outcome measures used were the patients' stated preference for continuous infusion versus oral therapy, frequency of readmission to the hospital because of poor pain control, and the requirement for more invasive procedures. The cost calculations for the two types of infusion pump were based on a number of assumptions, which were not substantiated explicitly with any kind of data. One of the pumps was programmable, allowing a certain amount of patient-controlled analgesia in the form of bolus doses for breakthrough pain and requiring some education of the patients and their family as caregivers in how to use it. The other was a disposable infusion apparatus, which is discarded every 24 h. Its rate of infusion is fixed, which requires that the drug concentration is adjusted to this flow rate to meet the patient's analgesic requirement. Each infuser must be prepared by a pharmacist, and the daily time requirement for this was estimated to be about 20 min. The disposable infusers also require some education of the patients and their caregivers, which was provided by nurses from the department.

All of the patients had poor pain control as the indication for the infusion, except for a few who were near death or had very high oral opioid requirements. The overall mean duration of infusion treatment was 68 days. A total of 18 patients died in hospital, while 42 were discharged and continued the infusion therapy for a mean of 94 days. The mean initial maintenance dose was almost three times higher than the dose given before infusion was started. All but one of the patients and their families preferred the infusion therapy to the previous oral regimen. This is taken as indirect evidence of analgesic efficacy and improved quality of life. Of the 42 patients discharged, 12 had to be readmitted because of poor pain control or because of unacceptable side effects from the infusion; 20% of the patients experienced serious toxic effects or complications.

---

[3] These 60 patients came from a complete series of 481 patients seen in a neuro-oncologic consultation for cancer pain, i.e., the incidence of patients eligible for continuous subcutaneous administration was only 12%, which is much lower than reported by Bloor et al. (1994) above. The rest of the patients could be managed by adjustment of oral opioids and adjuvant analgesic doses.

The daily operating costs of the programmable infusion pump are less than half of the costs of the disposable pump, but taking into account the initial cost of purchasing the programmable pump (around $ 3800), the breakeven point between the two systems is 236 days, i.e., after this period, the programmable pump becomes cheaper to operate. This is a much longer period than the mean duration of infusion therapy seen in the patients in the case series, making the disposable pump preferable from a cost-minimization point of view. This conclusion is reinforced when taking into account the fact that it will often be necessary for the patients to purchase at least two pumps because of variations in their analgesic requirements. With a requirement of two programmable pumps per patient, the breakeven point is postponed to around 16 months of use, compared to the mean of just over 3 months in the home for patients discharged from hospital observed in the case series used in the study.

Economic Evaluations of Alternatives in Palliative Care

As mentioned above, the growing interest in hospices as an alternative to hospital care for terminally ill (cancer) patients led to the initiation of a large cooperative research effort, the National Hospice Study, the main results of which were reported in a series of papers in 1986. Greer et al. (1986) reported the results of the analysis of the differential impact of hospices on the quality of life of the patients and their families and on the costs of care. Data were collected for 1754 hospice and nonhospice patients selected by predetermined criteria from a population of over 12,000 terminally ill cancer patients identified in 40 hospices and 14 conventional care settings from 1981 to 1983. The study sites were not chosen randomly, as about two thirds of the hospices were special demonstration projects chosen among 233 applicants. Non-demonstration hospices were chosen by the evaluators to resemble the others in their organizational structure. Two main categories were used for the hospices, i.e., those with beds (hospital based) and those without beds (home care). Conventional care sites were selected from among those providing good care on the advice of "knowledgeable" local physicians. Of the selected hospice patients, 3% refused to participate, while the refusal rate was 21% among the patients in conventional care.

Eligibility for the study was a confirmed cancer diagnosis with distant metastases, presence of a primary caregiver, and a requirement for assistance in daily activities. Personal interviews with the patients and their primary caregiver were conducted at study entry, 7 days later, and subsequently at 2-week intervals. In addition to the patient interview, at each session the primary caregiver provided information on personal attitudes and on the patient's condition and use of health care resources. Three to 4 months after the patient's death, a bereavement interview was conducted with the primary caregiver in order to assess the outcome for him or her and to summarize records of health care resource utilization. Four outcome areas were assessed, each of which had multiple domains and measures. In addition to the pattern of care and resource utilization and costs, these were patient and family outcome, each of which was based on the primary caregiver's report, and concerning overall quality of life, social quality of life, pain and symptoms, and satisfaction with care. The cost calculations concern only direct health care costs and not overall societal costs, and the total costs calculated combine cost and charge data, because for a number of services only charges were available.

The analytical approach is adequate, taking into consideration the quasi-experimental design of the study, making it very susceptible to the potentially confounding effect of selection bias. For instance, patients in either type of hospice were significantly less likely than conventional care patients to experience one of the intensive medical interventions or to have diagnostic blood tests or X-rays, while they received more analgesics and were reported to have significantly less pain during the last few weeks before death. It is clearly recognized that patients and families may have chosen settings that reflect their values and desire for palliative care and that the physicians have also chosen to practice in or in conjunction with such settings, so that the treatment differences observed may largely be attributed to selection bias.

Quality of life for the patients was judged to be similar in each setting. The primary caregivers of patients in both types of hospice care were more satisfied with where the patient died, while there were no differences in patient-reported levels of satisfaction with care, which were uniformly high. There were no significant differences between the three settings with respect to almost all the measures used for family outcomes, while the only difference observed in the bereavement interviews with the primary caregivers was a significantly higher level of emotional stress in the relatives of patients in home care than in the other two groups. The total cost per study day was almost equal for in-hospital hospices and conventional care and about a third lower for home care hospices. However, seen from the perspective of Medicare, the home care hospice patients incurred lower costs than the conventional care patients only in the last 2 months of life, while in earlier months the conventional care patients had lower costs than the patients in either type of hospice care.

Gray et al. (1987) attempted a comparison of the total costs incurred by the patients in an Australian home care hospice service, providing care for patients dying in their own home and support for family and friends during the terminal illness and the subsequent bereavement, and patients in more conventional terminal care. Health services used and expenditure during the last 90 days of life were compared for the patients and controls. There was no attempt to assess any differences in outcome, e.g., with respect to quality of life for the patients and their relatives. All hospice patients registered as dying within a given year (1983) were included. It is clearly acknowledged that, due to the self selection problem, it was not possible to obtain a control group which matched the hospice group precisely on all factors of relevance for the outcome of the study. Rather, the home care group was compared with a group of patients in conventional care who died in the same year and were matched on the basis of primary cancer site, age, and sex, on the assumption that patients thus matched would present similar clinical problems.

Data for this observational study came from a number of sources. The services provided, such as investigations and procedures performed, were taken from the patients' medical records, although these were estimated to be rather incomplete, especially with respect to services delivered by paramedical staff. Especially for the patients in conventional care, there were serious limitations in data availability, making it necessary to base the calculations on a number of assumptions. Similarly, the unit cost figures used for the calculations were derived from a number of different sources or were based on assumptions. For the hospice group, a correction of the final figure derived was made, based on the argument that the workload during the period of estimation was extraordinarily low. Services provided by general practitioners outside hospitals, nursing homes, or hospices were not included due to the lack of data. Also excluded were outpatient visits, ambulance services, and drug costs due to the lack of completeness in recording and the complexity of grouping the items.

The groups were equal in marital status and de facto living relationships, and there were no significant differences in social status, which is taken to indicate that there were no differences in the amount of home-based support and no financial constraints upon the selection of care for each group. However, the authors themselves warn about the risk of selection bias, which is present in all observational studies, and about the risk of not having identified the most appropriate matching criteria. The hospice patients were referred to traditional institutions at various points of their illness, but 59% died at home versus 16% of the controls. The hospice patients spent an average of 19 days in various institutions during the last 90 days of life. Their mean period of time under hospice care was 39 days, but the majority of services were provided during the last 12 days of life. Adding these to the number of days spent in institutional care resulted in a total of 31 days spent in intensive nursing and medical care by this group, compared to 28 days in institutional care for the control group. This difference is not statistically significant, and the mean cost in the two groups was also calculated to be equivalent when allowance was made for the temporary overcapacity of the hospice care service during the period of calculation.

Koopmanschap et al. (1992) provided estimates of the costs of home care for patients with advanced breast and cervical cancer. According to the authors, the results should be able to be generalized to other cancers, as they claim that several studies have shown that, in case of advanced cancer, the site from which the metastases originate does not significantly influence the amount of care and costs. The calculated costs were briefly compared with some previous publications to which two of the authors contributed containing calculations of the average total costs for hospitalized patients with advanced breast and cervical cancer. Advanced cancer was defined as starting when metastases were clinically detected and terminating when the patient died, a period lasting on average 21 months in breast cancer and 11 months in cervical cancer patients. The terminal episode was defined as the last 3 months before the patient's death, while the period up until then was called the initial episode.

Data for home care in the terminal episode were based on a Dutch experiment called the Intensive Home Care Project (IHP), directed at patients who would otherwise have been in need of hospital or nursing home care and for whom informal care was available. For these patients, the amount of informal and professional care was registered daily. The data used were taken from 1988 for 65 patients with advanced breast cancer. For terminally ill patients staying at home and receiving only "regular" care, two different data sources were used, resulting in very similar estimates. One set was collected for participants in the IHP before entry, while the other came from a study carried out by district nurses. Data about home care in the initial episode were derived from representative samples taken in several successive years by the district nurses' association. Included in these databases are data about home help, while there is no information about services provided by general practitioners, private nurses, or informal caregivers. There is no attempt at evaluating the outcomes, e.g., by measuring the degree of satisfaction expressed by the patients and their relatives.

For the various types of professional care, the relevant salaries for 1990 were used in the calculations, taking into account the relation between patient time and total working time, the costs of indirect personnel, allowances for overtime, and equipment costs. In order to value informal care, the price of the least qualified professional help (the cheapest home help) was used as a shadow price. The results of the calculations are reported in great detail, but only a few will be mentioned here.

The average total costs per patient with advanced disease were calculated as about 8500 and 7200 guilder for breast and cervical cancer, respectively.[4] District nursing and home care accounted for the majority of costs, while informal care (primarily based on an assumption of 45 h per week during the terminal episode) accounted for only 10%. For breast cancer patients, about 30% of the calculated costs were incurred during the initial episode, while 85% of the costs of cervical cancer were incurred during the terminal episode. The main difference between intensive and regular home care in the terminal episode was in the amount of district nursing and private nursing per week, which was five times higher in intensive care. The calculated total costs for patients with advanced disease were also compared to previously published calculations of the average total costs for inpatient treatment of the same types of patients, which were 42,200 guilder for breast cancer and 29,000 guilder for cervical cancer, i.e., four to five times higher, even taking into consideration some imputed costs for informal care provided in the patients' home.

Concluding Remarks

The economic assessments described above concerning pain management and hospice versus conventional terminal care are summarized in Table 1.

[4] With the 1990 PPPs, this is equivalent to about US$ 5000 and $ 4300, respectively.

Table 1. Main characteristics of economic assessments concerning pain management and terminal care in hospices versus conventional institutions

Reference	Disease category	Treatments examined	Main characteristics of the study
Bloor et al. (1994)	"Typical" cancer patient, both inpatient and outpatient	Various ways of administering opioids, oral, subcutaneous, transdermal	Cost-identification and cost-minimization analysis Hospital perspective Calculations for four types of patients based on assumptions about personnel time, typical doses of morphine, and necessary number of general practitioner and nurse visits; unit costs are hospital acquisition prices and median wages Oral outpatient treatment cheapest, in-hospital parenteral most expensive; however, half the patients eventually cannot tolerate oral treatment; potential savings by transdermal administration every 3 days, due to savings in personnel time and on costs of supplies and equipment, exact savings depend on the comparator
Moulin (1992)	Cancer patients requiring continuous subcutaneous infusion of opioids	Two types of infusion pumps, one allowing a certain patient control, the other with fixed rate of infusion	Cost-minimization analysis Perspective not stated explicitly Assessment of treatment outcome for series of 60 patients; outcomes are patients' preferences (oral vs. infusion), readmission because of poor pain control, and frequency of more invasive procedures; cost calculations based on several assumptions, e.g., personnel time requirements for preparation of pumps and education of patients For 42 patients discharged home (the others died in hospital), mean duration of infusion is 94 days; daily operating cost for pump allowing patient control is far lower, but acquisition price is much higher; breakeven point, where pump with patient control becomes less expensive, is 9 months, but the patients live much shorter
Greer et al. (1986)	Terminal cancer patients	Hospice (institution or home-based) vs. nonhospice	Observational study comparing outcomes and costs of the various types of terminal care Third-party payer perspective (Medicare) Data assembled for 1754 hospice and nonhospice terminal cancer patients selected by predetermined criteria; institutions not selected at random; pattern of care and resource utilization and costs registered in addition to patient and family outcome concerning quality of life, pain and symptoms, and satisfaction with care Quality of life for the patients judged to be the same and no differences in patient satisfaction with care; almost all measures used for family outcomes equal, but higher emotional stress on relatives of patients dying in their home; total costs per study day equal in conventional care and institutional hospice, a third lower in home care; for Medicare, home care patients only less costly in the last 2 months, before this more costly than conventional care patients

Table 1 (continued)

Reference	Disease category	Treatments examined	Main characteristics of the study
Gray et al. (1987)	Terminal cancer patients	Home care hospice service vs. conventional care	Observational study of total costs of each type of care for terminal patients Perspective not explicitly stated All hospice patients registered as dying within a given year (1983); control group of patients in conventional care recorded with respect to year of death, cancer site, age, and sex; registration of all health services uses and expenditure during last 90 days of life; data on care and procedures provided based on medical charts, but incomplete data, so assumptions are added; unit cost figures used from several sources, in addition to assumptions; general practitioner services, outpatient visits and services, and drug costs are excluded; no attempt to assess outcomes, e.g., quality of life 59% of hospice patients and 16% of controls died at home; the average total costs for the two groups are not different, and the actual number of days spent in intensive nursing and medical care of the two groups is not significantly different, although a little higher in the hospice group
Koopmanschap et al. (1992)	Patients with advanced breast and cervical cancer	Home care during advanced disease, including the terminal episode (last 3 months)	Determination of the costs of home care of patients with advanced cancer (assumed to be independent of cancer site) Societal perspective aimed at (e.g., including imputed costs for informal care by relatives) Data for home care in terminal episode from Dutch experiment with daily registration; data on home care in initial episode (from clinical detection of metastases till 3 months before death) from district nursing reports; evaluation of personnel costs by relevant salaries and imputed cost for informal care; no attempt to evaluate the outcomes, e.g., by patient/relative satisfaction Average total costs for advanced patients in home care found to be about equal for the two groups, with district nursing and home care accounting for the majority and informal care for only 10%; 70% of the costs for breast cancer patients and 85% for cervix cancer incurred in the terminal phase; compared to previous calculations of average total costs for inpatient treatment of same types of patients, home care is around four to five times less costly

The study of the potential cost savings due to transdermal, subcutaneous administration of opioids (Bloor et al. 1994) was based on an assumption of equal pain control and ignoring the costs of treating side effects, as the incidence of these was considered to be independent of the route of administration. However, there are indications that the transdermal route may lead to clearly reduced adverse effects. Thus a randomized cross-over study involving 202 patients and using a daily patient diary and a battery of questionnaires has shown that, for the same degree of pain control as slow-release morphine, the transdermal route was associated with significantly less constipation, nausea, and daytime drowsiness. In addition, significantly more patients preferred the transdermal path to oral administration (Ahmedzai and Brooks 1997).

However, the authors did not try to quantify or value the important potential disadvantage associated with transdermal administration that additional analgesics and patient monitoring may be required when starting patients on this form of treatment and titrating the dosage to match the pain. After stabilization, there may also be a need for additional analgesics to control breakthrough pain. The importance of these cost items is not known at present, but it is suspected that a number of clinicians hesitate to use this new technology because of the perceived difficulties in managing the patients during dose titration.

The possibility of cost containment was probably not an important factor for the original initiators of the hospice movement. The impetus was rather a dissatisfaction with conventional care facilities, a feeling that they were not capable of giving sufficient attendance to psychological, social, and existential factors in patient distress, and that there was a need for more attention to broader issues with regard to symptom control and family-based care. It was felt that there was ample evidence that many oncologists and centers did not feel a need to modify many patients' feelings of unnecessary suffering and unacceptable symptoms.

However, two of the three studies reported here estimate that home-based hospice care is less costly than conventional care, while there is no difference between the latter and institutional hospice care. The suspicion that such cost savings may just be a result of a marked and unmeasured cost shifting to the patients' families is at least partly refuted by the Dutch study, because this includes imputed values for the costs of family caregiving (which only accounted for around 10% of total costs). However, the problem of patient selection bias in observational studies such as the three reported here remains an important obstacle to more definitive assessments of the relative costs of the various forms of terminal care (see also Goodwin 1993). Even if the cost factor supports some form of hospice care, an important remaining issue is whether the outcomes for the patients and their families are actually better. The Dutch study did not include any outcome assessments, while the National Hospice Study did not find any significant differences.

Conclusion

In this report, a comprehensive survey of papers dealing with the economics of cancer treatments has been provided, while excluding interventions aiming at prevention, early detection, and screening. This should allow an overall assessment of the state of the art concerning the analysis designs and methods used in the papers surveyed and the practical usefulness of the information provided. A precondition for the results of the individual studies comprising this overview being relevant for practical decision making is of course that the study designs and the methods of analysis used are sound and that considerable care is shown in employing these methods. These requirements include that the data used should be pertinent and reliable. The subsequent necessary question for a given decision maker is whether results obtained in the specific settings of a particular study will be obtainable in his or her own setting. However, the methodological questions involved in determining the extent to which the results of a specific study can be generalized are rather complex and this still largely unsettled issue will not be pursued further here.

The first distinction may be made between studies which are orientated towards decision making and those which are not, or at least only in a very remote sense. The latter group comprises cost-of-illness (COI) studies and other attempts at determining the economic (or broader) impact of cancer on an aggregate, societal level. The number of studies concerned with determining the economic burden of cancer is rather limited, and the popularity of this analytical approach seems in general to be vanishing compared to the early days of the development of health economics as a subdiscipline. The published studies often have the appearance of rough and ready computations made in response to a usually not very well defined question and are as a rule limited to using readily available secondary data (often collected for administrative purposes).

Whatever legitimate criticisms may be raised against the study designs and methods and data employed in the published studies included in this section of the survey (see the chapter on "The Economic Burden of Cancer"), their results seem to converge in two respects. Rather unsurprisingly, the development of direct health care costs for the individual cancer patient typically follows a U-shaped curve. This development of costs over the course of disease has been found for all cancers investigated. The costs are high in the initial phase of diagnosis, staging and grading, patient workup, and primary treatment and then again in the terminal phase, mostly because of the high costs of hospital stays (the health care services provided in the terminal phase are rarely found to be very costly, as the aim is mainly to provide best supportive care or palliation). The direct costs in the intermediate phase between diagnosis and terminal care are usually very moderate, normally limited to periodic follow-up visits with ever increasing intervals in between as long as no recurrence or metastatic disease has appeared at the clinical level. High-cost procedures such as bone marrow transplantation (BMT) for relapsing patients with advanced disease do not seem to carry much weight in these aggregate cost calculations, probably because these procedures were still not used more or less as a matter of routine in the time period covered by most of these studies.

The vague speculations often heard about an increasing future economic burden of cancer due to the general aging of the population and (perhaps) an increasing incidence per se may be given some flesh and blood by the type of approach used by Koopmanschap et al. (1994). In this study, expected future costs were determined using a modeling technique which combines estimates of the development over time of the direct costs for the individual patient with assumptions about future changes in incidence and in the duration of the various phases of disease, especially the disease-free interval. Examining various possible future scenarios with a model of this kind by changing its parameters and assumptions may at least serve the useful purpose of anchoring the often alarmist speculations about future "explosions" in health care costs due to a rising incidence and prevalence of cancer.

The other result which emerges as an established fact of the macroeconomic studies is that the economic burden of cancer for society is disproportionately low compared to the share of mortality and morbidity attributed to the disease and the associated grief and dread. As argued in the chapter on "The Economic Burden of Cancer," it must be expected that this result would change considerably if such calculations were to include even a rough, minimal estimate of intangible costs, which until now no study has attempted. Presumably, quite another picture would also emerge if one were instead to examine the share of all medical research allocated to cancer research.[1]

Cancer's share of the direct health care costs of the countries in which these calculations have been made is found to be in the range of 5%–10%. This should probably not be considered as an indication of undertreatment. A more reasonable interpretation is that the cancer treatment regimens in common use at the time of data collection for these studies have been comparatively "cheap," resulting in very moderate costs even though the patients

[1] This, however, is nothing but an unsubstantiated guess, as it has not been possible to find any reliable and precise national or international statistics bearing on this issue. The measurement problems involved in such an exercise would of course also be formidable, e.g., with respect to the allocation of the funds for basic research. In the Biomedical and Health Research program of the EU, the share of funds dedicated to cancer research is more than 20%.

have most likely been given any treatment which might conceivably help. The picture may have changed during the last 5–10 years due to the increasing cost-consciousness in the health care systems worldwide and the simultaneous emergence and strong promotion of a number of new tumor treatment regimens and supportive care therapies with very high acquisition prices. However, there are as yet no data available which might corroborate or falsify such an hypothesis.

According to welfare economic theory, the correct approach to measuring the economic burden of a disease would rather be to investigate what the population at large, either as current or potential future patients or relatives of patients, would be willing to sacrifice in terms of other valuable goods or activities in order to diminish the incidence and/or the consequences of the disease. As far as it is known, this kind of willingness to pay approach has not yet been applied in the field of cancer, neither as a whole disease "entity" nor in connection with any evaluations of specific treatment alternatives. Neither should such an exercise be given very high priority, as it would still be difficult to see for what purposes the information obtained could sensibly be used or have any practical importance for decision making.

The papers surveyed in the chapter on "Breast Cancer" and in those following it have been categorized under the broad heading of cost analysis and economic evaluations of treatment alternatives for certain well-defined groups of cancer patients. At least one of the important intentions of carrying out such economic evaluations is to provide decision makers with information on the relative value of two or more treatment alternatives for specific conditions. Included in this group of papers are a number of studies in which only a single treatment regimen has been costed without considerations of the outcome of treatment or about any alternative treatments. These studies provide some preliminary cost calculations for a later full economic evaluation, and they definitely belong more naturally to this group of micro-level studies than to the above-mentioned aggregate studies at the societal level.

The most commonly used methods of economic evaluation, cost-effectiveness analysis and cost-utility analysis, are essentially *comparative techniques*, the results of which, expressed as the incremental costs per unit of effectiveness or utility (e.g., a quality-adjusted life-year, QALY), can only be interpreted meaningfully by being compared with something else. This something with which to compare and interpret the results of an individual study may be an externally determined standard, such as "society's willingness-to-pay" for the gain of 1 QALY. Alternatively, it may be other treatments with comparable effects on the health of the patients (whether these effects are measured in natural, biological units or in units such as QALYs). In contrast to this, cost-benefit analysis aims at determining the net benefits (benefits minus costs) of each individual treatment, by assessing both the costs and the benefits with the same yardstick, their pecuniary value. This allows a comparison of the net benefit of disease treatment in various groups of patients as well as a comparison with activities outside the health care sector.

The decision criterion in cost-benefit analysis is to prefer the one or more options offering the largest positive net benefits, and treatments resulting in negative net benefits should be abandoned.

The majority of the papers described and discussed in this survey belong to the cost-effectiveness and cost-utility variety of economic evaluation methods. A proper interpretation of the results of the individual studies thus requires that they be compared either with an externally determined standard for the acceptable costs per unit of effectiveness or utility or with the results of other studies of treatments resulting in comparable effects. Given that no externally determined standard for the level of acceptable costs actually exists,[2] it might seem natural to try to summarize the studies surveyed, or as many of them as at all possible, by establishing a listing of their main result expressed in a common ratio form.

The establishment of such rank-ordered listings of different treatments according to the costs per unit of outcome, often referred to as cost-effectiveness or cost-utility *league tables*, has attracted considerable research interest and is sometimes considered the ultimate purpose of performing economic evaluations of diverse interventions in health care. The interest in measuring and expressing treatment outcomes in terms of a single and common unidimensional quantity such as utilities derives, at least in part and implicitly, from an intention to make such rankings possible by making the outcomes of the interventions fully comparable. The establishment of such league tables is considered by some to be a valuable tool for decision making, e.g., in deciding which treatments should be offered in a health care system with limited resources and a strict budget constraint.[3]

In the cancer field, an approximate cost-utility league table was provided by Smith et al. (1993) in a paper with the significant subtitle "Rational Allocation of Resources Based on Decision Analysis." This table is reproduced as Table 1. It is implied that rational resource allocation requires that the supply of treatments is prioritized according to increasing cost-effectiveness ratios, i.e., treatments with a low cost per unit of effectiveness should be provided in preference to treatments with a higher cost per unit of effectiveness. Preferably, the unit of effectiveness used in studies intended to contribute to such league tables should be life-years gained adjusted for health-related

[2] It may be argued that any such standard implicitly used may be determined by analyzing a number of actual decisions. However, as pointed out already in the early analyses of public regulation written by economists (e.g., Lave 1981), one should not expect to find any consistency in the standards used in this implicit way, inter alia because many other factors greatly influence real-world decision making.

[3] The state of Oregon in the United States has gone furthest in this direction after passing the Oregon Basic Health Services Act in 1989. In 1990, a first priority list of health care services to provide, exclusively based on cost-effectiveness calculations, was published, but was met with strong criticism from both citizens and physicians. Consequently, the list was withdrawn and a new one produced, based on a number of other criteria in addition to cost-effectiveness. It was decided not to allow Medicaid to cover the financing of the 122 treatments considered least important (out of a total of 709). A 5-year trial period starting in the autumn of 1991 was decided on, so this experiment is currently up for evaluation.

Table 1. Efficacy and cost-effectiveness of cancer treatments

Intervention	Benefit	Costs in US$ per QALY
Intravenous IgG for CLL	0.8 days	7,100,000
Routine monitoring of CEA after colon cancer	0.1% increase in OS	31,000–6,600,000
Diagnosis and treatment of unknown primary cancer	11% increase in OS	2,400,000
Autologous BMT for all relapsed Hodgkin's disease patients	8 years	421,000
Second-line chemotherapy for NSCLC	Not stated	238,000
Autologous BMT for limited metastatic breast cancer	6.0 months	115,800
Chemotherapy for AML	Not applicable	80,300
Chemotherapy for metastatic gastric cancer	2–4 months	60,000–80,000
Chemotherapy for NSCLC	Not stated	38,300
Adjuvant tamoxifen for premenopausal, ER^- women	0.2–0.4 months	57,000–214,000
Transfusion of white blood cells against infection in AML	Mortality decreased from 23% to 10%	37,000
Autologous BMT for Hodgkin's disease, second relapse only	10.3 years	26,200
Adjuvant tamoxifen+chemotherapy in breast cancer, ER^+ women	1.2–2.1 months	14,000–33,000
Chemotherapy vs. allogeneic BMT for AML	21%–48% increase in OS	12,500
Two different chemotherapies for NSCLC	7–15 weeks	–8400 to +20,000
Adjuvant chemotherapy in breast cancer, 45-year-old women	9.2–10.7 months	4900
Two different chemotherapies for SCLC	1.6 months	4600
Tamoxifen for advanced breast cancer	Not stated	810
Interferon-α_{2b} for hairy cell leukemia	2-year mortality rate decreased from 37% to 8%	–13,800

From Smith et al. (1993).
OS, overall survival; AML, acute myeloblastic leukemia; CLL, chronic lymphocytic leukemia; CEA, carcinoembryonic antigen; BMT, bone marrow transplantation; ER, estrogen receptor; SCLC, small cell lung cancer; NSCLC, non-small-cell lung cancer.

quality of life in order to ensure comparability with all other activities within the health care sector which compete for the same limited resources.[4]

However, if the establishment of cost-effectiveness or cost-utility league tables is to be taken seriously, it is an extremely taxing task, because it is very difficult to establish the true comparability of the studies to be included in the list. Estab-

[4] In theory, cost-benefit analysis makes it possible to perform intersectorial comparisons by determining the net benefits in pecuniary terms of each of the activities competing for the same limited resources, whether real (e.g., manpower) or budgetary. By this means, the net benefits of health care activities might be compared to the net benefits of activities in any other sector, such as education or the military.

lishing real comparability will usually require that large amounts of additional data are collected and analyzed in detail. Because of limited research resources within any single institutional setting, league tables must, to a certain extent, necessarily be based on secondary analysis of studies performed by other research teams. It will probably only rarely or never be possible to ensure study comparability in the strictest sense with respect to both the effect measures used and the principles guiding the calculation of costs. In practice, the necessary data for performing a good, standardized secondary analysis of a number of independent studies will not be available from the primary studies even if direct access to the data collected and used is provided, thus impeding the possibility of ensuring real comparability of the individual studies.

In the general methodological discussions about economic evaluation of health care interventions and in relation to the issue of league tables in particular, most of the critical attention has been focused on variations and possible incompatibilities in the effect measures used. However, equal attention ought to be given to the costing issues, as problems concerning the methods used for cost calculations may be equally damaging for the objective of ensuring comparability between several studies as effect measurement problems. Until now, however, issues in costing (e.g., unclarity or inconsistencies in the perspective and time span of the analysis, which is of paramount importance for the cost items to include and the unit costs to choose) have been relatively neglected, despite the fact that one often sees inconsistent costing principles being used even within individual studies. When several such studies are being used for the purpose of establishing a rank ordering or league table, these inconsistency problems will of course be exacerbated, and major reanalysis may be necessary if meaningful comparisons are to result from the efforts.

Unless some means are found for ensuring true comparability among any number of economic evaluations in health care, the full potential of cost-effectiveness, and in particular cost-utility analysis, for providing support for decision making in health care will not be realized. This does not of course diminish the value of the methods used in individual studies to provide information of relevance for the choice between the treatments directly compared, and this will arguably remain the most useful role for economic evaluations for some time to come. Several efforts with the general aim of facilitating comparisons across studies are under way,[5] but, even if successful, these efforts will require considerable time to make a real impact on the studies performed and published.[6]

[5] Many countries have established so-called guidelines for conducting economic evaluations to be used as inputs for regulatory decision making (e.g., about reimbursement of a new pharmaceutical). Under the Biomedical and Health Research program of the EU, a project called HARMET (The Harmonisation by Consensus of the Methodology for Economic Evaluation of Health Care Technologies in the European Union) is under way, with many of the leading European researchers in the field as participants.

[6] Consensus about principles is obviously not of much value if they are not adhered to in the practical conduct of analyses. There has never been any dispute about the importance of stating explicitly the viewpoint of the analysis and all the assumptions used, but numerous published studies are seriously lacking in these respects. This is true for economic evaluations of cancer as for evaluations of any other health care interventions.

It should be clear from the detailed descriptions given of the individual studies in this survey that establishing a reliable league table of cancer treatments would be almost impossible, even if the effort was limited to studies using strictly the same outcome measures. Rendering the cost comparisons fully comparable with respect to the viewpoint and the time perspective chosen and ensuring consistency in the methods used for calculating the costs would require a considerable effort in supplementary data collection and analyses, but despite such an effort a substantial uncertainty about the validity of the data would remain. However, as stated by Smith et al. (1993), the results of such studies are probably correct within an order of magnitude, so if a gross comparison shows a substantial difference, it is likely that this will not be turned around by a more refined analysis.

The attempt at making comparisons "across the board" inevitably implies that almost all of the attention is centered on a single number, the cost-effectiveness or cost-utility ratio, at the expense of all the detailed descriptions and analyses going into the calculation of this final number. However, at present, the main value of the body of literature surveyed in this report lies in the details provided by individual studies on specific treatment choices for well-specified patient groups. The best of these studies provide decision makers with a wealth of pertinent and valuable information that certainly has the potential to contribute to improved decision making. By giving a precise description of the treatment context and by being clear and explicit about all the steps taken and assumptions made in the analysis, these studies provide local decision makers with the optimal means of assessing the possibility of transferring the study results to their local circumstances and of the possible need for adapting assumptions and values of variables to the local setting.

General Methodological Issues in Economic Evaluations of Health Care

As alluded to before, the study designs and methods to be chosen for carrying out an optimal economic evaluation of health care interventions is not a settled issue, and the evaluations performed in practice are usually very far from any such an ideal, however defined. A few of the many contentious methodological issues will be briefly discussed in the following.

Relevance of Outcome Measures

There are reasons to be concerned with the outcomes measures chosen because certain outcome measures are sometimes used in a very mechanistic and unthinking way, which may lead to erroneous conclusions. One example is the use of quality-adjusted survival as the outcome measure in a comparison of antiemetic treatments. This is a classic example of a treatment which may have only a limited influence on the length of survival (and then only indirectly, by allowing the patients to be able to follow the scheduled treatment regimen to a higher degree than otherwise and thereby achieving a better survival result), while it is assumed to improve quality of life considerably.

The improvement in quality of life may be very substantial, but if it is assessed by merely multiplying a point estimate of the difference in quality of life with and without an emetic episode by the mean duration of emetic episodes or something similar, the potential gain in the final outcome measure will become almost imperceptible. Almost regardless of the price of an effective antiemetic drug, this will result in a very high cost-utility ratio, which will make the treatment appear quite unacceptable when compared to some of the standard "thresholds" often cited in the literature.[7] Such a result appears intuitively wrong, given the common fear of chemotherapy-induced emesis and its alleged effect on some patients' ability to follow the scheduled treatment regimen. Accordingly, there seems to be a need for a more flexible approach to measuring changes in quality of life. Strictly from an economic theoretical point of view, it would be preferable using a measure of the patients' willingness-to-pay for an improved probability of not experiencing an emetic episode and the associated substantial, although brief, reduction in quality of life.

Costs or Charges?

A large number of the studies surveyed do not explicitly adopt a specific viewpoint or time span for the cost calculations performed. This often leads to inconsistencies in the calculations, especially in the form of inclusion of cost items or use of unit prices which are incorrect or irrelevant seen from the implicit viewpoint for the analysis. Another problem is the use of charge data instead of costs, which often appears to be done without any awareness of the problems inherent in this procedure. Charges are only unproblematical, however, if the adopted viewpoint of the analysis is that of a third-party payer paying the full official charges without any discounts. This viewpoint is not the most commonly chosen (explicitly), and most analyses are performed (at least implicitly) from the viewpoint of the health care provider.

Charges are determined by health care providers in a manner which is intended primarily to ensure that the provider's expenses will be covered and, possibly, that a profit will be earned (in profit-making institutions). They are not intended to reflect the actual costs of the various activities performed. The complex accounting systems used by providers in health care systems, where the provider institutions' only source of income are charges, are therefore designed to shift costs to activity centers, where charges may be levied, rather than being intended to track real resource utilization. The use of charges for cost calculations is often justified by the argument that charges are at least not lower than the actual costs, because the survival of the institution depends on having the total costs covered. However, this is only true

[7] The standard example of a threshold for acceptability is kidney transplantation, for which the cost-utility ratio is often indicated to be around $ 35,000/QALY.

at the aggregate level, and the charges for individual procedures or service may certainly be lower (sometimes substantially so) than the real costs. An extensive use of what economists refer to as cross-subsidization (i.e., where some services are provided at a price below cost, while the prices of others are higher than costs) is to be expected.

In the United States, so-called cost-to-charge ratios have been calculated and published for many years both at the level of the individual institutions and at more aggregate levels, even the national level. Such cost-to-charge ratios are commonly employed in economic evaluations emanating from the United States and are habitually postulated to give a more accurate picture of the actual costs compared to charges. This presumption should not be too readily accepted, however, partly because of the problems with aggregation mentioned above,[8] partly because the determination of the "real costs" to be used for calculating such ratios is usually poorly documented.

Should Data Be Collected in Clinical Trials?

About 10 years ago, it was suggested that the collection of cost data for economic evaluations of health care interventions should be linked more closely to controlled clinical trials (see Drummond and Stoddart 1984) and that in some cases the economic evaluation should be an integral part of new prospective randomized trials. The idea was that in this way one could ensure that the relevant and necessary economic data were collected prospectively and with the same rigor as the clinical data. This notion quickly won widespread approval, and it soon became an accepted dogma that the most valid and acceptable way of performing economic evaluations in health care was by using the economic data collected for patients participating in randomized clinical trials and relating them to efficacy data collected in the same trials (see, e.g., Morris and Goddard 1993; Morris et al. 1994).

Part of the explanation for the rapid acceptance of this idea was undoubtedly a widespread frustration with the haphazard way in which data for economic evaluations of health care interventions were often collected, using data availability and accessibility as the most important criteria. The models constructed for modeling studies are frequently perceived as impenetrable "black boxes," and the way data are chosen is often not justified in a satisfactory way. On the other hand, the randomized clinical trial is generally seen as the closest possible approximation to an ideal model for scientific experiments that is possible with human subjects and as the only truly valid way of estimating the relative efficacy of alternative interventions by minimizing the threats to the internal validity of the study design. Thus it seems evident

[8] If a cost-to-charge ratio calculated for the individual institution is used, this ratio will be an average for the institution as a whole, although the relation between the costs and charges for individual services may well diverge considerably. When more aggregate cost-to-charge ratios are used, this problem will of course be exacerbated.

that data for economic evaluations should ideally be collected in randomized clinical trials, although it is usually conceded that there may often be a conflict with regard to the length and comprehensiveness of follow-up needed for the economic and purely clinical evaluation, respectively.

More recently, some skepticism towards this position has increasingly often been expressed (see, e.g., Rittenhouse 1995; Rittenhouse and O'Brien 1996). This is not the place to provide any thorough discussion of these questions, but many of the issues may be considered as an expression of an inherent and unavoidable trade-off between the internal and external validity of scientific (quasi-)experiments.[9] As mentioned above, the primary virtue of the prospective randomized, controlled design is that it minimizes (but does not eliminate) the numerous threats against the internal validity of a scientific experiment, thereby providing the optimal conditions for drawing valid inferences about cause–effect relations. However, this is achieved at the expense of a greatly diminished external validity, as it may be very difficult to generalize the results of randomized, controlled experiments outside the specific settings of the experiment. Retrospective, observational studies, on the other hand, are perceived as giving a much more truthful description of the practical reality, but this design is plagued with selection bias problems and is usually considered to be without value in drawing inferences about cause–effect relations.

The critics of the strategy of basing economic evaluations exclusively on data collected in clinical trials argue, inter alia, that patients and physicians (hospitals) participating in clinical trials cannot be considered a random sample of the large majority of patients and treatment providers that will be using the treatment in daily practice.[10] Using clinical trials as the primary means of data collection for economic evaluations has to rest on the argument that such evaluations are limited to document *the potential for* a significant difference in cost-effectiveness or cost-utility of the treatments compared. It may be argued that, as it is not the absolute amounts but the differences between the treatments that counts in economic evaluations, it is of no consequence whether the absolute amounts observed in ordinary daily practice will differ, even considerably, from those observed in the trial, as long as the difference between the treatments is maintained. However, this will remain an unsubstantiated assumption until the relevant data to confirm or falsify it has been collected and analyzed. This would have to be done in each individual case, as there seems to be no basis for establishing a general rule concerning this relation.

---

[9] See Cook and Campbell (1979) for the original formulation of the problem using these terms, which are now standard in the evaluation literature. The terms are not used in the same way by analysts who have not been trained in the tradition of social evaluation, and this causes some confusion.

[10] Selection bias occurs in yet another form, because the patients consenting to participate in a clinical trial cannot be considered a random sample of "any useful population to which we might wish to generalise results" (see Senn 1990)

Another problem concerns the aggregation of resource utilization data from multiple centers, which will be necessary in most large clinical trials, as these are usually performed as international, multicenter trials. The clinical data from such trials are habitually analyzed by aggregating the data across the study centers in order to determine whatever are the outcomes chosen for comparison, e.g., the rate of 5-year survival in a cancer trial. However, can the amounts of resources used in each center for each treatment meaningfully be aggregated in the same way, e.g., in order to determine the average amount of physician time used in each treatment?

This seems to be a doubtful proposition, considering the fact that there may be large differences between the institutions in qualifications and competency of personnel, in staffing levels, in the available equipment and its quality, and in clinical care "traditions." Numerous studies have uniformly shown large inter- and intranational differences in patient handling between various hospitals, and simple aggregation of resource utilization data seems to be an untenable "solution." In already published evaluations, the most common procedure is to base the cost calculation on the resource utilization in a single center, but this "solution" is not consistent with one of the arguments for integrating the collection of economic data in clinical trials, i.e., to ensure agreement between the clinical and economic data.

The increasing use of economic evaluation instruments during the last 20 years has been accompanied by many methodological discussions and developments. At first, these discussions mainly concerned the proper methods for outcome assessment with the attempts at integrating quantity and quality of survival, e.g., by estimating global utility measures such as QALYs. Later on, the discussions were extended to include issues in costing methods, the appropriate statistical handling of economic data partly collected in clinical trials and partly based on other sources, and the proper ways of collecting data for these evaluations. Without trying to makes prophecies about the future development, it seems to be a fair bet that data collection through clinical trials and modeling based on other sources and assumptions will have to complement each other. By a skillful combination of these two methods of collecting the necessary data (as discussed, e.g. by Simpson 1994), it should be possible to obtain valid results that are relevant to the local context in which a decision about using treatment A or B or about the level of reimbursement for a new treatment has to be made.

An explicit statement of all assumptions made and a discussion and justification of all the choices made in the performance of the analysis will therefore continue to be an essential requirement for an analysis of good quality. Unfortunately, as mentioned above, this obvious requirement for a good-quality study which enjoys unanimous approval in methodological discussions has not been adhered to convincingly in the economic evaluations published so far. Few evaluations of cancer treatments meet this requirement, and this is one of the most obvious ways of improving the current standard - and, so it would seem, the easiest to implement. Analyses not meeting this requirement will always be regarded with some suspicion of "a hidden agenda."

Final Remarks

Secondary analyses of published economic evaluations and quality-of-life evaluations in health care appear regularly, making assessments of the state of the art, and, just as regularly, they conclude that the large majority of published evaluations fall short of the methodological requirements on which there is general agreement in the research community. The present survey of economic evaluations and cost analyses of cancer treatments is no exception in this regard.

The interest in carrying out economic evaluations in the cancer field has been limited and has developed slowly compared to the interest for many other important diseases. One of the reasons for this may be the high mortality rate associated with the disease and the fact that it is much dreaded by the general population, making treatment "at any cost" a natural priority. In practice, however, this may mean that large amounts of resources are used rather indiscriminately, both on interventions that greatly benefit patients and on ones that do patients little or no good at all. Another explanation, which is favored here, is that the number of treatment alternatives has been quite limited for many types of cancer patients. This makes it less of a priority to attempt careful and formal evaluations of their relative costs and benefits for the patients.

This situation is changing, however. As a result of large investments in research and development, many new treatment possibilities, whether as antitumor therapy or as supportive therapy, have already appeared or will soon be launched on the markets, thereby increasing the number of alternatives between which the clinical decision makers may choose. Whatever their therapeutic benefits relative to existing options, the innovative interventions will often have a relatively high acquisition price, at least until more or less close equivalents appear on the market as competitors (see, e.g., Lønning 1995). Simultaneously, the growth in resources made available for health care has been reduced or even, in some countries, stopped.

Economic evaluation is an instrument which may improve decision making by allowing better-informed decisions by taking into account the full consequences of the alternatives in terms of both costs and therapeutic benefits. In an environment in which health care systems all over the world are under pressure to contain expenditure on health care and to ensure that the available resources are actually used where they are expected to do the most good, the need for evaluation studies enabling better-informed decisions is becoming more obvious. If properly and conscientiously applied, economic evaluations may make a major contribution to enabling informed decisions to be taken, although they can never dictate the professionals' decisions on specific issues nor be a substitute for professional judgment.

Currently, rather the opposite is the case, however. The general judgment resulting from several studies (see Johannesson 1996) is that economic evaluations have only very little influence on practical decision making. This may be due to the often poor methodological quality of the studies carried out and published, which makes them unconvincing for the decision makers. It may also be caused by a perception of the field of economic evaluation as an immature scientific discipline with insufficiently strict standards and incessant quarrels about methodological issues. Arguably, this methodological debate has more than merely an intellectual interest and has resulted in great improvements in state-of-the-art "standards" for good-quality studies, but the practical evaluations carried out have not convincingly observed even long established standards.

A more fundamental problem may be the institutional structure of health care systems and the existing incentive mechanisms for the providers of care and other decision makers. Unless the place and importance of economic evaluations for decisions (e.g., about reimbursement or adoption of a new intervention as a standard treatment protocol) are somehow stipulated and imposed on decision makers, the impact of economic evaluations will continue to be uncertain and probably strictly limited. Demanding such regulatory stipulations would, however, be in blatant contradiction to the economists' usual credo, which is that such evaluations should only be considered as a guide to making better-informed decisions. Health insurance bodies (public or private) may be expected to increasingly demand economic evaluations as the direct basis for making decisions. From the analysts' viewpoint, however, it seems evident that the proper response should rather be to provide better evaluations and to raise the decision makers' awareness about the fundamental principles and aims guiding economic evaluations as properly conducted.

References

Ahmedzai S (1997) New approaches to pain control in patients with cancer. Eur J Cancer 33 [Suppl 6]:S8–S14

Ahmedzai S, Brooks D (1997) Transdermal fentanyl versus sustained release oral morphine in cancer pain: preference, efficacy and quality of life. J Pain Symptom Manage 13:254–261

Arrow K (1963) Uncertainty and the welfare economics of medical care. AER 53:941–973

ASCO (1994) American Society of Clinical Oncology recommendations for the use of hematopoetic colony-stimulating factors: evidence-based, clinical practice guidelines. J Clin Oncol 12:2471–2508

ASCO (1996) Update of recommendations for the use of hematopoietic colony-stimulating factors: evidence-based clinical practice guidelines. J Clin Oncol 14:1957–1960

Baker M, Kessler L, Smucker R (1989) Site-specific costs for cancer: an analysis of the Medicare continuous history sample file. In: Scheffler R, Andrews N (eds) Cancer care and cost – DRGs and beyond. Health Administration Press Perspectives, Ann Arbor

Baker M, Kessler L, Urban N et al. (1991) Estimating the treatment costs of breast and lung cancer. Med Care 29:40–49

Balducci L, Benson K, Lyman G et al. (1993) Cost-effectiveness of white cell-reduction filters in treatment of adult acute myelogenous leukemia. Transfusion 33:665–670

Balfour J, Faulds D (1993) Oral ciprofloxacin. A pharmacoeconomic evaluation of its use in the treatment of serious infections. PharmacoEconomics 3:398–421

Ballatori E, Roila F, Berto P et al. (1994) Cost and cost effectiveness analysis of ondansetron versus metalopramide regimens; a hospital perspective from Italy. PharmacoEconomics 5:227–237

Baniel J, Roth B, Foster R et al. (1995) Cost and risk benefit in the management of clinical stage II nonseminomatous testicular tumors. Cancer 75:2897–2903

Baranko P (1994) A cost comparison of laboratory charges in treating childhood leukemia. Am J Ped Hematol/Oncol 16:102–103

Beard M, Inder A, Allen J et al. (1991) The costs and benefits of bone marrow transplantation. 104:302–304

Bennett C, Armitage J, Armitage G et al. (1995) Costs of care and outcomes for high-dose therapy and autologous transplantation for lymphoid malignancies: results from the University of Nebraska 1987 through 1991. J Clin Oncol 13:969–973

Berdel W, Clemm C, Hartenstein R et al. (1987) Benefit and costs of follow-up programs in nonseminomatous germ cell tumor of the stages IIb–IV: The Munich experience. Oncology 44:273–278

Biermann W, Cantor R, Fellinn F et al. (1991) An evaluation of the potential cost reductions resulting from the use of clodronate in the treatment of metastatic carcinoma of the breast to the bone. Bone 12:S37–S42

Black W, Armstrong P, Daniel T (1988) Cost effectiveness of chest CT in T1N0M0 lung cancer. Radiology 167:373–378

Bloor K, Leese B, Maynard A (1994) The costs of managing severe cancer pain and potential savings from transdermal administration. Eur J Cancer 30A:463–468

Blumberg N, Heal J, Krikley S et al. (1995) Leukodepleted-AB0-identical blood components in the treatment of hematologic malignancies: a cost analysis. Am J Hematol 48:108–115

Brice P, Godin S, Marolleau J et al. (1995) Effect of Lenograstim on the cost of autologous bone marrow transplantation. PharmacoEconomics 7:283–241

Brodin H, Stalfelt A (1993) Treating acute leukaemias – a venture into economic uncertainty? Acta Oncol 332:501–505

Brown M (1990) The national economic burden of cancer – an update. J Nat Cancer Inst 82:1811–1814

Brown M, Fintor L (1994) The economic burden of cancer. In: Greenwald P, Kramer B, Weed E (eds) Cancer prevention and control. Dekker, New York

Brown M, Nayfield S, Shibley L (1994) Adjuvant therapy for stage III colon cancer: economic returns to investment and cost-effectiveness of treatment. J Nat Cancer Inst 86:1994

Bryson H, Plosker G (1993) Tamoxifen: a review of pharmacoeconomic and quality-of-life considerations for its use as adjuvant therapy in women with breast cancer. PharmacoEconomics 4:40–66

Butler J, Furnival C, Hart R (1995) Estimating treatment cost functions for progressive diseases: a multiproduct approach with an application to breast cancer. J Health Econ 14:361–385

Buxton M, O'Brien B (1992) Economic evaluation of ondansetron: preliminary analysis using clinical trial data prior to price setting. Br J Can 66:S64–S76

Cancer Care Inc. (1973) The impact: costs and consequences of catastrophic illness on patients and families. Cancer Care Inc. and the National Cancer Foundation Inc., New York

Carlsson P, Hjertberg H, Jönsson B et al. (1989) The cost of prostatic cancer in a defined population. Scan J Urol Nephrol 23:93–96

Ciatto S, Cionini S, Pacini P (1986) Cost-effectiveness of chest x-ray follow-up of patients treated for seminoma of the testis. Tumori 72:405–408

Cook D, Guyatt G, Laupacis A et al. (1992) Rules of evidence and clinical recommendations on the use of anti-thrombotic agents. Chest 102 [Suppl]:305S–311S

Cook T, Campbell D (1979) Quasi-experimentation: design and analysis issues for field settings. Houghton Mifflin, Boston

Covens A, Boucher S, Roche K et al. (1996) Is paclitaxel and cisplatin a cost-effective first-line therapy for advanced ovarian carcinoma? Cancer 77:2086–2091

Cox F, Hirsch J (1993) Ondansetron: a cost-effective advance in anti-emetic therapy. Oncology 50:186–190

Coy P, Schaafsma J, Schofield J et al. (1994) Comparative costs of lung cancer management. Clin Invest Med 17:577–587

Crawford J, Ozer H, Stoller R et al. (1991) Reduction by granulocyte colony-stimulating factor of fever and neutropenia induced by chemotherapy in patients with small-cell-lung cancer. N Engl J Med 325:164–170

Culyer A, Jönsson B (1993) Ought cancer treatments to be immune from socio-economic evaluation? An epilogue. Eur J Cancer 29A [Suppl 7]:S31–S32

Cunningham D, Gore M, Davidson N et al. (1993) The real costs of emesis – an economic analysis of ondansetron vs. metaclopramide in controlling emesis in patients receiving chemotherapy for cancer. Eur J Cancer 29A:303–306

Desch C, Lasala M, Smith T et al. (1992) The optimal timing of autologous bone marrow transplantation in Hodgkin's disease patients after a chemotherapy relapse. J Clin Oncol 10:200–209

Desch C, Hillner B, Smith T et al. (1993) Should the elderly receive chemotherapy for node-negative breast cancer? A cost-effectiveness analysis examining total and active life-expectancy outcomes. J Clin Oncol 11:777–782

DeVita V, Hellman S, Rosenberg S (eds) (1993) Cancer; principles and practice of oncology, 4th edn. Lippincott-Raven, Philadelphia

DeVita V, Hellman S, Rosenberg S (eds) (1997) Cancer; principles and practice of oncology, 5th edn. Lippincott-Raven, Philadelphia

Dranitsaris G, Tran T (1995) Economic analysis of toxicity secondary to anthracycline-based breast cancer chemotherapy. Eur J Cancer 31A:2174–2180

Dranitsaris G, Tran T, McGeer A et al. (1995) Pharmacoeconomic analysis of empirical therapy with ceftazidime alone or combination antibiotics for febrile neutropenia in cancer patients. PharmacoEconomics 7:49–62

Drummond M, Davies L (1994) Economic evaluation of Lenograstim for prophylaxis of chemotherapy-induced neutropenia in patients with small cell lung cancer. PharmacoEconomics 6 [Suppl 2]:44–52

Drummond M, Stoddart G (1984) Economic analysis and clinical trials. Control Clin Trials 5:118–128

Early Breast Cancer Trialists' Collaborative Group (1990) Treatment of early breast cancer, vol. I. Worldwide evidence 1985–90. Oxford Medical Publications, Oxford

Eddy R (1989) Cost-effectiveness of CT scanning compared with mediastinoscopy in the preoperative staging of lung cancer. J Can Assoc Radiol 40:189–193

Eisenberg J, Koffer H, Glick H et al. (1987) What is the cost of nephrotoxicity associated with aminoglycocides? Ann Intern Med 107:900–909

Eisenberg P (1994) Further profile of granisetron (Kytril): effect on quality of life and pharmacoeconomics. Semin Oncol 21 [Suppl 5]:26–29

Etzioni R, Urban N, Baker M (1996) Estimating the costs attributable to a disease with application to ovarian cancer. J Clin Epidemiol 49:95–103

Evans W, Le Chevalier T (1996) The cost-effectiveness of navelbine alone or in combination with cisplatin in comparison to other chemotherapy and best supportive care in stage IV non-small cell lung cancer. Eur J Cancer 32A:2249–2255

Faulds D (1996) Using Filgrastin efficiently. PharmacoEconomics 9:466–468

Faulds D, Lewis N, Milne R (1992) Recombinant granulocyte colony-stimulating factor (rG-CSF); pharmacoeconomic considerations in chemotherapy-induced neutropenia. PharmacoEconomics 1:231–249

Frampton J, Faulds D (1996) Filgrastim – a reappraisal of pharmacoeconomic considerations in the prophylaxis and treatment of chemotherapy-induced neutropenia. PharmacoEconomics 9:76–96

Freifeld A, Pizzo P (1995) Colony-stimulating factors and neutropenia: intersection of data and clinical relevance. J Nat Cancer Inst 87:78–79

GAO (1994) Bone marrow transplantation: international comparisons of availability and appropriateness of use. US General Accounting Office, Washington DC

Gelber R, Goldhirsch A, Cavalli F (1991) Quality-of-life-adjusted evaluation of adjuvant therapies for operable breast cancer. Ann Intern Med 114:621–628

Gibbs J, Newman J (1982) Studies of health services used and cost incurred during the last six months of a terminal illness. Final report to US Department of Health and Human Services. Blue Cross and Blue Shield Association, Research and Development Department, Chicago

Glaspy J, Jakway J (1993) Cost considerations in therapy with myeloid growth factors. Am J Hosp Pharm 50 [Suppl 3]:S19–S26

Glaspy J, Bleecker G, Crawford J et al. (1993) The impact of therapy with filgrastim (recombinant granulocyte colony-stimulating factor) on the health care costs associated with chemotherapy. Eur J Cancer 29A [Suppl 7]:S23–S30

Glimelius B, Hoffman K, Graf W et al. (1995) Cost-effectiveness of palliative chemotherapy in advanced gastrointestinal cancer. Ann Oncol 6:267–274

Goddard M, Drummond M (1991) The economic evaluation of cancer treatments and programmes. Eur J Cancer 27:1191–1196

Gold M, Russell L, Siegel J et al. (1996) Cost effectiveness in health and medicine. Oxford University Press, Oxford

Goldhirsch A, Gelber R, Simes J et al. (1989) Costs and benefits of adjuvant therapy in breast cancer: a quality-adjusted survival analysis. J Clin Oncol 7:36–44

Goodwin P (1993) Economic factors in cancer palliation – methodological considerations. Cancer Treat Rev 19 [Suppl A]:59–65

Goodwin P, Feld R, Evans W et al. (1988) Cost-effectiveness of cancer chemotherapy: an economic evaluation of a randomized trial in small cell lung cancer. J Clin Oncol 6:1537–1547

Graham P, Boyages J (1993) Economic and quality of life aspects of treating small cell lung cancer. PharmacoEconomics 3:446–453

Gray D, MacAdam D, Boldy D (1987) A comparative cost analysis of terminal cancer care in home hospice patients and controls. J Chron Dis 40:801–810

Greer D, Mor V, Morris J et al. (1986) An alternative in terminal care: results of the national hospice study. J Chron Dis 39:9–26

Gulati S, Bennett C (1992) Granulocyte-macrophage colony-stimulating factor (GM-CSF) as adjunct therapy in relapsed Hodgkin disease. Ann Intern Med 116:177–182

Hall R (1994) Superficial bladder cancer. Br Med J 308:910–913

Henriksson P, Edhag O (1987) Cost-effectiveness comparison of estrogen therapy and orchidectomy in patients with prostatic cancer. Int J Tech Assessm Health Care 3:523–529

Henriksson P, Stege R (1991) Cost comparison of parenteral estrogen and conventional hormonal treatment in patients with prostatic cancer. Int J Tech Assessm Health Care 7:220–225

Hillner B (1993) Financial costs, benefits, and patient risk preferences in node-negative breast cancer: insights from a decision analysis model. In: Recent results in cancer research, vol 127. Springer, Berlin Heidelberg New York

Hillner B, Smith T, Desch C (1992) Efficacy and cost-effectiveness of autologous bone marrow transplantation in metastatic breast cancer. JAMA 267:2055–2061

Hillner B, Smith T, Desch C (1993) Assessing the cost-effectiveness of adjuvant therapies in early breast cancer using a desicion analysis model. Breast Cancer Res Treat 25:97–105

Hillner B, Smith T, Desch C (1994) Cost-effective uses of autologous bone marrow transplantation; few answers, many questions, and suggestions for future assessments. PharmacoEconomics 6:114–126

Hillner B, McLeod D, Crawford D et al. (1995) Estimating the cost effectiveness of total androgen blockade with flutamide in M1 prostate cancer. Urology 45:633–640

Hodgson T (1994) Costs of illness in cost-effectiveness analysis. PharmacoEconomics 6:536–552

Hoyalake T, Franklin I (1994) Bone marrow transplants from peripheral blood. Set to transform medical oncology. Br Med J 309:4–5

Hunt M, Woodhouse C (1987) Cost-effectiveness of investigations for invasive bladder cancer. J Roy Soc Med 80:1443–444

Hurley S, Suggins R, Snyder R et al. (1992) The cost of breast cancer recurrences. Br J Can 65:449–455

Jaakkimainen L, Goodwin P, Pater J et al. (1990) Counting the costs of chemotherapy in a National Cancer Institute of Canada randomized trial in non-small cell lung cancer. J Clin Oncol 8:1301–1309

Jefferson T, Mugford M, Gray A et al. (1996) An exercise on the feasibiility of carrying out secondary economic analyses. Health Economics 5:155–165

Jobet I, Zygue, S, Prugnaud J (1995) Economic evaluation of anti-5HT3s: development of an economic model for cost minimization study. J Pharmacol Clin 14:55–63

Johannesson M (1996) Theory and methods of economic evaluation of health care. Kluwer, Dordrecht

Johannesson M, Jönsson B (1991) Economic evaluation in health care: is there a role for cost-benefit analysis. Health Policy 17:1–23

Johannesson M, Jönsson B, Karlsson G (1996) Outcome measurement in economic evaluation. Health Econ 5:279–296

Johnson N, Bosanquet N (1995) Cost-effectiveness of 5-hydroxytryptamine$_3$ receptor antogonists: a retrospective comparison of ondansetron and granisetron. Anticancer Drugs 6:243–249

Jones A, Lee G, Bosanquet N (1992) The budgetary impact of 5-HT3 receptor antagonists in the management of chemotherapy-induced emesis. Eur J Cancer 29A:51–56

Jönsson B, Karlsson G (1992) Economic evaluation of cancer treatments. In: Williams C (ed) Introducing new treatments for cancer: practical, ethical and legal problems. Wiley, Chichester

Jönsson B, Karlsson G (1993) Outcome measurement in economic evaluations of growth factors. Eur J Cancer 29A [Suppl 7]:S19–S22

Kay H, Lawler S, Powles R et al. (1980) Cost of bone marrow transplants in acute myeloid leukaemia. Lancet:1067–1069

Kennedy W, Reinharz D, Tessier G et al. (1995) Cost utility of chemotherapy and best supportive care in non-small cell lung cancer. PharmacoEconomics 8:316–323

Kievit J, van de Velde C (1990) Utility and cost of carcinoembryonic antigen monitoring in colon cancer follow-up evaluation; a Markov analysis. Cancer 65:2580–2587

Koopmanschap M, Rutten F (1993) Indirect costs in economic studies: confronting the confusion. PharmacoEconomics 4:446–454

Koopmanschap M, Ineveld M, Miltenburg T (1992) Costs of home care for advanced breast and cervical cancer in relation to cost-effectiveness of screening. Soc Sci Med 35:979–985

Koopmanschap M, von Roijen L, Bonneaux L et al. (1994) Current and future costs of cancer. Eur J Cancer 30A:60–65

Koopmanschap M, Rutten F, van Inefeld B et al. (1995) The friction cost method for measuring indirect costs of disease. J Health Econ 14:171–189

Lannin D, Silverman J, Pories W et al. (1986) Cost-effectiveness of fine needle biopsy of the breast. Ann Surg 203:474–480

Launois R, Reboul-Marty J, Henry B et al. (1996) A cost-utility analysis of second-line chemotherapy in metastatic breast cancer. Docetaxel versus paclitaxel versus vinorelbine. PharmacoEconomics 10:504–521

Lave L (1981) The strategy of social regulation: decision frameworks for policy. Washington

Le Corroller A, Moatti J-P, Detournay B et al. (1994) L'évaluation économiques du G-CSF en thérapeutique cancerologique: deux exemples d'études françaises. Presse Med 23:1105–1109

Leese B (1993) The costs of treating febrile neutropenia in six UK hospitals. Eur J Cancer 29A [Suppl 7]:S15–18

Leese B, Collin R, Clark D (1994) The costs of treating febrile neutropenia in patients with malignant blood disorders. PharmacoEconomics 6:232–239

Leivonen M (1987) Costs and benefits of breast cancer diagnosis. Acta Oncol 26:257–260

Levine M, Drummond M, Labelle R (1985) Cost-effectiveness in the diagnosis and treatment of carcinoma of unknown primary origin. Can Med Assoc J 133:977–986

Licht M, Klein E (1994) Early hospital discharge after radical retropubic prostatectomy: impact on cost and complication rate. Urology 44:700–704

Lindgren B (1990) The costs of nontreatment. In: Teeling-Smith G (ed) Measuring the benefits of medicines; the future agenda. OHE, London

Lobo P, Powles R, Hanrahan A et al. (1991) Acute myeloblastic leukaemia - a model for assessing value for money for new treatment programmes. Br Med J 34:323–326

Lønning P (1995) Paclitaxel and Docetaxel; innovation, but at what cost? PharmacoEconomics 8:1–4

Luce B, Singer J, Weschler J et al. (1994) Recombinant human granulocyte-macrophage colony-stimulating factor after autologous bone marrow transplantation for lymhoid cancer. PharmacoEconomics 6:49–56

Lyman G, Lyman C, Sanderson R et al. (1993) Decision analysis of hematopoietic growth factors in patients receiving cancer chemotherapy. J Natl Cancer Inst 85:488–493

Mapelli V, Graf v.d. Schulenberg M, Laaser U et al. (1994) Economic evaluation of Lenograstim (glycosylated rHuG-CSF) in the treatment of inflammatory breast cancer for Germany and Italy. PharmacoEconomics 6 [Suppl 2]:27–35

Marie J-P, Wdowik T, Bisserbe S et al. (1992a) Cost of complete remission induction in acute myeloblastic leukaemia: evaluation of the cost-effectiveness of a new drug. Leukemia 6:720–722

Marie J-P, Bisserbe S, Bouaziz C et al. (1992) Programme de médicalisation des systèmes d'information. Validité du calcul des coûts directs pour le traitement initial de la leucémie aigü myéloblastique. Presse Méd 21:1364–1368

Markman M (1988) An argument in support of cost-effectiveness analysis in oncology. J Clin Oncol 6:937–939

Maynard A (1993) Economic aspects of cancer care. Eur J Cancer 29A [Suppl 7]:S6–S9

Mayordomo J, Rivera F, Cortes-Funes H (1995a) Colony-stimulating factors for adjunctive therapy of infections in neutropenic cancer patients. Support Care Cancer 3:84–85

Mayordomo J, Rivera F, Diaz-Puente M et al. (1995b) Improving treatment of chemotherapy-induced neutropenic fever by administration of colony-stimulating factors. J Natl Cancer Inst 87:803–808

McEwan A, Amyotte G, McGowan D et al. (1994) A retrospective analysis of the cost-effectiveness of treatment with Metastron® (^{89}SR-chloride) in patients with prostate cancer metastatic to bone. Nucl Med Commun 15:499–504

McGuire W, Hoskins W, Brady M et al. (1996) Cyclophosphamide and cisplatin compared with paclitaxel and cisplatin in patients with stage III and stage IV ovarian cancer. N Engl J Med 334:1–6

McQuay H, Moore A (1994) Need for rigorous assessment of palliative care. Br Med J 309:1315–1316

Messori A, Trippoli S, Becagli P et al. (1996) Pharmacoeconomic profile of paclitaxel as a first-line treatment for patients with advanced ovarian carcinoma. Cancer 78:2366–2373

Montero M, Valdivia M, Carjaval E et al. (1994) Economic study of neutropenia induced by myelotoxic chemotherapy. Pharm World Sci 16:187–192

Morris J, Goddard M (1993) Economic evaluation and quality of life assessment in cancer clinical trials: the CHART trial. Eur J Cancer 29A:766–770

Morris J, Goddard M, Coyle D et al. (1994) Evaluating emerging technologies: a case study in the assessment of quality of life and resource use alongside clinical trials of radiotherapy for cancer. Working paper. Centre for Health Economics, University of York, York

Munro A, Warde P (1991) The use of a Markov process to simulate and assess follow-up policies for patients with malignant disease: surveillance of stage I nonseminatous tumors of the testis. Med Decision Making 11:131–139

Nichols C, Fox E, Roth B et al. (1994) Incidence of neutropenic fever in patients treated with standard-dose combination chemotherapy for small-cell lung cancer and the cost impact of treatment with granulocyte colony-stimulating factor. J Clin Oncol 12:1245–1250

Nicol D, Heathcote P, Kately G et al. (1993) Advanced prostate cancer. The role of high priced hormone therapy. Med J Aust 16–19

Norum J, Angelsen V, Wist E et al. (1996) Treatment costs in Hodgkin's disease: a cost-utility analysis. Eur J Cancer 32A:1510–1517

O'Brien B, Rusthoven J, Rocchi A et al. (1993) Impact of chemotherapy-associated nausea and vomiting on patients' functional status and on costs: survey of five Canadian centers. Can Med Assoc J 149:296–301

O'Brien B, Drummond M, Labelle R et al. (1994) In search of power and significance: issues in the design and analysis of stochastic cost-effectiveness studies in health care. Med Care 32:150–163

Oesterling J (1993) Using PSA to eliminate the staging radionuclide bone scan. Significant economic implications. Urol Clin North Am 20:705–711

Oesterling J (1995) Using prostate-specific antigen to eliminate unnecessary diagnostic tests: significant worldwide economic implications. Urology 46:26–33

Olsen J (1994) Production gains: should they count in health care evaluations? Scot J Polit Econ 41:69–84

Ozer H, Golomb H, Zimmerman H et al. (1989) Cost-benefit analysis of interferon alfa-2b in treatment of hairy cell leukaemia. J Natl Cancer Inst 81:594–602

Pashko S, Jacobs J, Santorsa J (1991) The cost-effectiveness of idarubicin/cytosine arabinoside versus daunorubicin/cytosine arabinoside in the treatment of adults with acute myeloid leukemia. Clin Ther 13:353–360

Persson U, Ragnarsson Tenvall G, Andersson S et al. (1992) Cost-effectiveness analysis of treatment with liposomal amphotericin B versus conventional amphotericin B in organ or bone transplant recipients with systemic mycoses. PharmacoEconomics 2:500–508

Peters W, Rogers M (1994) Variation in approval by insurance companies for coverage for autologous bone marrow transplantation for breast cancer. N Engl J Med 330:473–477

Phillips M, Richards S, Chessels J (1991) Acute myeloid leukaemia in childhood: the costs and benefits of intensive treatment. Br J Haematol 77:473–477
Plosker G, Benfield P (1996) Granisetron. A pharmacoeconomic evaluation of its use in the prophylaxis of chemotherapy-induced nausea and vomiting. PharmacoEconomics 9:357–374
Plosker G, Milne R (1992) Ondansetron: a pharmacoeconomic and quality-of-life evaluation of its antiemetic activity in patients receiving cancer chemotherapy. PharmacoEconomics 2:285–304
Potosky A, Riley G (1992) SEER-Medicare data base linking project; analysis plan and project results. Report to NCI. Applied Research Branch, NCI, Bethesda
Potosky A, Riley G, Lubitz J et al. (1993) Potential for cancer related health services register using a linked Medicare-Tumor registry database. Med Care 31:732–748
Rees G (1985) Cost-effectiveness in oncology. Lancet:1405–1407
Reiffers J (1993) PBPC support after high-dose chemotherapy. Helix 3:20–27
Rice D, Hodgson T (1981) Social and economic implications of cancer in the United States. Vital and Health Statistics, series 3, no 20. US Government Printing Office, Washington (DHSS publ no PHS 81-1404)
Rice D, Hodgson T, Kopstein A (1985) The economic costs of illness: a replication and update. Health Care Financing Rev 7:61–80
Richards M, Braysher S, Gregory W et al. (1993) Advanced breast cancer: use of resources and cost implications. Br J Cancer 67:856–860
Riley G, Potosky A, Lubitz J et al. (1995) Medicare payments from diagnosis to death for elderly cancer patients by stage at diagnosis. Med Care 33:828–841
Rimm A et al. (1991) Use of a clinical data registry to evaluate medical technologies – experience from the International Bone Marrow Transplant Registry. Int J Tech Assessm Health Care 7:182–193
Rittenhouse B (1995) The relevance of searching under a clinical-trial lamppost: a key issue. Med Decision Making 15:348–357
Rittenhouse B (1996) Designing and conducting cost-minimization and cost-effectiveness analysis. In: Spilker B (ed) Quality of life and pharmacoeconomics in clinical trials, 2nd edn. Lippincott-Raven, Philadelphia
Rittenhouse B, O'Brien B (1996) Threats to the validity of pharmacoeconomic analyses based on clinical trial data. In: Spilker B (ed) Quality of life and pharmacoeconomics in clinical trials, 2nd edn. Lippincott-Raven, Philadelphia
Robbins L (1932) An essay on the nature and significance of economic science. Macmillan, London
Rosenthal M, Webster P, Gebski V et al. (1992) The cost of treating small cell lung cancer. Med J Aus 156:605–610
Rubens R (1990) Auditing palliative cancer chemotherapy. Eur J Cancer 26:1023–1025
Rubens R (1993) Cost effectiveness in the treatment of advanced solid tumors. Eur J Cancer 29A:604–605
Ruckdeschel J (1990) Is chemotherapy for metastatic non-small cell lung cancer "worth it"? J Clin Oncol 8:1293–1296
Rutqvist L, Wilking N (1992) Analogues of LHRH versus orchidectomy: comparison of economic costs for castration in advanced cancer. Br J Cancer 65:927–929
Sackett D (1989) Rules of evidence and clinical recommendations on the use of anti-thrombotic agents. Chest 95 [Suppl]:2S–4S
Sagmeister M, Horisberger B, Gessner U (1992) Assessment of the costs of side effects in cancer chemotherapy: method and result of a multinational study. In: Chytil M, Duru G, Eimeren W et al. (eds) Healthcare. Omnipress, Prague
SBU (Statens Beredning för Utvärdering av medicinsk metodik) (1991) Bone marrow transplantation (in Swedish). SBU, Stockholm
Schapira D (1993) Breast cancer surveillance – a cost-effective strategy. Breast Cancer Res Treatment 25:107–111
Schapira D, Studnicki J, Bradham D et al. (1993) Intensive care, survival, and expense of treating critically ill cancer patients. JAMA 269:783–786

Schug S, Large R (1993) Economic considerations in pain management. PharmacoEconomics 3:260–267

Scotto J, Chiazze L (1976) Third National Cancer Survey: hospitalizations and payments to hospitals. US Department of Health, Education and Welfare, Washington (publ no NIH 76-1094)

Senn S (1990) Clinical trials and epidemiology. J Clin Epidemiol 43:628–632

Sharda N, Kinsella T, Ritter M (1996) Adjuvant radiation versus observation: a cost analysis of alternate management schemes in early-stage testicular seminoma. J Clin Oncol 14:2933–2939

Shibley L, Brown M, Schuttinga J et al. (1990) Cisplatin-based combination chemotherapy in the treatment of advanced stage testicular cancer: cost-benefit analysis. J Natl Cancer Inst 82:186–192

Simpson K (1994) Problems and perspectives on the use of decision analysis models for prostate cancer. J Urol 152:1888–1893

Smith P (1985) The costs of intravesical chemotherapy. In: Schroeder F, Richards B (eds) EORTC Genitourinary Group monograph 2, part B: superficial bladder tumors. Liss, New York

Smith T, Hillner B (1993) The efficacy and cost-effectiveness of adjuvant therapy of early breast cancer in premenopausal women. J Clin Oncol 11:771–776

Smith T, Hillner B, Desch C (1993) Efficacy and cost-effectiveness of cancer treatment: rational allocation of resources based on decision analysis. J Natl Cancer Inst 85:1460–1474

Smith T, Hillner B, Neighbors D et al. (1995) Economic evaluation of a randomized clinical trial comparing vinorelbine, vinorelbine plus cisplatin, and vindesine plus cisplatin for non-small cell lung cancer. J Clin Oncol 13:2166–2173

Souêtre E, Qing W (1994) Economic analyses of Lenograstim in the correction of neutropenia following chemotherapy for non-Hodgkin's lymphoma. PharmacoEconomics 6 [Suppl 2]:36–43

Souêtre E, Qing W, Pénelaud P (1996) Economic analysis of the use of recombinant human granulocyte colony stimulating factor in autologous bone marrow transplantation. Eur J Cancer 32A:1162–1165

Taplin S, Barlow W, Urban N et al. (1995) Stage, age, comorbidity, and direct costs of colon, prostate, and breast cancer care. J Natl Cancer Inst 87:417–426

Tennvall G, Persson U, Nilsson B (1994) The economic costs of acute myeloid leukaemia in Sweden. Int J Tech Ass Health Care 10:683–694

Uyl-de-Groot C (1995) Economic evaluation of cancer treatments. iMTA, Rotterdam

Uyl-de-Groot C, Richel D, Rutten F (1994) Peripheral blood progenitor cell transplantation mobilised by r-metHuG-CSH (Filgrastim); a less costly alternative to autologous bone marrow transplantation. Eur J Cancer 30A:1631–1635

Uyl-de-Groot C, Okhuijsen, Hagenbeck A et al. (1995) Costs of introducing autologous BMT in the treatment of lymphomas and acute leukaemia in the Netherlands. Bone Marrow Transplant 15:605–610

Uyl-de-Groot C, Vellenga E, Rutten F (1996a) An economic model to assess the savings from a clinical application of haematopoetic growth factors. Eur J Cancer 32A:57–62

Uyl-de-Groot C, Huijgens P, Rutten F (1996b) Colony-stimulating factors and peripheral blood progenitor cell transplantation. Benefits and costs. PharmacoEconomics 10:23–35

Vahrenhorst E, Carlsson P, Pedersen K (1994) Clinical and economic considerations in the treatment of prostate cancer. PharmacoEconomics 6:127–141

Walker A, Whynes D (1990) The costing of nursing care: a study of 65 colorectal cancer patients. J Adv Nurs 15:1305–1309

Walker A, Whynes D, Chamberlain J et al. (1991) The hospital costs of diagnostic procedures for colorectal cancer. J Clin Epidemiol 44:907–914

Weeks J, Tierney M, Weinstein M (1991) Cost-effectiveness of prophylactic intravenous immune globulin in chronic lymphocytic leukaemia. N Engl J Med 325:81–86

Welch G, Larson E (1989) Cost-effectiveness of bone marrow transplantation in acute nonlymphocytic leukaemia. N Engl J Med 321:807–812

Williams A (1990) EuroQol – a new facility for the measurement of health related quality of life. The EuroQol Group. Health Policy 16:199–208
Whinney I, Bass M, Donner A (1994) Evaluation of a palliative care service: problems and pitfalls. Br Med J 309:1340–1342
WHO (1990) Cancer pain relief and palliative care. WHO Technical Report Service, no. 804. World Health Organization, Geneva
Whynes D, Walker A (1995) On approximations in treatment costing. Health Econ 4:31–39
Whynes D, Walker A, Chamberlain J et al. (1993) Screening and the costs of colorectal cancer. Br J Cancer 68:965–968
Wiernikowski J, Rothney M, Dawson S et al. (1991) Evaluation of home intravenous antibiotic program in pediatric oncology. Am J Pediat Hematol/Oncol 13:144–147
Yarbro J (1991) Changing cancer care in the 1990s and the cost. Cancer 67 [Suppl]:1718–1727
Zbrozek A, Cantor S, Cardenas M et al. (1994) Pharmacoeconomic analysis of ondansetron versus metoclopramide for cisplatin-induced nausea and vomiting. Am J Hosp Pharm 51:1555–1563
Zittoun R, Mandelli F, Willemze R et al. (1995) Autologous or allogeneic bone marrow transplantation compared with intensive chemotherapy in acute myelogenous leukemia. N Engl J Med 332:217–223

MIX
Papier aus verantwortungsvollen Quellen
Paper from responsible sources
FSC® C105338

If you have any concerns about our products,
you can contact us on
ProductSafety@springernature.com

In case Publisher is established outside the EU,
the EU authorized representative is:
Springer Nature Customer Service Center GmbH
Europaplatz 3, 69115 Heidelberg, Germany

Printed by Libri Plureos GmbH
in Hamburg, Germany